PAEDIATRIC PSYCHOLOGY

Paediatric Gastrointestinal Disorders
A psychosocial perspective

Edited by

CLARISSA MARTIN

Consultant Paediatric Clinical Psychologist
Head of Child Health (Paediatrics), Midlands Psychology CIC
Stafford, UK

and

TERENCE DOVEY

Senior Lecturer in Psychology
School of Social Sciences
Brunel University
Uxbridge, UK

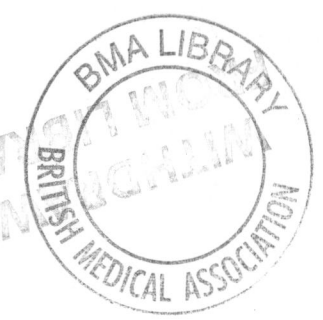

Series Editors
Angela Southall and Clarissa Martin

Foreword by
Douglas A Drossman, MD
Professor Emeritus of Medicine and Psychiatry, University of North Carolina
President, The Rome Foundation
President, Center for Education and Practice of Biopsychosocial Care
Drossman Gastroenterology, PLLC
Chapel Hill, North Carolina, USA

Radcliffe Publishing
London • New York

Radcliffe Publishing Ltd
St Mark's House
Shepherdess Walk
London N1 7BQ
United Kingdom

www.radcliffehealth.com

British Library Cataloguing in Publication Data

A catalogue record for this book is available from the British Library.

ISBN-13: 978 184619 995 0

The paper used for the text pages of this book
is FSC® certified. FSC (The Forest Stewardship
Council®) is an international network to promote
responsible management of the world's forests.

Typeset by Darkriver Design, Auckland, New Zealand
Printed and bound by TJI Digital, Padstow, Cornwall, UK

Contents

Series introduction

Whenever a child receives a diagnosis of a medical condition, numerous considerations are immediately brought to the fore, many of which are unique to children, including, of course, developmental, family and parenting issues. A child's cognitive, emotional, behavioural and social functioning may be significantly affected by his or her illness. Most significantly, just as the child is affected by his or her illness, so is the course of the illness affected by the child. This simple understanding and the success of paediatric psychologists in communicating and demonstrating it has led to the growth of paediatric psychology in children's wards, outpatient departments, community clinics and health centres around the world. Indeed, it is the propensity of the paediatric psychology team to make a difference to the child and his or her treatment that has led to widespread acknowledgement of the value that paediatric psychology brings.

Paediatric psychology is essentially the application of psychological theory, research and practice to children with medical conditions and health-related concerns. It takes a 'whole child' approach and is developmentally focused.

Practice is most often multidisciplinary and focuses on the understanding of physical, psychosocial and neuropsychological aspects of health and illness, and how these affect one another. The scope of paediatric psychology is extensive and encompasses many treatment areas ranging from adjustment to illness, coping with invasive medical procedures and pain management to adherence to treatment, children with chronic conditions and palliative care, to name just a few, as well as the prevention of illness among healthy children (Roberts *et al.*, 1984).

As a specialty, paediatric psychology has a surprisingly long history. Soon after the emergence of psychology as a discipline in the nineteenth century, it was suggested that psychologists and paediatricians would benefit from mutual collaboration (Witmer, 1907). These psychologists worked alongside paediatricians and shared with them a developmental perspective; they came to be described as 'paediatric psychologists' (Wright, 1967). These early paediatric psychologists helped establish that children with health and developmental problems had significant needs, which, although similar to one another, were different to those with psychiatric diagnoses. In the United States, the Society of Pediatric Psychology was founded to meet those needs (Wright, 1967). In the United Kingdom, paediatric psychology developed out of the discipline of clinical psychology and continues to be located within the category of clinical child psychologists working in medical healthcare settings, under the auspices of the British Psychological Society.

Recent policy emphases in the United Kingdom have highlighted the needs of children and young people with long-term conditions and the importance of providing them with good mental health input to maximise emotional well-being and minimise problems.[1] These policies emphasise that such support should be an integral part of the service a child receives in hospital and high-light the imperative on hospitals to ensure staff have an understanding of how to assess the emotional well-being of children and address any needs that are identified.[2] Elsewhere in Europe, mental health has also come to be empha-sised as an essential ingredient in health and well-being, not just for children but for everyone. This is perhaps best exemplified by the European Union's slogan, 'There is no health without mental health' (Lavikainen *et al.*, 2000).

The Paediatric Psychology series to which this book belongs was conceived as a way of sharing with readers salient ideas from applied research and practice that would be experienced as helpful to others in their own practice. A series of books was planned, each focusing on a different topic within paediatric psy-chology, with the overall aim of raising awareness among health professionals of the concomitant psychological and psychosocial aspects of child ill health and chronic illness.

The series has a deliberately international focus, which reflects the paedi-atric psychology community and brings together material that is otherwise unavailable in this form. The accompanying electronic toolkit offers practical, usable support to practitioners, as well as an opportunity to contribute to the developing knowledge base. It is our hope that the books will prove to be an inspiring and reliable resource for day-to-day paediatric practice.

Angela Southall
Clarissa Martin

REFERENCES

Lavikainen J, Lahtinen E, Lehtinen V, editors. *Public Health Approach on Mental Health in Europe*. Helsinki: National Research and Development Centre for Welfare and Health, STAKES Ministry of Social Affairs and Health; 2000.

Roberts MC, Maddux JE, Wright L. Developmental perspectives in behavioral health. In: Matarazzo JD, Miller NE, Weiss SM, *et al.*, editors. *Behavioral Health: a handbook of health enhancement and disease prevention*. New York, NY: Wiley; 1984.

Witmer L. Clinical psychology. *Psychol Clinic*. 1907; **1**(1): 1–9.

Wright L. The pediatric psychologist: a role model. *Am Psychol*. 1967; **22**(4): 323–5.

---

1 See Standard 6, 'Children and young people who are ill', from the Department of Health's *National Service Framework for Children, Young People and Maternity Services* (London: DoH; 2004).

2 See Standard 7, 'Children in hospital', from the Department of Health's *National Service Framework for Children* (London: DoH; 2003).

Dedicated to Dr J Houghton PhD

This *series* is dedicated to Dr Judith Houghton PhD,
Consultant Clinical Psychologist and first elected chair
(2001–2006) of the British Psychological Society-Paediatric
Psychology National Committee (BPS-PPNC) in gratitude
for and acknowledgement of her outstanding contribution
to the development of Paediatric Psychology in the UK

Foreword

You cannot reason with a hungry belly ... it has no ears.

—Greek Proverb, BCE

Man should strive to have his intestines relaxed all the days of his life.

—Moses Maimonades (Rambam), 13th Century

Affectes and passions of the minde ... annoye the body, and shorten the lyfe.

—Sir Thomas Elyot, 16th Century

A good set of bowels is worth more to a man than any quantity of brains.

—Josh Billings (Henry Wheeler Shaw), 19th Century

The development of the Biopsychosocial medical model is posed as a challenge for both medicine and psychiatry. For despite the enormous gains which have accrued from biomedical research, there is a growing uneasiness among the public as well as among physicians and especially among the younger generation that health needs are not being met. ...

—George L. Engel MD, 20th Century (1977)

Throughout recorded history poets, historians and physicians have recognized the close linkage between mind and gut, and why not? From the time of conception, the neural plate of the embryo serves as the anlage from which the central nervous system, spinal cord and myenteric plexi grow and differentiate, and so this linkage is hardwired and forever connected. Thus it comes as no surprise to this readership that understanding the reciprocal relationship between psychosocial and gastrointestinal functioning in health and disease is critical to understanding and caring for our patients, young and old. But why, less than 40 years ago, would George Engel the physician icon of the Biopsychosocial model write about this with such somber tones in his seminal paper? (Engel, 1977).

Answering this question requires a historical perspective on how the relationship of mind and body have been viewed over time (Drossman, 1998). Throughout most of Western history, beginning with the ancient Greeks there has existed the concept that mind and body were inseparable, and medical disease must take into account the entire person rather than just the diseased part. However, this changed, beginning in 1637, when Rene Descartes proposed that there is a separation of the thinking mind (res cogitans) from the body (res extensa). As he quotes: *'On the one hand I have a clear and distinct idea of myself, in so far as I am a thinking, non-extended thing; and on the other hand I have a distinct idea of body, in so far as this is simply an extended, non-thinking thing. And, accordingly, it is certain that I am really distinct from my body, and exist without it.'* (Drossman, 2006). This dualistic concept of separation of mind and body powerfully influenced scientific thinking and the practice of medicine. Notably the dissection of human cadavers, previously prohibited (because the spirit was thought to reside there), was now permitted, so what was seen (i.e. structural disease) was real and amenable to scientific study. In contrast symptoms, behaviors and illness without pathology was dismissed as insanity or at the time, possession by evil. These patients were ignored and/or relegated to the asylums. Over time this dualistic thinking morphed into the modern medical concept of continually seeking an 'organic' cause in an effort to frame the patient's reports of illness into something observable and real. When no cause is found, it is considered as 'functional' (not understood, a second class disease) and without reason presumed psychiatric.

Over the last three centuries the dualistic concept has permeated all sectors of society and it has relegated to second class the value of the teaching, learning and investigation of non-pathologically based disorders, in particular the functional somatic and GI diagnoses, and patients who have these disorders can be given negative attributions and labelled as being 'psychosomatic'.

Close to biomedical dualism is reductionism, i.e. the relegation of diseases to single causes that are both necessary and sufficient to explain the illness (also called linear causality). This is represented by Koch's 'germ theory' and has been important in understanding *acute* infectious disease. However, single-cause etiology has its limitations with chronic disease which is complex and multi-causal. Several years ago a notable gastroenterologist said at a symposium on IBS: *'Psychological issues are important, but finding the etiology (of IBS) will take care of the problem.'* This person acknowledged the importance of psychological factors, but his conceptualization was both reductionistic and dualistic.

Beginning in the late 1970s, educators were reporting that patients with structural diseases (e.g. inflammatory bowel disease, ulcer disease) varied in the illness experience from asymptomatic to severe given the same disease activity, and psychiatric and gastrointestinal disorders considered as functional now were found to have genetic determinants and biochemical and immunological correlates. Thus organic disease was being functionalized and functional disorders organified (Drossman, 2006). Then in 1977, Engel, being dissatisfied with the existing dualistic thinking of the time, proposed a multi-causal model that integrates mind and body: where biologic, psychological and social subsystems interact at multiple levels. This Biopsychosocial model reconciled the emerging research findings not explained by biomedicine, permitted the heterogeneity of medical illness and the various physiological components and clinical expressions of disease, and also opened the door to the concept of mind–body (e.g. brain–gut) disorders.

I believe the field of gastroenterology may be ahead of the curve in moving forward with these newer concepts; the organic and functional dichotomy within GI is disappearing through good research in neurogastroenterology and education (Drossman, 2006; Drossman 2005). I also believe that the Rome Criteria laid the foundation for upgrading our knowledge in the field by classifying functional GI disorders (Drossman *et al.*, 2006). This makes them identifiable and thus amenable to research which leads to more targeted treatments based on the diagnosis for clinical practice. Through this the disorders are also legitimized as 'real' entities. The Rome Foundation is proud to have recruited superb pediatric investigators and clinicians who have defined, classified and made recommendations for the care of patients with pediatric functional GI disorders.

Thus the Biopsychosocial model and the Pediatric Rome Criteria provide a template to aid in the elaboration of the science and art of pediatric gastrointestinal disorders; that work is well represented in this informative book by Drs Martin and Dovey. The editors who singularly have promoted this model for years have also joined to produce this book. *Paediatric Gastrointestinal Disorders: a psychosocial perspective* forges the way for a greater integration of knowledge in the field by bringing together a multidisciplinary team of pediatric GI clinicians, behaviorists, nutritionists and investigators to help educate clinicians on understanding and caring for the 'whole child'.

Their aim '*… to offer health professionals, students and health professionals in training, and members of the public a multidisciplinary perspective on the psychosocial considerations of children and young people with gastrointestinal disorders and their families'* is well handled in this book. Chapters initially address the definitional and classification aspects of FGIDs, models of care, specific psychological treatments such as CBT, social and family influences on the child, and nutritional aspects of care including home parenteral nutrition. Following this they provide information on the clinical aspects of care: autism spectrum, tube feeding, rumination syndrome, inflammatory bowel disorders, defecation disorders, as well as information on working with adolescents. The book ends with a section on various assessment measures and other practical material that might be of help in clinical practice.

I am most pleased to have been asked to contribute to this book and am hopeful that many others will benefit from this well written compendium of knowledge in the management of patients with pediatric GI disorders.

Douglas A. Drossman, MD
Professor Emeritus of Medicine and Psychiatry,
University of North Carolina
President, The Rome Foundation
President, Center for Education and Practice of
Biopsychosocial Care
Drossman Gastroenterology, PLLC
Chapel Hill, North Carolina, USA
March 2014

REFERENCES

Drossman DA. Presidential address: gastrointestinal illness and biopsychosocial model. *Psychosom Med.* 1998; **60**(3): 258–67.

Drossman DA. Functional GI disorders: what's in a name? *Gastroenterol.* 2005: **128**(7): 1771–2.

Drossman DA. Functional versus organic: an inappropriate dichotomy for clinical care. *Am J Gastroenterol.* 2006; **101**(6): 1172–5.

Drossman DA, Corazziari E, Delvaux M, *et al. Rome III: the functional gastrointestinal disorders.* 3rd ed. McLean: Degnon Associates; 2006.

Engel GL. The need for a new medical model: a challenge for biomedicine. *Science.* 1977; **196**: 129–36.

About the editors

Clarissa Martin is Consultant Clinical Psychologist in Paediatrics and the Head of Child Health (Paediatrics) at Midlands Psychology. During many years she has led a CAMHS Paediatric Psychology Specialty and has been involved in multidisciplinary clinics (diabetes and gastroenterology) at District General Hospitals helping children, young people and their families to adapt to the illness. She is a specialist in children's feeding disorders and has pioneered multidisciplinary intensive intervention for children with severe avoidant/ restrictive eating disorders in the general hospitals setting. She is also active in collaborative, interdisciplinary work in both community and acute settings. She has extensive experience of developing and delivering training to health professionals to support the enhancement of their skills in psychosocial aspects of paediatric care. She is known for her national and international conference contributions and is the author of a number of peer-reviewed papers in the area of diabetes and gastroenterology. She is co-editor, with Angela Southall, of this series in Paediatric Psychology, the first of its kind in the United Kingdom.

Dr Terence M Dovey, PhD, is a Senior Lecturer in Psychology in the Department of Psychology, School of Social Sciences, Brunel University (London, UK). His main areas of research are in the application of intervention strategies for children with avoidant/restrictive eating disorders (aka feeding disorders) and tube-dependency. He has written over fifty peer-reviewed papers and books on the topic from theoretical commentaries through basic research to designing applied interventions for children with a variety of difficulties with eating. Prior to coming to clinical practice, Dr Dovey wrote in the area of biological under-pinnings of appetite regulation. Currently he is also working as a Behavioural Therapist with Midlands Psychology.

List of contributors

Dr Chandran P Alexander
Paediatric Gastroenterologist
Penn State Hershey Pediatric
  Gastroenterology
Hershey, PA, USA

Dr Anthony Alioto, PhD
Department of Pediatrics
The Ohio State University
Section of Pediatric Psychology and
  Neuropsychology
Nationwide Children's Hospital
Columbus, OH, USA

Professor Marc Benninga, MD
Professor of Paediatrics
Department of Paediatric
  Gastroenterology and Nutrition
Emma Children's Hospital
Academic Medical Center
Amsterdam, The Netherlands

Jessica Boutilier, BA
Mount Saint Vincent University
Faculty of Education
Seton Academic Centre
Halifax, NS, Canada

Dr Christine T Chambers, PhD
Associate Professor of Pediatrics and
  Psychology
Departments of Pediatrics and
  Psychology
Dalhousie University
Halifax, NS, Canada

Dr Caroline E Danda, PhD
Volunteer Research Professor,
University of Kansas Medical Center
Prairie Village, KS, USA

Dr Amanda D Deacy, PhD
Associate Professor of Pediatrics
University of Missouri – Kansas City
  School of Medicine
 Clinical Director, Abdominal Pain
  Program
Children's Mercy Hospitals & Clinics
Kansas City, MO, USA

Dr Niranga Devanarayana, MD
Head, Department of Physiology
Faculty of Medicine
University of Kelaniya
Ragama, Sri Lanka

Dr Carlo Di Lorenzo, MD
Department of Pediatrics
The Ohio State University
Section of Pediatric Gastroenterology
Nationwide Children's Hospital
Columbus, OH, USA

Tania Emiliou, MSc
Assistant Psychologist (Paediatrics)
Midlands Psychology
Stafford, UK

Dr Douglas G Field, MD
Pediatric Gastroenterologist
Associate Professor of Pediatrics
Penn State College of Medicine
Chief of the Pediatric Gastroenterology
Milton S Hershey Medical Center
Hershey, PA, USA

Dr Shomik Ghosal, MD
Consultant Paediatric Gastroenterologist
Mid Staffordshire NHS Foundation Trust
Stafford, UK

Taigh Giles
Gastroenterology Services User
UK

Dr Wendy N Gray, PhD
Assistant Professor
Auburn University
Auburn, AL, USA

Dr Kevin A Hommel, PhD
Research Associate Professor of Pediatrics
Center for the Promotion of Treatment
  Adherence and Self-Management
Cincinnati Children's Hospital Medical
  Center
Division of Behavioral Medicine and
  Clinical Psychology
Department of Pediatrics
Cincinnati, OH, USA

Dr Ruth A Howard, PhD
Senior Academic Tutor
Clinical Psychology Doctorate Course
School of Psychology
University of Birmingham
Birmingham, UK

Dr Paul E Hyman, MD
Professor of Pediatrics
Division Head, Gastroenterology
Children's Hospital
New Orleans, LA, USA

Dr Sara King, PhD
Assistant Professor
Mount Saint Vincent University
Faculty of Education
Seton Academic Centre
Halifax, NS, Canada

Dr Colleen Lukens, PhD
Licensed Psychologist
Children's Mercy Hospitals and Clinics
Division of Developmental & Behavioral
  Sciences/Division of Gastroenterology
University of Missouri – Kansas City
  School of Medicine
Kansas City, MO, USA

Dr Michele H Maddux, PhD
Licensed Psychologist
Children's Mercy Hospitals and Clinics
Division of Developmental & Behavioral
  Sciences
Division of Gastroenterology
University of Missouri
Kansas City School of Medicine
Kansas City, MO, USA

Adrian G Martin, MRes
Teacher (PGCE), Swindon Academy
Beech Avenue
Swindon, UK

Tess Mobberley
Advanced Nurse Practitioner
Staffordshire General Hospital
Stafford, UK

Dr Ella Mozdiak, MB
Specialist Registrar
The Princess Royal Hospital
Telford, UK

Dr Michela I Parzanese
Department of Gastroenterology
IRCCS Istituto Clinico Humanitas
Milan, Italy

Dr Sue Protheroe, MD
Consultant Paediatric Gastroenterologist
Department of Gastroenterology and
  Nutrition
Birmingham Children's Hospital
Birmingham, UK

Dr Shaman Rajindrajith, MD
Consultant Paediatric Gastroenterologist
Department of Paediatrics,
Faculty of Medicine,
University of Kelaniya,
Ragama, Sri Lanka

Professor Jennifer V Schurman, PhD
Professor of Pediatrics
University of Missouri – Kansas City
  School of Medicine

Program Co-Director, Abdominal Pain
  Program
Director, GI Psychological Services &
  Programs
Children's Mercy Hospitals and Clinics
Kansas City, MO, USA

Dr Alan Silverman, PhD
Pediatric Psychologist
Associate Professor of Pediatrics
Pediatric Gastroenterology
Medical College of Wisconsin
Milwaukee, WI, USA

Angela Southall, MSc
Consultant Clinical Psychologist
Director of Services
Midlands Psychology CIC
Stafford, UK

Dr Gill Townson, MD
Consultant Gastroenterologist
The Princess Royal Hospital
Telford, UK

Dr Gary Urquhart-Law, PhD
Senior Academic Tutor
Lecturer in Clinical Psychology & Child
  Clinical Psychologist
School of Psychology
University of Birmingham
Birmingham, UK

Dr Sara E Williams, PhD
Assistant Professor of Pediatrics
Medical College of Wisconsin
Milwaukee, WI, USA

Dr Keith E Williams, PhD
Pediatric Neuropsychologist
Associate Professor of Pediatrics
Penn State College of Medicine
Director of the Feeding Program
Milton S Hershey Medical Center
Hershey, PA, USA

Introduction

Children and young people experiencing gastroenterological discomfort such as nausea, vomiting, diarrhoea, abdominal pain, gastro-oesophageal reflux disease, colic and constipation are common presenting problems at paediatric clinics. It is widely recognised that *gastroenterology* is a key component in general paediatric practice (Beattie, 2002), with its unique challenges such as the diversity in cognitive maturation found within paediatric population and the specific characteristics of the development of the gastrointestinal system in children (Chumpitazi and Nurko, 2008).

The need for specialists trained in paediatric gastroenterology has been given added impetus in recent years by increasing evidence of the profound impact that many chronic gastrointestinal diseases have on children's growth and development, as well as by the knowledge that certain gastroenterological conditions are specific to infants (Walker-Smith and Walker, 2003).[3] The practice of paediatric gastroenterology requires not only knowledge of all gastrointestinal problems and disorders but also a thorough understanding of the normal development and the maturation of the digestive system in infants (Hamilton, 1991).

The medical specialty of paediatric gastroenterology is focused on problems and disorders within the gastrointestinal tract, liver and pancreas of children from infancy until age 18. Centres of excellence for children with gastroenterological disorders began to emerge in Great Britain, the United States, Europe and Australia in the 1950s and 1960s. However, it was in the 1970s when paediatric gastroenterology became fully recognised as a sub-specialty of paediatrics in the United Kingdom, the United States and Europe (Walker-Smith and Walker, 2003).

Important milestones in the development of this specialty have been the establishment of the diverse paediatric gastroenterology societies around the globe. The *European Society for Paediatric Gastroenterology* (ESPG) led by Dolf Weijers (Utrecht) held its first meeting in Paris in 1968 with the aim to create a European forum for research in paediatric gastroenterology. Nutrition and hepatology specialties joined this group in 1976 and 1990, respectively, to create ESPGHAN, the *European Society for Paediatric Gastroenterology, Hepatology and Nutrition*. NASPGHAN, the *North American Society for Pediatric Gastroenterology, Hepatology, and Nutrition*, was established in 1973, and in 1978 both societies

---

3 Examples include the inborn errors in bilirubin metabolism and digestive and absorptive genetic defects.

(ESPGHAN and NASPGHAN) met for the first time in Paris. LAPSGAN, the *Latin American Society for Pediatric Gastroenterology and Nutrition*, was founded in October 1974 in Buenos Aires. The *Asian Pan Pacific Society of Paediatric Gastroenterology* (APPSPGN) was founded in Tokyo in 1993. BSPGHAN, the *British Society of Paediatric Gastroenterology, Hepatology and Nutrition*, was created in 1986 and the *Commonwealth Association of Paediatric Gastroenterology and Nutrition* (CAPGAN) was founded in 1994 in Hong Kong, with a focus on interaction between developing and developed communities. FSPGHAN, the *Federation of Societies of Pediatric Gastroenterology, Hepatology and Nutrition*, was established in 2000 to unite the paediatric gastroenterology specialty at global level. Although paediatric gastroenterology is now 40–50 years old and it has evolved rapidly, the field of gastrointestinal diseases in children is still in need of further research and development (Walker-Smith and Walker, 2003).

Under the umbrella of gastrointestinal disorders, several variable combinations with or without identified underlined pathophysiology are defined. Effectively, there are gastroenterological disorders that have a structural and/or congenital abnormality of the gastrointestinal tract. However, there is also a group of gastrointestinal disorders that are characterised by recurrent symptoms that cannot be explained by structural biochemical abnormalities. This last group are known as 'functional gastrointestinal disorders', or FGIDs (Drossman *et al.*, 1993; Nurko and Di Lorenzo, 2008). The term FGIDs is used to define chronic or recurrent gastrointestinal symptoms that do not have an identified underlying pathophysiology (Corazziari, 2004; Rasquin *et al.*, 2006). They are a challenging group of conditions that are frequently misdiagnosed in children and which encompass a major portion of gastroenterology practice. FGIDs are also associated with significant impaired health-related quality of life and increased medical costs (Drossman *et al.*, 1993, 1999).

Although attempts to create a classification for FGIDs may be found initially in the 1960s, exceptional specialists in gastroenterology led by Professor Drossman established the first criteria for FGIDs in 1990 – this date is a clear landmark for this group of disorders. This initial classification was reviewed and expanded, recognised as Rome I (1994), Rome II (1999) and then Rome III (2006) criteria, all of which have definitively changed the diagnostic approach towards FGIDs (Drossman *et al.*, 2006). A paediatric criterion was included within Rome II for the first time (Mostafa, 2008). The symposium on the multidisciplinary approach to childhood abdominal pain and irritable bowel syndrome took place in 2007 and brought together more than 350 specialists in paediatrics, gastroenterology, psychology and other paediatric specialties. It was acknowledged then that FGIDs did not fit into a medical pathophysiology model. Therefore, it would require a model able to integrate the complex interaction of observed biological, psychological and social variables found within those conditions. All of these contributive factors were widely recognised as interlinked within FGIDs, and the biopsychosocial model was accepted as a model of reference (Nurko and Di Lorenzo, 2008). Psychosocial factors have been recognised as significant in FGIDs, regarding their modulation on the experience of specific symptoms, their effects in the brain–gut interaction, their influence in illness behaviour, their impact on outcomes and their influence in the choice of therapeutic approach (Drossman *et al.*, 1999). The Rome III manual is also recognised as the most comprehensive and authoritative resource on FGIDs (Lucak, 2006), as it provides information on the epidemiology, pathophysiology, diagnosis and treatment of more than 20 FGIDs commonly seen in clinical practice (Pace, 2008). It included areas dedicated to neuro-gastroenterology, the role of gender and culture, and the psychological aspects of FGIDs (Sheth, 2007).

Children and adolescents are faced with the demands of normal development while at the same time they also have to deal with their illness. Physical sequelae such as delayed growth, inadequate nutritional status and pain may persist even after treatment of the disorder (Hyams *et al.*, 1996). Psychological development is affected because of these disorders interfering with normal developmental tasks such as independence and self-care behaviours, social relationships and the dynamics within the family (Moody *et al.*, 1999). Body image concerns caused by the treatment of the disorders (e.g. having an ostomy) or the medication side effects (e.g. mood swings from steroids prescribed for irritable bowel disease) affect peer relationships, school attendance and the confidence to participate in age-appropriate activities (Akobeng *et al.*, 1999). Evidence of psychological disturbances including depression and anxiety in children and young people with FGIDs such as rumination syndrome (e.g. Chial *et al.*, 2003), irritable bowel syndrome (e.g. Caplan *et al.*, 2003), cyclical vomiting syndrome (Loening-Baucke, 2000) and recurrent abdominal pain (e.g. Di Lorenzo *et al.*, 2005; Schurman *et al.*, 2008) has also been reported in the literature.

Psychological treatment approaches applied to paediatric FGIDs have been systematically reviewed (Brent *et al.*, 2009) and have shown to be effective for this population (Lackner, 2004). These include behavioural management (e.g. Hyman and Danda, 2004; Walia *et al.*, 2009), cognitive behavioural therapy (CBT) (e.g. Chambers *et al.*, 2004; Huertas-Ceballos *et al.*, 2008; Toner, 1994), distraction techniques (e.g. Walker *et al.*, 2006), relaxation training techniques (e.g. Blanchard *et al.*, 1993). The combination of psychological therapies (e.g. CBT, family intervention, problem-solving) and lifestyle recommendations has also shown efficacy (e.g. Bursch, 2008; Drossman *et al.*, 2000; Heymann-Mönnikes *et al.*, 2000).

The number of psychologists in paediatrics who are developing a specialty in gastrointestinal conditions is also increasing. In the United States, the *Pediatric Gastroenterology Special Interest Group* (PG-SIG) is an officially recognised group within the *Society of Pediatric Psychology* (Division 54 of the American Psychological Association). The PG-SIG began as an unofficial interest group in January 2010 and received official approval as a special interest group under the umbrella of the Society of Pediatric Psychology in February 2011. The inaugural meeting of the PG-SIG occurred at the American Psychological Association's national conference in August 2010 (in San Diego). The PG-SIG co-founders were Jennifer Verrill Schurman and Anthony Alioto. In the United Kingdom, the *Paediatric Psychology Gastroenterology Special Interest Group (PP Gastro SiG)* sits within the *Paediatric Psychology Network of the British Psychological Society (BPS-PPN)*. This group, convened by Kate Blakeley and Clarissa Martin, organised the symposia in psychological approaches to children and young people with gastrointestinal conditions at the first European Paediatric Psychology Conference, which took place in Oxford in June 2012. In the rest of the countries of the European Union, clinical and academic child health psychologists cover this specialty.

Taking into consideration the entire historical context cited here, it is clear that the specialty of *paediatric gastroenterology* is opening doors to future multidisciplinary research and development while looking for a 'whole child' approach. Therefore, a book with up-to-date research and clinical practice on psychosocial aspects of paediatric gastrointestinal conditions, which includes international specialists and experts in the field of paediatric gastroenterology, was paramount at this stage. It is within this context that this third book of the Paediatric Psychology series was conceived. Its aim is to offer health professionals, students and health professionals in training, and members of the public a multidisciplinary perspective on the psychosocial considerations of children and young people with gastrointestinal disorders and their families. The book, like the other books of the series, is divided into three parts. Part I is loosely focused on theoretical aspects and issues that underpin the casework that follows in Part II. Part III includes tools and examples that have proved to be useful for the clinical practice.

In Chapter 1, Rajindrajith, Devaranayana and Benninga introduce us to the definition of paediatric FGIDs, revisiting the Rome criteria. Their global perspective on prevalence and epidemiology data provides an awareness of the universal dimension of these disorders and provides a baseline for the rest of the book. In Chapter 2, Silverman and Williams describe the various models of integrated care commonly found within paediatric gastroenterology clinical practice settings. They review the empirical support for interdisciplinary services and describe the role of a psychologist working within gastroenterology services. They also advocate for coordination of clinical services as essential to the successful treatment of complex disorders in the field of paediatric gastroenterology. In Chapter 3, King, Boutilier and Chambers look at the application of CBT for recurrent abdominal pain. The authors review the strong evidence base and outline the core components of a CBT programme. In Chapter 4, Schurman and Deacy highlight the application of the social–ecological model to assess social–family–environmental contributory factors, and present intervention strategies from a social learning perspective. Adherence is the subject of Chapter 5. Hommel and Gray review and summarise the literature on adherence in paediatric irritable bowel disease and liver transplant and expand on intervention strategies aimed to improve adherence. In Chapter 6, Protheroe describes home parenteral nutrition and how this approach has helped children with chronic gastroenterological illness to survive. The importance of a multidisciplinary team approach is highlighted when planning the transition from hospital to home and from paediatric to adult services. Part I is rounded off by Dovey's critique of the biopsychosocial model (Chapter 7). His chapter revisits its historical context and challenges current interpretations and understanding of its application.

Part II begins with Danda and Hyman's Chapter 8, describing how children presenting with defecation disorders are common in paediatric gastroenterology practice but are not well understood. They also address the management of functional constipation including the combination of medication and comprehensive behavioural methods. Following this, in Chapter 9, Alioto, Di Lorenzo and Parzanese review the literature on physiological and psychological factors in the rare condition of rumination syndrome. They also describe their interdisciplinary inpatient programme sharing with us the lessons learnt. In Chapter 10, Williams, Field and Alexander revisit the current state of research and clinical practice on children with autism spectrum conditions that suffer gastrointestinal problems and the impact that these may have on the children's problematic behaviour. Chapter 11 focuses on young people with coeliac disease, as Howard and Urquhart-Law consider its impact on psychological well-being and quality of life. In Chapter 12, Townson helps us to appreciate the many challenges that adolescents living with Crohn's disease and their families face and how this illness affects their quality of life. In Chapter 13, Martin discusses various aspects of tube-feeding and tube-weaning feeding therapy. Finally, the last word goes to the patient: in Giles and Southall's Chapter 14, we hear how an undiagnosed gastrointestinal disorder affects the life of Taigh Giles as she grows up into a young woman. This chapter presents a powerful case for listening to, and learning from, the patient. Revisiting the narrative of personal experience makes it possible to reflect on some of the basic beliefs about medicine that govern what we do as healthcare professionals and challenges us to think differently about them.

Part III of the book is essentially the 'toolkit' for the interested practitioner. Ghosal and Martin begin this section, revisiting the unique characteristics of the anatomy and physiology of normal development and the maturation of the digestive system in infants. This section of the book includes a compendium of assessment measures compiled by the Assessment Working Group (Maddux, Deacy and Lukens) of the PG-SIG of the American Psychological Association, Division 54 (Pediatric Psychology). We have also included practical material such as flow charts, clinical interview schedules, handouts for parents and leaflets used in constipation clinics and shared by Mobberley, Danda and Hyman. We have also shared notes on cyclical vomiting syndrome, an example of a standard letter describing symptoms of recurrent abdominal pain and material from one of our cases that required tube-weaning feeding therapy in an inpatient setting. Information on tube types courtesy of CORPAK is also included.

Clarissa Martin and Terence Dovey
March 2014

REFERENCES

Akobeng AK, Suresh-Babu MV, Firth D, *et al*. Quality of life in children with Crohn's disease: a pilot study. *J Pediatr Gastroenterol Nutr.* 1999; **28**(4): S37–9.

Beattie RM. *Report of the British Society of Paediatric Gastroenterology, Hepatology and Nutrition Working Group to Develop Criteria for DGH Gastroenterology Hepatology and Nutrition Services.* British Society of Paediatric Gastroenterology Hepatology and Nutrition (BSPGHAN); 2002.

Blanchard EB, Greene B, Scharff L, *et al*. Relaxation training as a treatment for irritable bowel syndrome. *Biofeedback Self Regul.* 1993; **18**(3): 125–32.

Brent M, Lobato D, LeLeiko N. Psychological treatments for pediatric functional gastrointestinal disorders. *J Pediatr Gastroenterol Nutr.* 2009; **48**(1): 13–21.

Bursch B. Psychological/cognitive behavioral treatment of childhood functional abdominal pain and irritable bowel syndrome. *J Pediatr Gastroenterol Nutr.* 2008; **47**(5): 706–7.

Caplan A, Lambrette P, Joly L, *et al*. Intergenerational transmission of functional gastrointestinal disorders: children of IBS patients versus children with IBS, functional dyspepsia and functional abdominal pain. *Gastroenterology.* 2003; **124**(4 Suppl. 1): A533.

Chambers CT, Holly C, Eakins D. Cognitive-behavioural treatment of recurrent abdominal pain in children: a primer for paediatricians. *Paediatr Child Health.* 2004; **9**(10): 705–8.

Chial HJ, Camilleri M, Williams DE, *et al*. Rumination syndrome in children and adolescents: diagnosis, treatment, and prognosis. *Pediatrics.* 2003; **111**(1): 158–62.

Chumpitazi B, Nurko S. Pediatric gastrointestinal motility disorders: challenges and a clinical update. *Gastroenterol Hepatol (N Y).* 2008; **4**(2): 140–8.

Corazziari E. Definition and epidemiology of functional gastrointestinal disorders. *Best Pract Res Clin Gastroenterol.* 2004; **18**(4): 613–31.

Di Lorenzo C, Colletti RB, Lehmann HP, *et al*. Chronic abdominal pain in children: a technical report of the American Academy of Pediatrics and the North American Society for Pediatric Gastroenterology, Hepatology and Nutrition. *J Pediatr Gastroenterol Nutr.* 2005; **40**: 249–61.

Drossman DA, Li Z, Andruzzi E, *et al*. U.S. Householder survey of functional gastrointestinal disorders: prevalence, sociodemography and health impact. *Dig Dis Sci.* 1993; **38**(9): 1569–80.

Drossman DA, Creed FH, Olden KW, *et al*. Psychosocial aspects of the functional gastrointestinal disorders. *Gut.* 1999; **45**(2): 25–30.

Drossman DA, Creed FH, Olden KW, *et al*. Psychosocial aspects of the functional gastrointestinal disorders. In: Drossman DA, Corazziari E, Talley NJ, editors. *Rome II: the functional gastrointestinal disorders: diagnosis, pathophysiology and treatment; a multinational consensus.* 2nd ed. McLean, VA: Degnon; 2000. pp. 157–245.

Drossman DA, Corazziari E, Delvaux M, *et al*., editors. *Rome III: the functional gastrointestinal disorders.* 3rd ed. McLean, VA: Degnon; 2006.

Hamilton JR. Pediatric gastroenterorology: an emerging specialty. In: Walker WA, Durie PR, Hamilton JR, *et al*., editors. *Pediatric Gastrointestinal Disease.* Hamilton, ON: BC Decker; 1991. pp. 3–5.

Heymann-Mönnikes I, Arnold R, Florin I, *et al*. The combination of medical treatment plus multicomponent behavioral therapy is superior to medical treatment alone in the therapy of irritable bowel syndrome. *Am J Gastroenterol.* 2000; **95**(4): 981–94.

Huertas-Ceballos A, Logan S, Bennett C, *et al*. Psychosocial interventions for recurrent abdominal pain (RAP) and irritable bowel syndrome (IBS) in childhood. *Cochrane Database Syst Rev.* 2008;(1): CD003014.

Hyams JS, Burke G, Davis PM, *et al*. Abdominal pain and irritable bowel syndrome in adolescents: a community-based study. *J Pediatr.* 1996; **129**(2): 220–6.

Hyman PE, Danda CE. Understanding and treating childhood bellyaches: pediatric functional gastrointestinal disorders. *Pediatric Annals.* 2004; **33**(2): 97–104.

Lackner JM. Psychological treatments for irritable bowel syndrome: a systematic review and meta-analysis. *J Consult Clin Psychol.* 2004; **72**(6): 1100–13.

Loening-Baucke V. Aerophagia as cause of gaseous abdominal distention in a toddler. *J Pediatr Gastroenterol Nutr.* 2000; **31**(2): 204–7.

Lucak S. Rome III: the functional gastrointestinal disorders, third edition [book review]. *Functional Brain-Gut Research Group Newsletter.* 2006; **38**: 12.

Moody G, Eaden JA, Mayberry JF. Social implications of childhood Crohn's disease. *J Pediatr Gastroenterol Nutr.* 1999: **28**(4); S43–5.

Mostafa R. Rome III: the functional gastrointestinal disorders third edition, 2006. *World J Gastroenterol.* 2008; **14**(13): 2124–5.

Nurko S, Di Lorenzo C. Functional abdominal pain: time to get together and move forward. *J Pediatr Gastroenterol Nutr.* 2008; **47**(5): 697–715.

Pace F. The functional gastrointestinal disorders. *Dig Liver Dis.* 2008; **40**: 232–3.

Rasquin A, Di Lorenzo C, Forbes D, *et al.* Childhood functional gastrointestinal disorders: child / adolescent. *Gastreoenterology.* 2006; **130**: 1527–37.

Schurman JV, Danda CE, Friesen CA, *et al.* Variations in psychological profile among children with recurrent abdominal pain. *J Clin Psychol Med Settings.* 2008; **15**(3): 241–51.

Sheth AA. Rome III: the functional gastrointestinal disorders. *J Clin Gastroenterol.* 2007; **41**(9): 867.

Toner BB. Cognitive-behavioral treatment of functional somatic syndromes: integrating gender issues. *Cogn Behav Pract.* 1994; **1**: 157–78.

Walker LS, Williams SE, Smith CA, *et al.* Parent attention versus distraction: impact on symptom complaints by children with and without chronic functional abdominal pain. *Pain.* 2006; **122**(12): 43–52.

Walker-Smith J, Walker WA. The development of pediatric gastroenterology: a historical overview. *Pediatr Res.* 2003; **53**(4): 706–15.

Walia R, Mahajan L, Steffen R. Recent advances in chronic constipation. *Curr Opin Pediatr.* 2009; **21**(5): 661–6.

PART I

Understanding gastrointestinal disorders

Global prevalence and international perspective of paediatric gastrointestinal disorders

Shaman Rajindrajith, Niranga Devanarayana and Marc Benninga

INTRODUCTION

Functional gastrointestinal disorders (FGIDs) consist of a group of chronic gastrointestinal problems characterised by recurrent symptoms that cannot be explained by structural and biochemical abnormalities. The chronic and disabling nature of symptoms and their remarkably high prevalence across the globe has identified them as a concern for paediatric public health. Initial epidemiological data and hospital-based studies from the Western world provided a notion that these disorders were possibly a result of a 'Western lifestyle'. However, compelling data have emerged from Asia and Latin American countries indicating that functional gastrointestinal disorders have a global dimension in prevalence. They have come to challenge the already overstretched health budgets of both developed and developing countries and compete with other prioritised communicable and non-communicable diseases such as HIV, tuberculosis, malnutrition, obesity and malignancies. Moreover, the biology and pathophysiology of FGIDs are shown to be increasingly associated with psychological stress, early adverse life events, infections and urbanisation, all of which are common across the globe. In addition, certain categories of FGIDs are commonly seen among children living in deprived and disrupted societies such as those affected by war. These disorders are known to have deleterious ramifications on childhood functioning and health-related quality of life (QoL). This chapter reviews the current epidemiological trends and international perspectives of FGIDs in children.

CLASSIFICATION AND DEFINITIONS

Historical facts

Recurrent abdominal pain

In 1909 a British paediatrician, GF Still, wrote: 'I know of no symptom which can be more obscure in its causation than colicky abdominal pain in childhood' (Still, 1909). A century later, childhood abdominal pain remains a curious enigma. Recently, significant progress has been made to shed some light upon this subject.

The term 'recurrent abdominal pain' came into use in the 1950s, following John Apley's use of the term (Apley and Naish, 1958). The majority of children with recurrent abdominal pain had no recognisable organic cause for their symptoms and were thought to have abdominal pain of functional origin. However, Apley's diagnostic entity soon proved to be too general, as it transpired that up to 68% of children with recurrent abdominal pain could be classified as having irritable bowel syndrome (IBS) using established adult diagnostic criteria (Hyams *et al.*, 1996). In addition, constipation had come to be widely acknowledged as a common organic cause for abdominal pain. Previously, constipation had been recognised as an organic disorder that could cause harm through an accumulation of faeces in the body. Traditionally, medical staff regularly prescribed laxatives to 'decontaminate' the bowel, a practice that continued even up to the 1950s (Bongers, 2008). (*See* also Chapters 3 and 8.)

Classification of Functional gastrointestinal disorders (FGIDs)

The first internationally accepted classification system of adult FGID was known as the *Rome I* classification. This has since been iterated and updated (Drossman *et al.*, 1990), and it is currently the most widely accepted classification system for FGIDs.

The *Rome II* classification of FGIDs, introduced in 1999, was a historical landmark in paediatric gastroenterology (Rasquin-Weber *et al.*, 1999). For the first time, functional gastrointestinal diseases in children were formally recognised, establishing a foundation for future research and enabling researchers to link the historic 'recurrent abdominal pain' classifications to modern FGIDs.

Rome III criteria

The currently accepted diagnostic criteria for FGIDs are known as the *Rome III criteria*. These were introduced in 2006 and, as discussed, developed out of the two previous criteria (Rome I and Rome II). The classification includes two separate systems, one for infants and toddlers and the other for children and adolescents (Hyman *et al.*, 2006; Rasquin *et al.*, 2006). Table 1.1 gives the details of classification of functional gastrointestinal diseases in children and adolescents. The Rome III Committee has reduced the required duration of symptoms of most functional gastrointestinal diseases from 3 months to 2.

> **BOX 1.1** Limitations of the Rome II classification system
>
> Several studies have shown a significant percentage of children with non-organic recurrent abdominal pain to have functional gastrointestinal diseases. Walker *et al.* (2004) showed that 73% of children with 'full terminology of recurrent abdominal pain' can be classified into FGIDs such as IBS and functional abdominal pain using the Rome II criteria. A school-based study from Asia has shown that 73% of children with recurrent abdominal pain had functional gastrointestinal diseases (Devanarayana *et al.*, 2008). However, the Rome II criteria had limitations. A prospective study in school children demonstrated that at least 8% of children with chronic abdominal pain of a 3-month duration could not be assigned to a particular functional gastrointestinal disease group using Rome II criteria (Saps *et al.*, 2006). Another study found only a fair agreement between physicians and parents using Rome II criteria (Schurman *et al.*, 2005). Furthermore, two additional studies on defecation disorders illustrated that Rome II criteria for defecation disorders were too restrictive and would exclude a significant proportion of children when applied to clinical settings (Loening-Baucke, 2004; Voskuijl *et al.*, 2004). These findings paved the way for modifications of the Rome II criteria.

Furthermore, a threshold of symptom frequency of at least once a week has been introduced.[4]

TABLE 1.1 Classification of childhood functional gastrointestinal diseases (FGIDs) in Rome III criteria

1 Vomiting and aerophagia

    1a. Adolescent rumination syndrome

    1b. Cyclical vomiting syndrome

    1c. Aerophagia

2 Abdominal pain-related FGIDs

    2a. Functional dyspepsia

    2b. Irritable bowel syndrome

    2c. Abdominal migraine

    2d. Childhood functional abdominal pain

3 Constipation and incontinence

    3a. Functional constipation

    3b. Non-retentive faecal incontinence

---

4 The Rome III revised duration and symptom thresholds do not apply to abdominal migraine and cyclical vomiting syndrome.

In defecation disorders, functional faecal retention is excluded from current classification criteria as a separate diagnostic entity. However, several significant clinical characteristics of constipation have now been included, such as non-retentive faecal incontinence, with a frequency of occurrence of at least once a month. These modifications have made the Rome III criteria more inclusive and more useful in the diagnosis of functional gastrointestinal disease in children and more likely to positively diagnose the whole spectrum of functional gastrointestinal diseases than the previous Rome II criteria (Baber *et al.*, 2008; Devanarayana *et al.*, 2011a). However, much stills needs to be done to refine them and, more important, to convince paediatricians to use them in day-to-day clinical practice.

EPIDEMIOLOGY OF FUNCTIONAL GASTROINTESTINAL DISORDERS (FGIDS)

Vomiting and aerophagia

Aerophagia

Aerophagia is a functional gastrointestinal disease characterised by repetitive swallowing of air that leads to abdominal distension, excessive belching and/or flatus. Clinically, children with aerophagia present with a non-distended abdomen in the morning and gradual distension of the abdomen throughout the day. Excessive belching is noted during the day. In addition, frequency of passing flatus increases, especially during the night. On physical examination the abdomen shows gross distension and the percussion note is tympanic all over the abdomen. Although it seems benign, in severe cases aerophagia leads to serious complications such as pneumoperitoneum, volvulus and intestinal perforation (Basaran *et al.*, 2007; Hutchinson *et al.*, 1980; Trillis F Jr *et al.*, 1986).

Until recently, there were no studies assessing the epidemiology of aerophagia. Initially, aerophagia was believed to be more prevalent in children with chronic neurological conditions such as Rett's syndrome and autism (Morton *et al.*, 2000; Ramocki *et al.*, 2009). However, subsequent studies have found aerophagia in a significant percentage of otherwise healthy children. In a prospective study among 243 black American schoolchildren, attending a community primary care clinic, Uc and co-workers (Uc *et al.*, 2006) reported aerophagia in 2.4%. Only a few studies have assessed the community prevalence of aerophagia. Two recent school-based studies in 10- to 16-year-olds have reported this condition in 6.3% and 7.5%, respectively. In these studies there was no significant gender difference in prevalence (Devanarayana *et al.*, 2011b, 2012). Higher prevalence of aerophagia was observed in older children but there was no clear correlation with age. The identified risk factors were lower socio-economic status, large family size, having a working mother, living in an urban area and exposure to stressful life events. Furthermore, children with aerophagia had difficulty in sleeping and had missed school because of their symptoms.

Cyclical vomiting syndrome

Cyclical vomiting syndrome (CVS) is a clinical entity associated with recurrent episodes of severe nausea and vomiting that may last for hours to days with well-demarcated symptom-free intervals. The disorder is typically associated with negative laboratory, endoscopic and radiological test results. There is a stereotypical pattern of symptoms in most of the individuals with regard to time of day, duration and onset of symptoms. Vomiting begins late night or early morning with intense nausea, often triggered by psychological distress. Associated symptoms include pallor, listlessness, retching, abdominal pain, headache and photophobia (Rasquin *et al.*, 2006; Li *et al.*, 2008).

Data on the epidemiology of CVS in children are limited. A population-based survey from Aberdeen, Scotland, involving children aged 5–15 years, has shown the prevalence of cyclical vomiting to be 1.9% in the United Kingdom (Abu-Arafeh and Russell, 1995a), 2.3% in Australia (Cullen and Macdonald, 1963), 0.5% in Sri Lanka (Devanarayana and Rajindrajith, 2012) and 1.9% in Turkey (Ertekin *et al.*, 2006). Although overall sex ratio for the whole population was 1:1, cyclical vomiting was more common among boys in the younger age group of less than 7 years. The sex ratio reversed in children older than 7 years. Travel, stress, tiredness and lack of sleep were the recognised precipitating factors. In a prospective surveillance study in Ireland, the incidence of CVS was found to be 3.5/100 000 children per annum. In this study, the median age of diagnosis was 7.42 years and the median age of onset was 4 years. The majority of children missed school because of their symptoms, indicating the disabling nature of the disease (Fitzpatrick *et al.*, 2008). Current research is inconclusive, as there seems to be considerable heterogeneity and variability of the prevalence rates in different studies conducted in different geographical locations. (*See* also 'Notes on cyclical vomiting syndrome' in Part III.)

Rumination syndrome

Rumination syndrome is defined as effortless, repetitive, painless regurgitation of partially digested food into the mouth soon after the meal, which is subsequently re-chewed and re-swallowed or, in the alternative, expelled (Rasquin *et al.*, 2006). Rumination syndrome is thought to be common in children who are neurologically handicapped with developmental abnormalities and learning difficulties (Chatoor *et al.*, 1984; Rogers *et al.*, 1992). In clinical settings, rumination syndrome is frequently misdiagnosed as gastro-oesophageal reflux, gastroparesis and recurrent vomiting. These misconceptions and misdiagnoses and poor awareness among clinicians have led to underdiagnosis of this important and sometimes disabling disease in children. However, recent data show its increasing prevalence among otherwise healthy people with normal cognitive function (Khan *et al.*, 2000; Lee *et al.*, 2007).

Data for this disorder have been derived from case series from tertiary care referral centres and therefore include a bias towards severe cases. A recent small-scale epidemiological survey in Sri Lanka noted a prevalence of 4%

among 12- to 16-year-old children in a semi-urban school (Devanarayana and Rajindrajith, 2012). (*See also* Chapter 9.)

Abdominal pain-predominant functional gastrointestinal diseases
Functional dyspepsia

Functional dyspepsia is a disorder characterised by the presence of persistent or recurrent pain or discomfort that does not subside with defecation and which is localised to the central region of the abdomen above the umbilicus (Rasquin *et al.*, 2006). Epidemiology of functional dyspepsia has not been adequately studied across the world. A school-based study in Italy of children aged 6–19 years using Rome II criteria noted ulcer-like dyspepsia in 3.4% of children and dysmotility-like dyspepsia in 3.7% (De Giacomo *et al.*, 2002). A prospective survey from the same country and that included children of a much more diverse age range showed a prevalence of 0.3% (Miele *et al.*, 2004). A study from Asia has evaluated prevalence of abdominal pain-predominant functional gastrointestinal diseases in children and shown a prevalence of functional dyspepsia in 2.5% (Devanarayana and Rajindrajith, 2012). The prevalence was higher among girls than boys. A detailed symptom analysis showed that the majority of children have pain several times a week and the pain is short-lasting (less than 1 hour). Furthermore, children with functional dyspepsia also suffer from a range of intestinal-related symptoms such as bloating, loss of appetite, nausea, burping and flatulence, as well as extra-intestinal symptoms such as headaches, limb pains, headache, sleeping difficulties and light-headedness (Devanarayana *et al.*, 2011b).

Irritable bowel syndrome

IBS denotes the presence of abdominal pain that is relieved by defecation and/or associated with change in bowel frequency and/or consistency of the stool with the onset of pain. Even though epidemiology of IBS has been studied in detail in adults, research assessing this important disorder in children is sparse and limited. Early studies from the Western world led to the belief that IBS is a disease of affluent societies. Emerging data from Asia, both in children and adults, have suggested otherwise. Studies on prevalence of IBS in Europe and the United States are old, with many having been conducted nearly a decade ago. According to these studies prevalence of IBS among school children in the United Kingdom and the United States are 1.29% and 10.05%, respectively (Hyams *et al.*, 1996; Thompson and Dancey, 1996). In addition, a higher prevalence (20%) was observed in children in Russia (western Siberia) according to the Rome II criteria (Rashetnikov *et al.*, 2001). In contrast to this, a prospective study from Italy using the same criteria reported a much lower prevalence (0.21%) (Miele *et al.*, 2004). Wide variation in the age of the recruited in different studies may have contributed to these differences in reported prevalence of IBS. Two of the studies found that IBS is much more common among girls and prevalence increases as they grow older (Hyams *et al.*, 1996; Thompson and Dancey, 1996). To date, no study has used the sub-classification criteria of IBS.

In the last decade, however, the epidemiology of IBS has been well studied. Most of these studies have been fairly large and have included over 400 children, using Rome II or Rome III criteria to establish the diagnosis. The prevalence of IBS in Asian countries varies from 2.8%, in Sri Lankan children aged 10–16 years (Devanarayana *et al.*, 2011a), to 25.7%, in Korean girls (Son *et al.*, 2009). Furthermore, studies from other developed nations in Asia such as Japan have also shown high prevalence of IBS 14.6%–19% (Endo *et al.*, 2011). Prevalence in China varies between 13.25% and 20.72% (Dong *et al.*, 2005; Zhou *et al.*, 2010, 2011), and a study from Sri Lanka has shown a prevalence of 6.2% (Rajindrajith and Devanarayana, 2012). Figure 1.1 and Table 1.2 show the distribution and prevalence of epidemiological studies of IBS around the world.

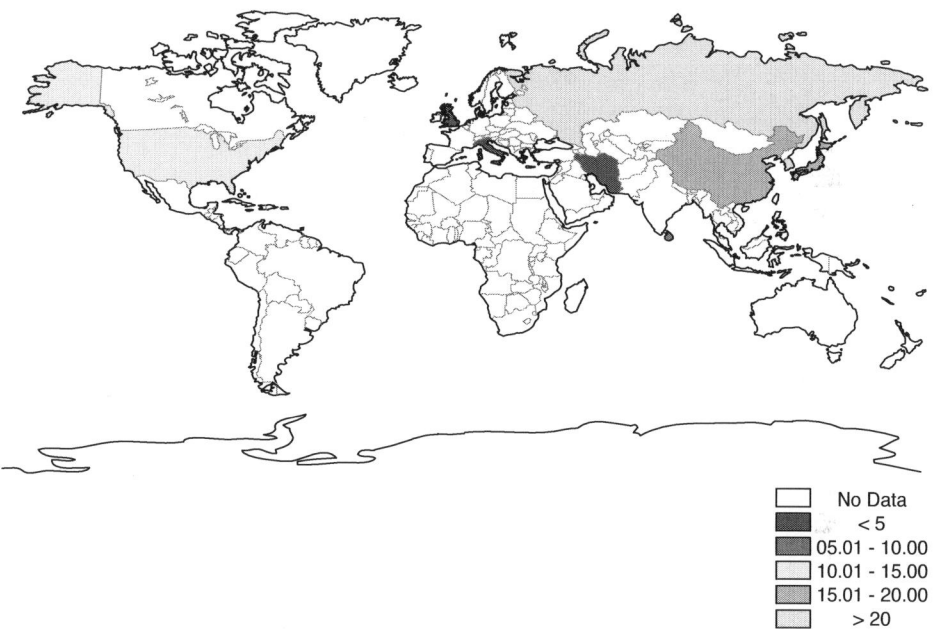

☐	No Data
■	< 5
▨	05.01 - 10.00
☐	10.01 - 15.00
▨	15.01 - 20.00
☐	> 20

FIGURE 1.1 Global distribution of irritable bowel syndrome in children

TABLE 1.2 Prevalence of irritable bowel syndrome in children in the world

Country	Year of publication	Age group (years)	Prevalence (%)
Sri Lanka	2012	10–16	6.2
Sri Lanka	2011	10–16	4.9
Sri Lanka	2010	12–16	7.0
Japan	2011	15	14.6
China	2011	12–18	19.9
China	2010	10–18	20.72
China	2005	6–18	13.25

(continued)

Country	Year of publication	Age group (years)	Prevalence (%)
Iran	2009	14–19	4.1
Korea	2007	15–17 (girls)	25.7
Italy	2004	0–12	0.21
Russia	2001	14–17	20.0
United States	1996	12–16	10.0
United Kingdom	1996	11–17	1.29
Italy	2004	0–12	0.7

Several researchers have studied subtypes of IBS in children using Rome criteria described for adults (Devanarayana *et al.*, 2011a; Dong *et al.*, 2005; Endo
et al., 2011; Longstreth *et al.*, 2006; Rajindrajith and Devanarayana, 2012; Son
et al., 2009; Thompson *et al.*, 1999; Zhou *et al.*, 2010, 2011). Classification of
IBS according to the bowel habits of the individual is extensively used in adult
studies and clinical trials. The following subtypes have been identified in this
classification: diarrhoea-predominant IBS, constipation-predominant IBS,
mixed IBS (alternating diarrhoea and constipation) and unsubtyped IBS (not
falling into any of the aforementioned categories depending on predominant
bowel habits). Using this sub-classification, in two studies Zhou *et al.* (2010,
2011) have shown that unsubtypable IBS predominates among Chinese children. Other countries such as Korea, Iran and Sri Lanka have shown wide
variations in distribution of subtypes of IBS (Rajindrajith and Devanarayana,
2012; Sohrabi *et al.*, 2010; Son *et al.*, 2009).

TABLE 1.3 Prevalence of subtypes of irritable bowel syndrome (IBS) in children

	Authors					
	Rajindrajith *et al.*	Devanarayana *et al.*	Zhou *et al.*	Zhou *et al.*	Sohrabi *et al.*	Son *et al.*
Country	Sri Lanka	Sri Lanka	China	China	Iran	Korea
Sample size	1717	417	3671	2013	1436	1517
Publication year	2012	2011	2011	2010	2010	2009
Diagnostic criteria for IBS	Rome III (child)	Rome III (child)	Rome III (adult)	Rome III (adult)	Rome II (adult)	Rome II (adult)
IBS-C (%)	27.1	26.7	20.14	20.14	52.5	34.6
IBS-D (%)	28.0	26.7	17.76	18.47	11.8	26.9
IBS-M/IBS-A (%)	27.1	33.3	10.27	10.31	18.6	38.5
IBS-U (%)	17.8	13.3	51.1	51.08	–	–

IBS-C, constipation-predominant IBS; IBS-D, diarrhoea-predominant IBS; IBS-M, mixed IBS; IBS-A,
alternating IBS; IBS-U, unsubtyped IBS.

Functional abdominal pain

Functional abdominal pain (*see* Chapter 3) according to the Rome III criteria is a different clinical entity compared with the recurrent abdominal pain described by Apley and Naish (1958). The definition includes persistent or recurrent pain episodes, at least once a week for 2 months, without the presence of organic diseases (Rasquin *et al.*, 2006). Epidemiology of this disorder is not well studied in children. A study carried out in Sri Lanka has shown a prevalence of 4.4% (Devanarayana *et al.*, 2008). Another study in Sri Lanka has also shown that functional abdominal pain has the highest prevalence rates among all of the FGIDs in children (Devanarayana *et al.*, 2011a).

Abdominal migraine

Abdominal migraine is a well-known cause for abdominal pain in children. In the current Rome III criteria, it is recognised as paroxysmal episodes of intense peri-umbilical pain lasting for more than 1 hour with associated symptoms such as nausea, anorexia, vomiting, headache, photophobia and pallor. Affected children are otherwise well between attacks and the period between episodes may last for weeks to months (Rasquin *et al.*, 2006). Abdominal migraine has been recognised as a common cause of recurrent abdominal pain in children in several hospital-based studies using Rome II or Rome III criteria (Devanarayana *et al.*, 2011a; Helgeland *et al.*, 2009; Walker *et al.*, 2004). In a study using the International Classification of Headache Disorders, 4.4% children evaluated for abdominal pain had abdominal migraine (Carson *et al.*, 2011). An epidemiological survey conducted in the United Kingdom, using International Headache Society criteria, noted 4.1% of children as having abdominal migraine (Abu-Arafeh and Russell, 1995b). In this study, the prevalence of abdominal migraine was higher among girls and attacks were associated with exposure to stressful events, travel, tiredness and consumption of certain food items. In a Sri Lankan school-based survey involving children aged 10–16 years, it was found that only 1% of children suffered from abdominal migraine according to the accepted criteria (Devanarayana *et al.*, 2011a). It was also noted that this disorder is associated with family- and school-related psychological stress. Other painful conditions such as headache and limb pains, photophobia, light-headedness and sleeping difficulties were commonly associated with abdominal migraine. In addition, other functional abdominal symptoms such as bloating, loss of appetite, flatulence, burping, nausea and vomiting were also associated with abdominal migraine (Devanarayana *et al.*, 2011b).

Functional defecation disorders

(For functional defecation disorders, *see* also Chapter 8.)

Functional constipation

Functional constipation is a cosmopolitan problem and with prevalence rates varying by geographical location and environmental considerations. Rates are high enough to be considered a public health issue. Epidemiology of functional constipation has been well studied in both the Western world and Asia using well-established criteria. Studies from Western countries during the first decade of the new millennium have shown a prevalence range from 0.7% in Italy to 16% in the United States (Uc *et al.*, 2006; Miele *et al.*, 2004). A significant number of studies have also been conducted in both developed and developing nations across Asia (Chung *et al.*, 2010; Devanarayana and Rajindrajith, 2010; Ip *et al.*, 2005; Lee, *et al.*, 2008; Sohrabi *et al.*, 2010; Wu *et al.*, 2011; Rajindrajith *et al.*, 2012a). In these studies, particularly among developed countries in the Asian region, prevalence of functional constipation is more or less close to the prevalence in the Western world (Chung *et al.*, 2010; Ip *et al.*, 2005; Lee, *et al.*, 2008; Wu *et al.*, 2011). Similarly, studies from South America, particularly in Brazil, have shown higher prevalence rates of functional constipation (20%–28%), similar to the developed nations in Asia (De Arajuo Sant'Anna and Calcado, 1999; Del Ciampo *et al.*, 2002). In addition, studies from Sri Lanka have revealed functional constipation as an emergent issue, with a prevalence rate ranging between 4.2% and 15.4% (Devanarayana *et al.*, 2011a; Devanarayana and Rajindrajith, 2010; Rajindrajith *et al.*, 2012a). Data from Asian countries constantly challenge the common paradigm that constipation is a disease of Western countries. Rapidly changing dietary habits, lifestyles and stressful events in the developing Asian economies such as Korea, China and Sri Lanka may have contributed to closing the gap in prevalence of constipation between different nations and regions of the world.

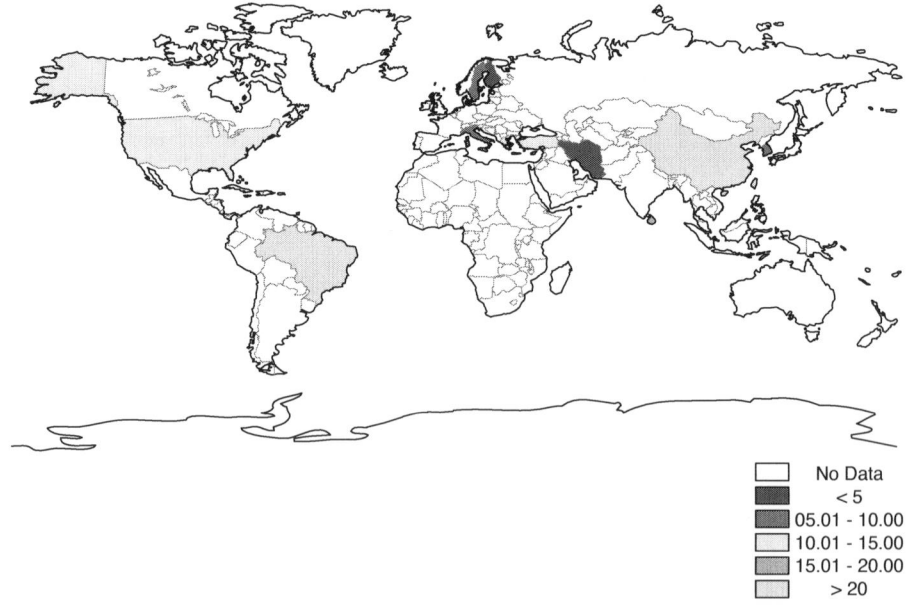

☐	No Data
■	< 5
▨	05.01 - 10.00
☐	10.01 - 15.00
▨	15.01 - 20.00
▨	> 20

FIGURE 1.2 Global distribution of constipation in children

TABLE 1.4 Prevalence of constipation in children in the world

Country	Year of publication	Age group (years)	Prevalence (%)
Taiwan	2012	6–15	12.2
Sri Lanka	2012	10–16	15.4
Taiwan	2011	7–12	32.2
Korea	2010	5–13	6.7
Iran	2010	14–19	2.5
The Netherlands	2010	2	12
United States	2009	5–8	10
Hong Kong/China	2008	3–5	28.8
Turkey	2007	7–12	7.2
Sweden	2006	2.5	6.5
Hong Kong/China	2005	3–5	29.6
Italy	2005	0–0.5	17.6
Italy	2005	0–12	2.6
Italy	2004	0–12	0.7
Finland	2004	10–11	1.5
Turkey	2003	10–11	12.4
Brazil	2002	1–10	26.8
Brazil	1999	8–10	20
Greece	1999	2–14	15
Greece	1999	2–14	6

Functional non-retentive faecal incontinence

Faecal incontinence is defined as passing stools in inappropriate places irrespective of the amount. It is a common problem in the paediatric age range and has significant social repercussions on affected children. Prevalence of functional faecal incontinence ranges from 0.8% to 4.1% in Western countries (Joinson *et al.*, 2006; Van der Wal *et al.*, 2005). Recent studies from Asia noted much higher prevalence ranging from 2% in Sri Lanka to 7.8% in Korea (Chung *et al.*, 2010; Rajindrajith *et al.*, 2010; Zhou *et al.*, 2011). Epidemiological studies on faecal incontinence have not attempted to differentiate between various types of functional faecal incontinence up until recently, although these subtypes have different pathophysiological mechanisms. A school-based survey conducted in Sri Lanka has shown that the majority of children suffering from functional faecal incontinence have constipation-associated faecal incontinence. Only 0.4% of them had functional non-retentive faecal incontinence. This study has also highlighted that the bowel habits of these children are quite different from children with constipation-associated faecal incontinence (Rajindrajith *et al.*, 2010).

GLOBAL PERSPECTIVE OF FUNCTIONAL GASTROINTESTINAL DISEASES

For decades, gastrointestinal infections in the developing world and inflammatory bowel disease in the West were considered to be the main causes of gastrointestinal-related morbidity and mortality. However, with the availability of oral rehydration therapy, vaccination against gastrointestinal infections, therapeutic advances such as immunosuppressants and monoclonal antibodies, the disease burden of gastrointestinal infections has been reduced and the natural history of inflammatory bowel disease has been modified. Against this backdrop, FGIDs in children are emerging as one of the most prevalent types of disorders and they are receiving greater attention in the twenty-first century.

Type and geographical distribution

In summary, the geographical burden of FGIDs is shifting from the West to the East, where the prevalence of most subtypes is increasing. Its fast-growing population will probably identify Asia as the epicentre of FGIDs in the future. Follow-up data with regard to the course of life and long-term prognosis of childhood functional gastrointestinal disorders are limited. The available data suggest that a significant percentage (25%–30%) of children with functional constipation and faecal incontinence grow up to be adults with persistent symptoms (Bongers *et al.*, 2010; Van Ginkel *et al.*, 2003). In addition, in a small retrospective study by Khan *et al.* (2007), childhood constipation appeared to be a predictor of IBS in adulthood.

Age distribution

Relationship between age and FGIDs has been evaluated to reveal a wide variation and heterogeneity in symptoms for all subtypes. The main reason for this is that different studies have recruited children in different age groups, varying from birth to 19 years. Therefore, a precise age distribution in epidemiology cannot be described with certainty. However, several trends have been highlighted. For example, a study among school children in Sri Lanka has illustrated a negative correlation between prevalence of abdominal pain-related FGIDs and age (Devanarayana *et al.*, 2008). A more descriptive analysis of IBS patients by the same group of researchers has found linear reduction of probability in developing IBS with age. On the other hand, three other epidemiological studies from the United States and China have noted a trend of increasing prevalence of IBS with age (Dong *et al.*, 2005; Endo *et al.*, 2011; Hyams *et al.*, 1996).

Similarly, the majority of previous studies have shown a reduction of prevalence of defecation disorders with age. Two epidemiological studies from Sri Lanka have demonstrated that both constipation and faecal incontinence show the highest prevalence at the age of 10 years and a decline with advancing age (Rajindrajith *et al.*, 2010, 2012a). A study from the Netherlands also noted a similar reduction in prevalence of faecal incontinence with age (Van der Wal *et al.*, 2005). It is likely that maturation provides better control over bodily functions, including bowel habits.

In contrast to this, the few available studies on aerophagia and rumination

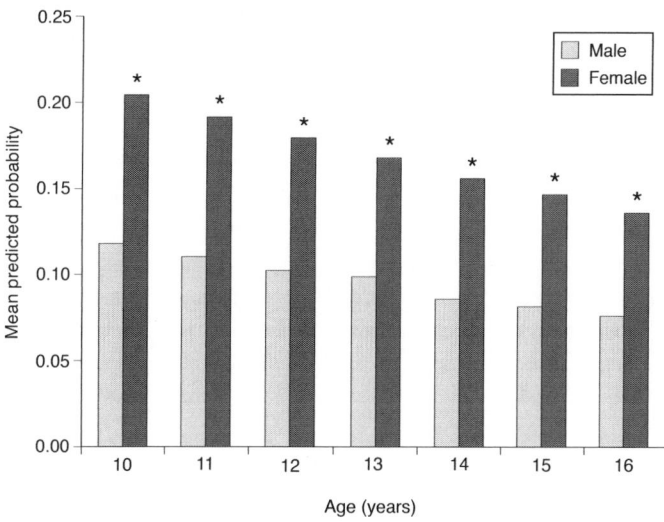

FIGURE 1.3 Age-related prevalence of abdominal pain-predominant FGIDs in children (adopted from Devanarayana *et al.* (2011b) with permission)

syndrome have not shown a significant relationship between their prevalence and age (Devanarayana and Rajindrajith, 2012; Fitzpatrick *et al.*, 2008). The mean age of developing cyclical vomiting is between 4.6 and 6.9 years (Yang, 2010). These contrasting findings need further epidemiological evaluation.

Sex differences studies among adults have clearly shown that several FGIDs, such as IBS and constipation, are found with higher frequency among females (Choung and Locke, 2011). In contrast, gender differences of most FGIDs are not clearly visible in children. Some previous studies have shown a clear female preponderance in development of abdominal pain-predominant FGIDs in children. These studies have shown a higher prevalence of functional dyspepsia and IBS in girls than in boys (Devanarayana *et al.*, 2011b; Hyams *et al.*, 1996; Rajindrajith and Devanarayana, 2012), which is comparable with previous adult studies conducted in IBS and functional dyspepsia around the world (Choung and Locke, 2011). Newly developed Asian economies, the Middle East and developing nations such as Sri Lanka also show a similar female preponderance in prevalence of IBS (Dong *et al.*, 2005; Endo *et al.*, 2011; Hyams *et al.*, 1996; Rajindrajith and Devanarayana, 2012; Zhou *et al.*, 2011). A convincing biological reason for this phenomenon has never been articulated. Effects of female sex hormones on gastrointestinal tract and brain–gut interactions have been suggested as a possible reason (Heitkemper and Jarrett, 2008). However, since most of the children included in previous studies are of young age and have not achieved menarche to acquire the fully mature hormonal profile of a female, the gender difference seen in the abdominal pain-predominant functional gastrointestinal diseases cannot be fully attributed to the effects of female sex hormones. It is also possible that factors other than gender-specific hormonal difference, such as biological differences between males and females, may play an important role in the natural history of the abdominal pain-predominant FGIDs that predispose girls to develop them. Sex-related biological differences in the integration, processing and modulation of pain may also be key mechanisms responsible for the greater female prevalence of many chronic pain disorders such as FGIDs. Psychosocial factors, including how boys and girls are socialised to express emotions differently, are also likely to play an important part in sex differences in prevalence. These considerations lie outside the scope of the present chapter.

Sex-specific prevalence of constipation is more complex and is currently unclear. A few large studies have shown a predilection of girls to develop constipation but the ratios are not statistically significant (Chung *et al.*, 2010; Ip *et al.*, 2005). Several other studies have noted almost equal prevalence between girls and boys (Iacono *et al.*, 2005; Inan *et al.*, 2007). A study from Sri Lanka noted higher prevalence of constipation in boys (Rajindrajith *et al.*, 2012a). This is in contrast to the data from adult studies, which show a clear, statistically significant female preponderance (Suares and Ford, 2011). Progesterone is known to increase transit time of the large and small bowel in women, and childbirth-associated physiological disruption of pelvic floor muscles may have contributed to the higher prevalence of functional constipation in the older population (Chiarelli *et al.*, 2000; Jung *et al.*, 2003). Lack of these physiological phenomena in children would have contributed to lack of gender difference in prevalence of constipation in children and adolescents. Several studies from both developed and developing countries have convincingly demonstrated that functional faecal incontinence is clearly more common among boys (Levine, 1975; Loening-Baucke, 1996; Van der Wal *et al.*, 2005).

The only available epidemiological study on aerophagia does not show a difference of prevalence between girls and boys (Devanarayana and Rajindrajith, 2012). Some recent studies on CVS have found no gender difference in prevalence (Fitzpatrick *et al.*, 2008; Haghighat *et al.*, 2007) while others have found that CVS has a higher prevalence rate among girls (Ertekin *et al.*, 2006; Fleisher and Matar, 1993). Finally, hospital-based data have illustrated a higher prevalence of rumination syndrome among females (Fernandez *et al.*, 2010; Green *et al.*, 2011).

Socio-demographic factors

Sociocultural influences on the development and persistence of a wide variety of functional gastrointestinal diseases are not evidently seen in the paediatric literature. Although studies on most of the functional gastrointestinal diseases do not show a significant influence by sociocultural factors, defecation disorders such as functional constipation and functional faecal incontinence are clearly more common among children from low socio-economic strata (Rajindrajith *et al.*, 2010; Rajindrajith and Devanarayana, 2012; Van der Wal *et al.*, 2005). Poor toilet facilities and large number of family members sharing the same toilet may lead to faecal withholding, which predisposes children to develop both constipation and functional faecal incontinence. In addition, delayed seeking of medical care for constipation may also contribute to the development of defecation disorders in children from disadvantaged socio-economic backgrounds. Furthermore, children living in socially disrupted environments, such as areas affected by war, have higher chances of developing functional defecation disorders (Burns, 1958; Rajindrajith *et al.*, 2011).

Growth

Paediatric obesity and overweight are rising global health problems. Apart from associations with many chronic diseases, including hypertension, hypercho-lesterolemia and non-alcoholic steatohepatitis, obesity in children seems to predispose them to develop abdominal pain-predominant functional gastroin-testinal diseases, although the mechanisms are not clear (Bonilla *et al.*, 2011; Teitelbaum *et al.*, 2009). Several other investigators have noted that functional defecation disorders, both constipation and faecal incontinence, are signifi-cantly more common in children with obesity (Fishman *et al.*, 2004). Obese children are known to have poor gastric accommodation (Hoffman and Tack, 2012). In addition, 10% of morbidly obese children have delayed colonic tran-sit time (Van der Baan-Slootweg *et al.*, 2011). These mechanisms may at least partly explain the increase in functional gastrointestinal diseases seen in obese children.

Psychological factors and child abuse

Psychological factors are well recognised as principal contributory factors to the development of FGIDs in children. Psychological stress is known to alter receptor functions of the central corticotropin-releasing factor signalling sys-tem, inducing acute and chronic stress-induced visceral hyperalgesia. This is thought to be a major pathophysiological mechanism for the development of functional gastrointestinal diseases (Mayer and Tillisch, 2011). Stressful life events have become a common problem in the day-to-day lives of children. A series of epidemiological investigations from Sri Lanka has shown that several FGIDs are associated with school- and home-related stress (Devanarayana *et al.*, 2011b; Rajindrajith and Devanarayana, 2012; Devanarayana and Rajindrajith, 2010). In addition, other studies on Asiatic populations have shown that fre-quency of IBS is increased in children exposed to stress (Endo *et al.*, 2011; Son *et al.*, 2009).

Child maltreatment is a major social welfare problem. Every year about 4%–16% of children are physically abused and one in ten is neglected or psychologically abused. Exposure to multiple types and repeated episodes of maltreatment increases the risk of severe psychological harm (Gilbert *et al.*, 2009). The association between being abused during childhood and the development of functional gastrointestinal diseases as an adult is well known (Koloski *et al.*, 2005). Emerging data show such associations also exist in chil-dren (Van Tilburg, 2011). A preliminary study, from Sri Lanka, has indicated that child abuse is associated with abdominal pain-predominant functional gastrointestinal diseases (Devanarayana *et al.*, 2012).

Infections

Gastrointestinal infections are a common health problem in children. It is estimated that each year 1 billion children in the world under the age of 5 years
suffer from gastroenteritis (Bern *et al.*, 1992). Although the majority recover
without consequence, a small percentage progress to develop FGIDs such as IBS
– known as post-infectious IBS (PI-IBS). PI-IBS is more common after infection
with *Campylobacter* species (Spiller and Garsed, 2009). Two studies have clearly
demonstrated an association between bacterial gastroenteritis and IBS in children. Saps *et al.* (2008) have reported a significant incidence of post-infectious
(bacterial) abdominal pain-related FGIDs. Preliminary investigations suggest
that 36% of children exposed to bacterial enteritis subsequently developed
FGIDs, with 31% diagnosed with PI-IBS. Paediatric data from the Walkerton
Health Study (Thabane *et al.*, 2010), demonstrated a higher incidence of IBS
after exposure to a bacterial gastroenteritis outbreak such as *Escherichia coli* and
Campylobacter species.

These studies have demonstrated that children are at risk of developing
IBS after gastrointestinal infections. Gastrointestinal infections are a common
occurrence in the developing world. It has been noted that a poorly nourished
child living in socially impoverished and cramped conditions without access
to proper sewage disposal and running water will have eight or more gastrointestinal infections a year when compared to a child living with better sanitary
facilities (O'Ryan *et al.*, 2005). These data imply that children living in the
developing world have a higher predilection to develop PI-IBS than children
in the developed world and that this will become a significant burden for these
low-income countries with comparatively small health budgets.

Diet and food allergies

Dietary habits have been studied as possible mechanisms for FGIDs in children. According to a recent retrospective study, 19% of children with cow's milk
protein allergy during infancy have developed abdominal pain-predominant
functional gastrointestinal diseases later on in life. IBS was reported to be the
most common functional gastrointestinal disease within this group of allergy
sufferers (Saps *et al.*, 2011). Similarly, constipation has also been associated
with cow's milk protein allergy in children. Furthermore, several studies have
reported improvement of symptoms of constipation with an elimination diet
(Daher *et al.*, 2001; Davis *et al.*, 1986; Iacono *et al.*, 1998). However, most of
these retrospective studies are limited by a lack of appropriate independent
allergy corroboration or diagnosis and significant recall bias. These limitations
have reduced the applicability of the results in general terms and careful clinical appraisal and laboratory confirmation are needed before recommending
a bovine milk-elimination diet for FGIDs in children.

Fibre is an important component in the human diet. It is recommended
that a child should take a reasonable amount of fibre-containing foods in his
or her diet (age + 5 g per day). Fibre is known to improve stool frequency, stool
volume and colonic transit time (Davis *et al.*, 1986). Several studies have shown

a low-fibre diet as a risk factor for developing constipation in children. Two studies from Asia noted low mean intake of dietary fibre in young children with functional constipation, especially in terms of fruits and vegetables (Chao *et al.*, 2008). In addition, another study has also shown an association between constipation and consumption of fast food, which is known to be low in fibre (Tam *et al.*, 2012). Therefore, a diet low in fibre is a significant risk factor for developing functional constipation in children.

Quality of life

Even though FGIDs are not life threatening, they are known to lead to a low-ered QoL for the children who have them. Significantly lower QoL scores have been reported in all four domains (i.e. physical, emotional, social and school functioning domains) (Varni *et al.*, 2006). Youssef *et al.* (2006) studied QoL in a group of children with functional abdominal pain and compared the results against those of children suffering from inflammatory bowel disease, children suffering from gastro-oesophageal reflux and healthy children. Children with functional abdominal pain had lower physical and emotional scores than healthy children. Furthermore, QoL scores of children with functional abdom-inal pain were comparable with children suffering from inflammatory bowel disease and gastro-oesophageal reflux. These two studies indicate clearly the low QoL in children with abdominal pain-predominant FGIDs. Moreover, the scores are similar to severe organic disorders such as inflammatory bowel disease, indicating a significant component of suffering in these children.

Several studies have shown poor QoL in children with functional consti-pation. According to one study from the United States, the mean QoL score of children with functional constipation was lower than that of children with organic disorders such as reflux oesophagitis (Youssef *et al.*, 2005). Another study, performed in Australia, also noted similar findings in children with slow transit constipation (Clarke *et al.*, 2008). In addition, both studies have clearly shown that QoL ratings on parent reports were significantly lower than that of child reports.

Co-morbid factors

A large number of co-morbid factors are known to be associated with FGIDs in children. Some studies from Sri Lanka have found extra-intestinal symptoms such as headache, limb pain, photophobia and sleeping difficulties occur more frequently in children with abdominal pain-predominant functional gastroin-testinal disease than in controls (Devanarayana *et al.*, 2011b). Similarly, Dong *et al.* (2005) noted an association between functional headache and IBS in Chinese children. Children with aerophagia were also noted to have an array of extra-intestinal symptoms (Devanarayana *et al.*, 2012). These symptoms can significantly contribute to the suffering and poor QoL of children who are already having pain and discomfort. In this light, extra-intestinal symptoms need to be addressed in the management of children with functional gastroin-testinal diseases.

Healthcare seeking

Although functional gastrointestinal diseases are a considerable problem in the community, healthcare-seeking patterns for this group of disorders in children are not well understood. Evaluating ambulatory healthcare data, one study reported that chronic constipation is a common cause for an ambulatory healthcare visit for children in the United States (Everhart and Ruhl, 2009). Two other studies have assessed the healthcare use of children with constipation in a single-birth cohort at different time points. The first study noted that children suffering from constipation have the highest number of medical appointments in comparison with all other gastrointestinal complaints (Chitkara *et al.*, 2007). The second study illustrated that children with constipation seek medical care more often than children with other illnesses such as bronchial asthma and migraine (Choung *et al.*, 2011). In contrast, another study from Sri Lanka has shown that despite higher prevalence rates, healthcare-seeking for chronic constipation remains very low (3.8%) (Rajindrajith *et al.*, 2012b). Younger age, family history of constipation and associated vomiting were significant predictive factors for visits to a doctor. Healthcare-seeking for other FGIDs in children have not been studied in depth in different parts of the world with different healthcare systems; therefore, further research into this important area would aid in the planning and allocation of healthcare resources for FGIDs at a global level.

SUMMARY

Prevalence of FGIDs has dramatically increased over the past decade and now represents a large global healthcare burden. With growing population trends and increasing predisposing factors such as obesity and psychological stress, it can be predicted that the incidence of FGIDs will increase further and become a significant healthcare problem. Although FGIDs are not life threatening, research shows that children suffering from FGIDs tend to have a lower QoL than their healthy peers and frequently miss school as a result of the disorders. In addition, many FGIDs such as constipation and IBS have high healthcare expenditure and are becoming a major challenge to already-overstretched healthcare budgets, both in developing and in developed countries, competing with other prioritised diseases. These factors suggest that functional gastrointestinal diseases need to be one of the main research focal points of the twenty-first century.

REFERENCES

Abu-Arafeh I, Russell G. Cyclical vomiting syndrome in children: a population-based study. *J Pediatr Gastroenterol Nutr.* 1995a; **21**(4): 454–8.

Abu-Arafeh I, Russell G. Prevalence and clinical features of abdominal migraine compared with those of migraine. *Arch Dis Chid.* 1995b; **72**(5): 413–17.

Apley J, Naish N. Recurrent abdominal pains: a field survey of 1,000 children. *Arch Dis Child.* 1958; **33**(168): 165–70.

Baber KF, Anderson J, Puzanovova M, *et al*. Rome II versus Rome III classification of functional gastrointestinal disorders in pediatric chronic abdominal pain. *J Pediatr Gastroenterol Nutr*. 2008; **47**(3): 299–302.

Basaran UN, Inan M, Aksu B, *et al*. Colonic perforation due to pathologic aerophagia in an intellectually disabled child. *J Paediatr Child Health*. 2007; **43**(10): 710–12.

Bern C, Martines J, de Zoysa I, *et al*. The magnitude of the global problem of diarrhoeal update: a ten-year update. *Bull World Health Org*. 1992; **70**(6): 705–14.

Bongers MEJ. *Childhood Constipation Treatment, Long-Term Prognosis and Quality of Life* [thesis]. Amsterdam, AM: University of Amsterdam: The Netherlands; 2008.

Bongers ME, Van Wijk MP, Reitsma JB, *et al*. Long-term prognosis for childhood constipation: clinical outcome in adulthood. *Pediatrics*. 2010; **126**(1): 156–62.

Bonilla S, Wang D, Saps M. Obesity predicts persistence of pain in children with functional gastrointestinal disorders. *Int J Obesity (Lond)*. 2011; **35**(4): 517–21.

Burns C. Childhood encopresis. *Med World*. 1958; **89**(6): 529–32.

Carson L, Lewis D, Tsou M, *et al*. Abdominal migraine: an under-diagnosed cause of recurrent abdominal pain in children. *Headache*. 2011; **51**(5): 707–12.

Chao HC, Lai MW, Kong MS, *et al*. Cutoff volume of dietary fiber to ameliorate constipation in children. *J Pediatr*. 2008; **153**(1): 45–9.

Chatoor I, Dickson L, Einhorn A. Rumination: etiology and treatment. *Pediatr Ann*. 1984; **13**(12): 924–9.

Chiarelli P, Brown W, McElduff P. Constipation in Australian women: prevalence and associated factors. *Int Urogynecol J Pelvic Floor Dysfunct*. 2000; **11**(2): 71–8.

Chitkara DK, Talley NJ, Weaver AL, *et al*. Incidence of presentation of common functional gastrointestinal disorders in children from birth to 5 years: a cohort study. *Clin Gastroenterol Hepatol*. 2007; **5**(2): 186–91.

Choung RS, Locke GR. Epidemiology of IBS. *Gastroenterol Clin N Am*. 2011; **40**(1): 1–10.

Choung RS, Shan ND, Chitkara D, *et al*. Direct medical costs of constipation from childhood to early adulthood: a population-based birth cohort study. *J Pediatr Gastroenterol Nutr*. 2011; **52**(1): 47–54.

Chung JM, Lee SD, Kang DI, *et al*. An epidemiologic study of voiding and bowel habits in Korean children: a nationwide multicenter study. *Urology*. 2010; **76**(1): 215–19.

Clarke MC, Chow CS, Chase JW, *et al*. Quality of life in children with slow transit constipation. *J Pediatr Surg*. 2008; **43**(2): 320–4.

Cullen KJ, Macdonald WB. The periodic syndrome: its nature and prevalence. *Med J Aust*. 1963; **50**(2): 167–73.

Daher S, Tahan S, Sole D, *et al*. Cow's milk protein intolerance and chronic constipation in children. *Pediatr Allergy Immunol*. 2001; **12**(6): 339–42.

Davis GJ, Crowder M, Reid B, *et al*. Bowel function measurement of individuals with different eating patterns. *Gut*. 1986; **27**(2): 164–9.

De Arajuo Sant'Anna AM, Calcado AC. Constipation in school-aged children at public schools in Rio de Janeiro, Brazil. *J Pediatr Gastroenterol Nutr*. 1999; **29**(2): 190–3.

Del Ciampo IR, Galvão LC, Del Ciampo LA, *et al*. Prevalence of chronic constipation in children at a primary healthcare unit [Portuguese]. *J Pediatr (Rio J)*. 2002; **78**(6): 497–502.

De Giacomo C, Valdambrini V, Lizzoli F, *et al*. A population-based survey on gastrointestinal tract symptoms and *Helicobacter pylori* infection in children and adolescents. *Helicobacter*. 2002; **7**(6): 356–63.

Devanarayana NM, de Silva DG, de Silva HJ. Aetiology of recurrent abdominal pain in a cohort of Sri Lankan children. *J Paediatr Child Health*. 2008; **44**(4): 195–209.

Devanarayana NM, Rajindrajith S. Association between constipation and stressful life events in a cohort of Sri Lankan children and adolescents. *J Trop Pediatr*. 2010; **56**(3): 144–8.

Devanarayana NM, Adhikari C, Pannala W, *et al*. Prevalence of functional gastrointestinal diseases in a cohort of Sri Lankan adolescents: comparison between Rome II and Rome III criteria. *J Trop Pediatr*. 2011a; **57**(1): 34–9.

Devanarayana NM, Mettananda S, Liyanarachchi C, *et al.* Abdominal pain-predominant functional gastrointestinal diseases in children and adolescents: symptomatology and association with stress. *J Paediatr Gastroenterol Nutr.* 2011b; **53**(6): 659–65.

Devanarayana NM, Rajindrajith S. Aerophagia among Sri Lankan children: Epidemiological patterns and symptom characteristics. *J Pediatr Gastroenterol Nutr.* 2012; **54**(4): 516–20.

Devanarayana NM, Rajindrajith S, Mettananda S, *et al.* Child abuse and abdominal pain – is there an association? *Ceylon Med J.* 2012; **57**: S25.

Dong L, Dingguo L, Xiaosing X, *et al.* An epidemiologic study of irritable bowel syndrome in adolescents and children in China: a school-based study. *Pediatrics.* 2005; **116**(3): e393–6.

Drossman DA, Thompson WG, Talley NJ, *et al.* Identification of sub-groups of functional gastrointestinal disorders. *Gastroenterol Int.* 1990; **3**: 159–72.

Endo Y, Shoji T, Fukuda S, *et al.* The features of adolescent irritable bowel syndrome in Japan. *J Gastroenterol Hepatol.* 2011; **26**(Suppl. 3): 106–9.

Ertekin V, Selimoglu MA, Altnkaynak S. Prevalence of cyclic vomiting syndrome in a sample of Turkish school children in an urban area. *J Clin Gastroenterol.* 2006; **40**(10): 896–8.

Everhart JE, Ruhl CE. Burden of digestive diseases in the United States part II: lower gastrointestinal diseases. *Gastroenterology.* 2009; **136**(3): 741–54.

Fernandez S, Aspirot A, Kerzner B, *et al.* Do some adolescents with rumination syndrome have 'supragastric vomiting'? *J Pediatr Gastroenterol Nutr.* 2010; **50**(1): 103–5.

Fishman L, Lenders C, Fortunato C, *et al.* Increased prevalence of constipation and fecal soiling in a population of obese children. *J Pediatr.* 2004; **145**(2): 253–4.

Fitzpatrick E, Bourke B, Drumm B, *et al.* The incidence of cyclic vomiting in children: population-based study. *Am J Gastroenterol.* 2008; **103**(4): 991–5.

Fleisher DR, Matar M. The cyclic vomiting syndrome: a report of 71 cases and literature review. *J Pediatr Gastroenterol Nutr.* 1993; **17**(4): 361–9.

Gilbert R, Widom CS, Browne K, *et al.* Burden and consequences of child maltreatment in high-income countries. *Lancet.* 2009; **373**(9657): 68–81.

Green AD, Alioto A, Mousa H, *et al.* Severe pediatric rumination syndrome: successful interdisciplinary inpatient management. *J Pediatr Gastroenterol Nutr.* 2011; **52**(4): 414–18.

Haghighat M, Rafie SM, Dehghani SM, *et al.* Cyclic vomiting in children: experience with 181 cases from south Iran. *World J Gastroenterol.* 2007; **13**: 1833–6.

Heitkemper MM, Jarrett ME. Update irritable bowel syndrome and gender differences. *Nutr Clin Pract.* 2008; **23**(3): 275–83.

Helgeland H, Flagstad G, Grotta J, *et al.* Diagnosing pediatric functional abdominal pain in children (4–15 years old) according to Rome III Criteria: results from a Norwegian prospective study. *J Pediatr Gastroenterol Nutr.* 2009; **49**(3): 309–15.

Hoffman I, Tack J. Assessment of gastric motor function in childhood functional dyspepsia and obesity. *Neurogastroenterol Motil.* 2012; **24**(2): 108–13.

Hutchinson GH, Alderson DM, Turnberg LA. Fatal tension pneumoperitoneum due to aerophagy. *Postgrad Med J.* 1980; **56**(657): 516–18.

Hyams JS, Burke G, Davis PM, *et al.* Abdominal pain and irritable bowel syndrome in adolescents: a community-based study. *J Pediatr.* 1996; **129**(2): 220–6.

Hyman PE, Milla PJ, Benninga MA, *et al.* Childhood functional gastrointestinal disorders: neonate/toddler. *Gastroenterology.* 2006; **130**(5): 1519–26.

Iacono G, Cavataio F, Montalto G, *et al.* Intolerance of cow's milk and chronic constipation in children. *N Engl J Med.* 1998; **339**(16): 1100–4.

Iacono G, Merolla R, D'Amico D, *et al.* Gastrointestinal symptoms in infancy: a population-based prospective study. *Dig Liver Dis.* 2005; **37**(6): 432–8.

Inan M, Aydiner CY, Tokuc B, *et al.* Factors associated with childhood constipation. *J Pediatr Child Health.* 2007; **43**(10): 700–6.

Ip KS, Lee WT, Chan JS, *et al.* A community-based study of the prevalence of constipation in young children and the role of dietary fiber. *Hong Kong Med J.* 2005; **11**(6): 431–6.

Joinson C, Heron J, Butler U, *et al*. Psychological differences between children with and without soiling problems. *Pediatrics*. 2006; **117**(5): 1575–84.

Jung HK, Kim DY, Moon IH. Effects of gender and menstrual cycle on colonic transit time in healthy subjects. *Korean J Intern Med*. 2003; **18**(3): 181–6.

Khan S, Campo JV, Bridge JA, *et al*. Long-term outcome of functional childhood constipation. *Dig Dis Sci*. 2007; **52**(1): 64–9.

Khan S, Hyman PE, Cocjin J, *et al*. Rumination syndrome in adolescents. *J Pediatr*. 2000; **136**(4): 528–31.

Koloski NA, Talley NJ, Boyce PM. A history of abuse in community subjects with irritable bowel syndrome and functional dyspepsia. *Digestion*. 2005; **72**(2–3): 86–96.

Lee H, Rhee PL, Park EH, *et al*. Clinical outcome of rumination syndrome in adults without psychiatric illness: a prospective study. *Gastroenterol Hepatol*. 2007; **22**(11): 1741–7.

Lee WT, Ip KS, Chan JS, *et al*. Increased prevalence of constipation in pre-school children is attributable to under-consumption of plant foods: a community-based study. *J Pediatr Child Health*. 2008; **44**(4): 170–5.

Levine MD. Children with encopresis: a descriptive analysis. *Pediatrics*. 1975; **56**(3): 412–16.

Li BU, Lefevre F, Chelimsky GG, *et al*. North American society for pediatric gastroenterology, hepatology and nutrition consensus statement on the diagnosis and management of cyclic vomiting syndrome. *J Pediatr Gastroenterol Nutr*. 2008; **47**(3): 379–93.

Loening-Baucke V. Encopresis and soiling. *Pediatr Clin North Am*. 1996; **43**(1): 279–98.

Loening-Baucke V. Functional fecal retention with encopresis in childhood. *J Pediatr Gastroenterol Nutr*. 2004; **38**(1): 79–84.

Longstreth GF, Thompson WG, Chey WD, *et al*. Functional bowel disorders. *Gastroenterology*. 2006; **130**(5): 1480–91.

Mayer EA, Tillisch K. The brain-gut axis in abdominal pain syndromes. *Annu Rev Med*. 2011; **62**: 386–92.

Miele E, Simeone D, Marino A, *et al*. Functional gastrointestinal disorders in children: an Italian prospective survey. *Pediatrics*. 2004; **114**(1): 73–8.

Morton RE, Pinnington L, Ellis RE. Air swallowing in Rett syndrome. *Dev Med Child Neurol*. 2000; **42**(4): 271–5.

O'Ryan M, Prado V, Pickering LK. A millennium update on pediatric diarrhoeal illness in the developing world. *Semin Pediatr Infect Dis*. 2005; **16**(2): 125–36.

Rajindrajith S, Devanarayana NM. Subtypes and symptomatology of irritable bowel syndrome in children and adolescents: a school-based survey using Rome III criteria. *J Neurogastroenterol Motil*. 2012; **18**(3): 298–304.

Rajindrajith S, Devanarayana NM, Adhikari C, *et al*. Constipation in children: an epidemiological study in Sri Lanka using Rome III criteria. *Arch Dis Child*. 2012a; **97**(1): 43–5.

Rajindrajith S, Devanarayana NM, Benninga MA. Constipation-associated and nonretentive fecal incontinence in children and adolescents: an epidemiological survey in Sri Lanka. *J Pediatr Gastroenterol Nutr*. 2010; **51**(4): 472–6.

Rajindrajith S, Devanarayana NM, Benninga MA. Children and adolescents with chronic constipation: how many seek healthcare and what determines it? *J Trop Pediatr*. 2012b; **58**(4): 280–5.

Rajindrajith S, Mettananda S, Devanarayana NM. Constipation during and after the civil war in Sri Lanka: a paediatric study. *J Trop Pediatr*. 2011; **57**(6): 439–43.

Ramocki MB, Peters SU, Tavyev YJ, *et al*. Autism and other neuropsychiatric symptoms are prevalent in individuals with MeCP2 duplication syndrome. *Ann Neurol*. 2009; **66**(6): 771–82.

Rashetnikov OV, Kurilovich SA, Denisova DV, *et al*. Prevalence of dyspepsia and irritable bowel syndrome among adolescents of Novosibirsk, western Siberia. *Int J Circumpolar Health*. 2001; **60**(2): 253–7.

Rasquin A, Di Lorenzo C, Forbes D, *et al*. Childhood functional gastrointestinal disorders: child/adolescent. *Gastroenterology*. 2006; **130**(5): 1527–37.

Rasquin-Weber A, Hyman PE, Cucchiara S, *et al.* Childhood functional gastrointestinal disorders. *Gut.* 1999; **45**(Suppl. 2): II60–8.

Rogers B, Stratton P, Victor J, *et al.* Chronic regurgitation among persons with mental retardation: a need for combined medical and interdisciplinary strategies. *Am J Ment Retard.* 1992; **96**(5): 522–7.

Saps M, Lu P, Bonilla S. Cow's-milk allergy is a risk factor for the development of FGIDs in children. *J Pediatr Gastroenterol Nutr.* 2011; **52**(2): 166–9.

Saps M, Pensabaene L, Di Martino L, *et al.* Post-infectious functional gastrointestinal disorders in children. *J Pediatr.* 2008; **152**(6): 812–16.

Saps M, Sztainberg M, Di Lorenzo C. A prospective community-based study of gastroenterological symptoms in school-age children. *J Pediatr Gastroenterol Nutr.* 2006; **43**(4): 477–82.

Schurman JV, Friesen CA, Danda CE, *et al.* Diagnosing functional abdominal pain with the Rome II criteria: parent, child, and clinician agreement. *J Pediatr Gastroenterol Nutr.* 2005; **41**(3): 291–5.

Sohrabi S, Nouraie M, Khademi H, *et al.* Epidemiology of uninvestigated gastrointestinal symptoms in adolescents: a population-based study applying the Rome III questionnaire. *J Pediatr Gastroenterol Nutr.* 2010; **51**(1): 41–5.

Son YJ, Jun EY, Park JH. Prevalence and risk factors of irritable bowel syndrome in Korean adolescent girls: a school-based study. *Int J Nurs Stud.* 2009; **46**(1): 77–84.

Spiller R, Garsed K. Infection, inflammation, and the irritable bowel syndrome. *Dig Liver Dis.* 2009; **41**(12): 844–9.

Still GF. *Common Disorders and Diseases of Childhood.* London: Oxford University Press; 1909.

Suares NC, Ford AC. Prevalence of, and risk factors for, chronic idiopathic constipation in the community: systematic review and meta-analysis. *Am J Gastroenterol.* 2011; **106**: 1582–91.

Tam YH, Li AM, So HK, *et al.* Socio-environmental factors in family, school and lifestyle associated with childhood constipation: the first territory-wide survey in Hong Kong Chinese children using Rome III criteria. *J Pediatr Gastroenterol Nutr.* 2012; **55**: 56–61.

Teitelbaum JE, Sinha P, Micale M, *et al.* Obesity is related to multiple functional abdominal disease. *J Pediatr.* 2009; **154**(3): 444–6.

Thabane M, Simunovic M, Akhtar-Danesh N, *et al.* An outbreak of acute gastroenteritis is associated with an increased incidence of irritable bowel syndrome in children. *Am J Gastroenterol.* 2010; **105**(4): 933–9.

Thompson S, Dancey CP. Symptoms of irritable bowel syndrome in children: prevalence and psychological effects. *J Pediatr Health Care.* 1996; **10**: 280–5.

Thompson WG, Longstreth GF, Drossman DA, *et al.* Functional bowel disorders and functional abdominal pain. *Gut.* 1999; **45**(Suppl. 2): II43–7.

Trillis F Jr, Gauderer MW, Ponsky JL, *et al.* Transverse colon volvulus in a child with pathologic aerophagia. *J Pediatr Surg.* 1986; **21**(11): 966–8.

Uc A, Hyman PE, Walker LS. Functional gastrointestinal diseases in African American children in primary care. *J Pediatr Gastroenterol Nutr.* 2006; **42**(3): 270–4.

Van der Baan-Slootweg OH, Liem O, Bekkali N, *et al.* Constipation and colonic transit times in children with morbid obesity. *J Pediatr Gastroenterol Nutr.* 2011; **52**(4): 442–5.

Van der Wal MF, Benninga MA, Hirasing RA. The prevalence of encopresis in multicultural population. *J Pediatr Gastroenterol Nutr.* 2005; **40**(3): 345–8.

Van Ginkel R, Reitsma JB, Buller HA, *et al.* Childhood constipation: longitudinal follow-up beyond puberty. *Gastroenterology.* 2003; **125**(2): 357–63.

Van Tilburg M. Child abuse is not only a case of bruises and broken bones: role of abuse in unexplained GI symptoms in children. *J Pediatr Gastroenterol Nutr.* 2011; **33**: S40–1.

Varni JW, Lane MM, Burwinkle TM, *et al.* Health-related quality of life in pediatric patients with irritable bowel syndrome: a comparative analysis. *J Dev Behav Pediatr.* 2006; **27**(6): 451–8.

Voskuijl WP, Heijmans J, Heijmans HS, *et al.* Use of Rome II criteria in childhood defecation disorders: applicability in clinical and research practice. *J Pediatr.* 2004; **145**(2): 213–17.

Walker LS, Lipani TA, Greene JW, *et al*. Recurrent abdominal pain: symptom subtypes based on the Rome II Criteria for pediatric functional gastrointestinal disorders. *J Pediatr Gastroenterol Nutr.* 2004; **38**(2): 187–91.

Wu TC, Chen LK, Pan WH, *et al*. Constipation in Taiwan elementary school students: a nationwide survey. *J Chinese Med Ass.* 2011; **74**(2): 57–61.

Yang HR. Recent concepts on cyclic vomiting syndrome in children. *J Neurogastroenterol Motil.* 2010; **16**(2): 139–47.

Youssef NN, Langseder AL, Verga BJ, *et al*. Chronic childhood constipation is associated with impaired quality of life: a case-controlled study. *J Pediatr Gastroenterol Nutr.* 2005; **41**(1): 56–60.

Youssef NN, Murphy TG, Langseder AL, *et al*. Quality of life for children with functional abdominal pain: a comparison study of patients' and parents' perceptions. *Pediatrics.* 2006; **117**(1): 54–9.

Zhou H, Li D, Cheng G, *et al*. An epidemiologic study of irritable bowel syndrome in adolescents and children in south China: a school-based survey. *Child Care Health Dev.* 2010; **36**(6): 781–6.

Zhou H, Yao M, Cheng GY, *et al*. Prevalence and associated factors of functional gastrointestinal disorders and bowel habits in Chinese adolescents: a school-based study. *J Pediatr Gastroenterol Nutr.* 2011; **53**(2): 168–73.

CHAPTER 2

Multidisciplinary team approach and the role of psychologists in gastroenterology services

Alan Silverman and Sara E Williams

INTRODUCTION

In traditional psychological practice settings, therapy is conducted in weekly hour-long sessions involving an individual client and a singular therapist. Many successful therapeutic practices have been built on this model, which is often referred to as *individual outpatient care*. While this model capitalises on a therapeutic process that has been shown to be efficacious for the treatment of a variety of problems, some clinical populations, including medically complex patients and/or clinical issues involving children, may have better clinical outcomes when an interdisciplinary care model is employed (Sampson, 1999). Gastroenterology, the branch of medicine focused on the digestive system and its disorders, provides a good example of an area of medicine in which integrated treatment teams work to provide care. Individual disciplines working within gastroenterology may include, but are not limited to, gastroenterologists, advanced practice nurses, dietitians, speech and language pathologists, occupational therapists, social workers and psychologists (Kedesdy and Budd, 1998b).

This chapter describes the various models of integrated care commonly found within paediatric gastroenterology clinical practice settings, describes the specific role of a psychologist working in gastroenterology (*see* also Chapter 7), reviews the empirical support for interdisciplinary services in paediatric gastroenterology, and provides guidelines for structuring successful integrated care clinics. Case examples are used throughout this chapter to illustrate key concepts.

INTEGRATED TEAM MODELS

Multidisciplinary treatment, or perhaps more accurately called *integrated treatment*, is the practice of healthcare that involves multiple disciplines working in a coordinated fashion to promote the best health outcome for the patient (Kedesdy and Budd, 1998a). The most common configurations of integrated treatment are:

- co-treatment
- multidisciplinary
- interdisciplinary
- transdisciplinary.

While each of these treatment approaches involves multiple professional approaches working in tandem (Armstrong, 2009), the magnitude of collaboration differs and warrants further consideration.

Co-treatment

Co-treatment or interdisciplinary collaboration is a form of integrated care in which two or more disciplines work towards a common therapeutic goal. The co-treatment collaborators are specifically matched to address the clinical needs of the family (Kedesdy and Budd, 1998a). Typically, providers have separate appointments and practise out of different settings. One common example of co-treatment is the collaborative treatment of a general practice physician who refers to a specialist to provide care for a condition that the physician is overseeing medically. Co-treatment is the most common integrated approach, as it is typically the easiest to provide, and as such it is the most readily available to families. Relative advantages of co-treatment for the family include greater availability of providers, greater flexibility of scheduling of appointments, and the ability to select individual providers with whom the family would like to work. This model lends itself particularly well to conditions that involve one discipline more intensively than another, or when one of the disciplines is acting primarily as a consultant (e.g. psychological consultation to assess psychosocial factors affecting a medical condition). The major disadvantages to co-treatment are associated with the difficulties of care coordination across practice settings. These difficulties may include differences in treatment philosophies, which may lead to conflicting treatment recommendations and/or confusion in treatment planning, and logistical difficulties associated with multiple appointments and sharing documentation across practice settings.

Multidisciplinary

Multidisciplinary care involves separate visits with providers of differing disciplines who work within the same practice setting or clinic. In multidisciplinary settings, appointments with providers typically occur as individual appointments, but the team of treatment providers has an established and formalised working relationship (Bithoney *et al.*, 1991; Walter, 1994). Typically the organisational infrastructure includes an administrative structure and clinical support system to facilitate care delivery within the same practice setting. Similar to co-treatment, patients are seen by each discipline in separate appointments, but providers typically share access to the same documentation, have opportunities to *staff* cases collaboratively, and generally have fewer barriers associated with working in a coordinated fashion. An example of multidisciplinary care is a gastroenterologist working closely with a paediatric psychologist and a dietitian in the care of a child with coeliac disease. Each discipline has separate visits but works together to keep the child healthy and growing by focusing on different aspects of care. Relative advantages of the multidisciplinary care model include increased access to specialist providers, easier coordination of clinical visits, and relatively fewer instances of conflicting care recommendations. Disadvantages of multidisciplinary care stem from separate visits with providers, which may reduce treatment efficiency and increase family frustration. Furthermore, true multidisciplinary clinics are less common than co-treatment clinics and may be more difficult for families to find outside of larger metropolitan areas.

Interdisciplinary

Interdisciplinary care is the provision of clinical services in a fully integrated clinical setting. Interdisciplinary care expands upon the advantages of multi-disciplinary care by having all providers present in a singular appointment and collaborating in real time (Armstrong and Drotar, 2000). There are many advantages to the interdisciplinary model. Interdisciplinary care enhances treatment team ability to process the information together and generate uni-form impressions, which helps the team allocate treatment resources efficiently (Guralnick, 2000). Furthermore, all providers are typically using the same documentation systems, which further improves collaboration efforts. Once therapy begins, disciplines continue to work together in real time to ensure that all clinical needs are met and that treatment recommendations by specific disciplines are not conflicting with any of the other disciplines working on the clinical team. Another relative advantage is that interdisciplinary treatment teams are able to focus clinical attention to specific objectives until a patient is ready for other clinical activities. Disadvantages associated with interdiscipli-nary care are similar to those in the multidisciplinary care settings, including limited access to clinics, additional logistical demands (including expense and difficulties in coordination and administration) and greater limitations to confidentiality for the patient and the patient's family, given shared docu-mentation systems.

Transdisciplinary

In transdisciplinary care settings, an individual provider practises across dis-ciplines, providing education, consultation and treatment recommendations that are beyond the scope of the provider's terminal degree(s) (Armstrong and Reaman, 2005). Given limitations of access to multidisciplinary and interdis-ciplinary clinics, transdisciplinary care is attractive to families, as it is often readily available. One example of transdisciplinary care may be a psychologist who has a practice specialising in the treatment of children who have soiling disorder. Frequently, these families will seek medical advice about laxatives and nutrition advice regarding fluid and fibre goals from such an individual, as laxatives and dietary supplements are readily available in pharmacies without a prescription. Unfortunately, a well-intentioned provider may give recommendations that may be inefficacious or, worse, may complicate care or delay a family from seeking appropriate help. Thus, clinical services outside of the scope of providers' practices are best left to individuals well trained and licensed to provide those services.

CASE STUDY: AVIVA – MULTIDISCIPLINARY, INTERDISCIPLINARY AND TRANSDISCIPLINARY CARE

Case Study 1: background

Aviva is a 7-year-old female with feeding problems since her birth. She has a significant history of silent aspiration, recurrent pneumonias and pulmonary infarcts. Aviva's oral feedings were discontinued early in life, causing her to miss feeding milestones. Aviva's family attempted to reintroduce feeding at 1 year of life but had great difficulties with behavioural resistance, prompting the family to seek the community speech and language pathologist for feeding intervention in which providers were practising in a transdisciplinary model, providing psychological behavioural intervention as well as feeding therapy. Unfortunately, Aviva made little progress in this model of outpatient care, which prompted that provider to refer the family to a comprehensive feeding and swallowing centre when she was 18 months old.

The interdisciplinary centre included gastroenterology, dietetics, speech–language pathology and psychology. The centre's first step was to identify other health concerns warranting further attention. At that time, Aviva had persistent feeding intolerance and eczema, so the feeding centre went on to refer Aviva to an asthma and allergy centre for further evaluation, where she was diagnosed with multiple food allergies, including allergies to peanuts, tree nuts, dairy, eggs, fish and soy. In further gastrointestinal investigation through the interdisciplinary feeding team, she was also diagnosed with eosinophilic esophagitis, a condition of inflammation of the oesophagus that leads to dysmotility of the oesophagus, pain, and feeding and swallowing difficulties. This case illustrates the complexity of patient care when a child has multiple medical conditions.

Now with a clear picture of her medical diagnoses, Aviva's community and school providers collaborated with the interdisciplinary treatment team who were providing care in coordination with an independent clinic. Essentially, the family was receiving traditional treatment (e.g. co-treatment), multidisciplinary treatment and interdisciplinary treatment simultaneously. Each of these treatment partners had a distinctly defined roll and treatment objectives in Aviva's care with the community and school providers working most frequently with the family, the interdisciplinary feeding team providing ongoing assessment and directing care, and the multidisciplinary collaborations with the allergy clinic helping to ensure the safety of treatment recommendations.

After 5 years of outpatient care coordination, Aviva's medical conditions stabilised, including successful allergy challenges to all foods other than egg whites and dairy. She no longer had any evidence of aspirations and appeared to be developing adequate chewing and swallowing skills to manage a variety of textures and liquids. She was admitted to the hospital to complete a comprehensive feeding treatment programme with family-specified goals of gastrostomy tube wean and increased intake of age-appropriate textures. Aviva spent 10 days in hospital with the psychology team providing treatment sessions at breakfast, lunch and dinner. The medical team monitored health status during daily rounds, monitoring weight, hydration, blood glucose levels and urine ketones. Dietitians monitored weight loss to ensure that no acute nutrition problems developed (weight loss >5% of weight at time of admission), and helped the psychologists work towards an oral daily nutrition and fluid goal. Speech and language pathologists provided recommendations regarding texture and continued to assess chewing and swallowing skills. By the end of the programme, Aviva had improved nutrition status with increased intake of chewable solids, she had minimal behavioural resistance to feeding, her parents consistently demonstrated skills for management of behavioural refusals, and ongoing monitoring needs were well understood by the parents and were shared with community providers and the school.

Follow-up appointments scheduled to continue care post tube wean. Aviva was discharged on all oral feedings within continued care by her community speech and language therapist and ongoing assessment by the feeding and swallowing centre and the asthma and allergy clinic. Recently, her gastrostomy tube was removed and she eats a variety of foods similar to same-age peers. Her family hopes to successfully complete egg and dairy challenges in the next few years.

In summary, coordination of clinical services is essential to the successful treatment of complex disorders, especially in the field of paediatric gastroenterology. The psychologist who works within an integrated clinical setting works not only with the patient and the family but also with the treatment team at large. Interdisciplinary and multidisciplinary care models are widely believed to be the most efficient and efficacious treatment approaches. Unfortunately, few families have access to these clinics. When these clinical approaches are not readily available, it is essential that co-treating therapists coordinate their practices with all other providers as much as possible.

INTEGRATED CARE AND THE ROLE OF THE PSYCHOLOGIST

In the specialty field of paediatric psychology, the psychologist has training in the psychological aspects of illness and general clinical child psychopathology.

Paediatric psychologists work in inpatient and outpatient settings, providing consultation, assessment and/or treatment to address psychosocial issues of health and illness. A recent survey found that 63% of paediatric psychologists work in hospital settings (Opipari-Arrigan *et al.*, 2006), and it is likely that many of those providers work as part of a multidisciplinary or interdisciplinary team. As such, the psychologist works with other healthcare providers to achieve medical objectives, such as improving psychological adjustment to a medical condition, helping families improve adherence to medical regimens, and assessing the long-term cognitive and emotional effects of having a chronic condition. In this section, three major paediatric psychology provider roles are reviewed:
1. consultation-liaison
2. assessment and evaluation
3. treatment.

The challenges presented to the psychologist in each role are considered and a case example of a psychologist working in each of three roles is provided to illustrate key concepts.

Consultation-liaison

In an inpatient setting, it is common for a paediatric psychologist to serve a *consultation-liaison* role. In this role, the medical team is the 'client' and the psychologist is called on as a consultant to the team to assess the paediatric patient in the context of the presenting medical problem (Carter and Von Weiss, 2004). The focus for a psychologist working in this setting is to answer a specific question or questions affecting the presenting medical problem. The psychology consultant then makes recommendations to the medical treatment team for acute management to facilitate integrated treatment (Buckloh and Greco, 2009). While this model is typically employed in inpatient medical settings, psychologists can also fill consultation-liaison roles in outpatient settings. In the outpatient treatment environment, the psychologist would similarly be employed by a primary medical team to engage in brief assessment of acute issues, with a focus on making recommendations to the team for treatment and follow-up care (Carter and Von Weiss, 2004).

Evaluation of the consultation-liaison approach has found many benefits of having a psychologist as part of an integrated medical team. Froese and colleagues (1976–77) were among the first groups to identify the benefit of a consultation-liaison psychologist. Their descriptive analysis concluded that a psychologist serving on an integrated treatment team provided an opportunity for disciplines to learn from each other, contributed a 'unified approach to the emotional and social needs of the patient', and promoted 'a forum for informal consultations and interdisciplinary meetings' (Froese *et al.*, 1976–77, p. 47).

Assessment and evaluation

A common role for a psychologist is to provide *assessment and evaluation*. A psychologist providing assessment may function as part of a co-treatment, multidisciplinary or interdisciplinary team. Often the medical team will refer a child to a paediatric psychologist for evaluation to answer a specific question that affects treatment planning or recommendations or which may answer questions about a child's response to treatment.

Assessment typically starts by the psychologist interviewing the paediatric patient and family members. The interview focuses on collecting information about current medical problems (e.g. adjustment to illness), current functional ability (e.g. level of disability associated with illness) and assessment of any co-morbid psychological issues (e.g. anxiety, depression). Many psychologists also employ formal assessment practices, such as a battery of psychological or neuropsychological tests to assess cognitive, behavioural or psychosocial factors with objective measures (*see* also 'Assessment resources' in Part III, 3.1). After synthesising the information, the psychologist makes treatment recommendations. Depending on the treatment model, the psychologist either works with other providers to present feedback to the patient and family or presents information directly to the patient and family and later communicates that information to other providers. For instance, a psychologist working in a multidisciplinary or interdisciplinary model works with other members of the treatment team to synthesise assessment information and formulate a treatment plan, whereas a psychologist in a co-treatment setting may communicate with other providers but does not involve them in feedback or treatment planning.

Treatment

After the initial assessment, many psychologists then take on the *treatment* role. Treatment consists of the psychologist working directly with the patient and family to engage in empirically based treatment of problems identified through previous consultation or assessment. Once again, depending on the treatment model, treatment can be carried out independently (e.g. co-treatment and transdisciplinary treatment) or in conjunction with the rest of the team (e.g. multidisciplinary and interdisciplinary treatment).

Challenges and benefits

Although the role of a psychologist within the team can vary, there are several key factors that remain important to the psychologist's success regardless of the role. First, communication with team members is arguably the most important factor in successful teamwork (Carter and Von Weiss, 2004). Whether in consultation, assessment or treatment, the degree of success that the psychologist has in working with the patient and family depends in large part on close communication with the rest of the team. The psychologist bears the responsibility not only of communicating with the team about psychological aspects of treatment but also to ensure that team members are communicating effectively with one another. Providers who collaborate to deliver a unified message to the family have the greatest likelihood of eliciting every team member's positive treatment goals for paediatric patients and their families.

Psychologists themselves also benefit by working as part of a multidisciplinary treatment team (Froese *et al.*, 1976–77). Children with medical illnesses are a challenging population. When a paediatric psychologist is part of a larger treatment team, the psychologist can be assured that all aspects of a child's health are being properly looked after by a group of trusted colleagues. Receiving support for difficult cases from colleagues can be of great service to all members of the team.

While there are many benefits to integrated care models there are also challenges for the psychologist. Traditionally, psychologists' work with their clients is of a confidential nature, which is essential to building a therapeutic working relationship, eliciting trust and working through difficult problems in a non-judgemental, supportive environment (Koocher and Keith-Spiegel, 2008). Confidentiality in the team environment is a significant challenge. When working as part a team, the psychologist must be clear with children and families about what information will be shared with the team and whether they can elect to keep any information private. Ethical practice requires breaching confidentiality regardless of the family's requests if there are safety concerns involved (Koocher and Keith-Spiegel, 2008). It is the responsibility of the psychologist to clearly inform families about limitations to confidentiality in the team setting. Families should be reassured that the psychologist will share only the information that is most pertinent to the care of the child and family (Rae *et al.*, 2009). Another challenge of working in a team is when providers attempt to work outside of their discipline (e.g. transdisciplinary care). This can be a unique challenge for a psychologist encountering a non-psychologist colleague acting as an 'armchair therapist'. Finally, while the different training background of team members provides strength to comprehensive care delivery, it can also be a challenge when opinions differ on the nature of the problem or the course of treatment (Froese *et al.*, 1976–77). Good communication among team members and establishing clear team roles helps to ensure that all providers are practising within their areas of training and keeping the best interests of the patient and family in mind.

CASE STUDY: A PSYCHOLOGIST IN MULTIPLE ROLES

To illustrate the multiple roles a psychologist can serve on a team, a case will be presented of an 11-year-old boy, 'Charlie', who has a diagnosis of cyclical vomiting syndrome (CVS) (*see* also Chapter 1 and 'Notes on cyclical vomiting syndrome' in Part III, 3.3). CVS is a functional gastrointestinal disorder characterised by recurrent, severe, stereotypical spells of vomiting with periods of normal or baseline health between episodes (Li and Balint, 2000). Children with severe bouts of vomiting are frequently hospitalised to receive fluids and intravenous medications in an attempt to break the episode.

Case Study 2: background

Charlie was hospitalised for a CVS episode. First, the primary medical team (paediatric gastroenterology) called for a consultation–liaison psychologist with the referral problem of:

> patient was recovering from vomiting episode until the team started discussing discharge from the hospital, at which point he appeared to become anxious and relapsed into another vomiting episode, and was unable to be discharged home.

The psychologist was asked to help the medical team assess the role of stress and anxiety in prolonging the medical problem (acute vomiting) and make recommendations on how the team could best support the patient to return him to his baseline state of health so he could be discharged home successfully.

The psychologist conducted a bedside interview with Charlie and his parents, at which point a history of stress and anxiety triggering CVS episodes was obtained. The psychologist provided psychoeducation to the team and family on the common role of stress-triggering episodes among CVS patients and the high incidence of anxiety disorders in this population (Tarbell and Li, 2008). The specific triggers that led to Charlie going into another episode when discharged from the hospital were discussed. The psychologist worked with the team to create a plan of delivering information to the patient that would not increase his anxiety. In this case, the psychologist suggested that instead of just telling the patient that he would be discharged, the team should involve the patient in a discussion of the course of his hospitalisation and allow him to exert some control over the situation by stating what he needed to be in place before going home. With this recommendation, the team worked with the patient and family to make a specific discharge plan and Charlie was allowed to voice his concerns about specific aspects of his medical status improving prior to being sent home (e.g. feeling less nauseous and being able to tolerate meals). After this intervention, Charlie quickly improved, recovered from his episode and was successfully discharged home within a 24-hour period. The team was grateful for the support and recommendations of the psychologist, and the whole team recommended further psychological evaluation and treatment for follow-up.

Subsequent to discharge from the hospital, the family followed through with the psychological recommendations. A paediatric psychologist in a multidisciplinary outpatient paediatric gastroenterology clinic saw Charlie for an assessment. At the first visit, the psychologist evaluated Charlie through interview with him and his parents. A standardised assessment of anxiety and depression symptoms was also obtained, along with a more thorough history of his illness, adjustment, functioning, anxiety and depression. The psychologist consulted with the medical team and in agreement with them, provided feedback to the family that Charlie met criteria for an anxiety disorder and would benefit from treatment, especially to help lessen the effect of anxiety on triggering CVS episodes.

Finally, the psychologist provided biofeedback and cognitive behavioural treatment to Charlie to address the symptoms of anxiety and its connection to CVS. The patient was bright and motivated to engage in treatment. First, psychoeducation was provided regarding the connection between stress and illness to provide a rationale for why psychological coping skills would benefit health, specifically making the link between anxiety and vomiting. Next, relaxation skills were taught (e.g. diaphragmatic breathing, progressive muscle relaxation and guided imagery) with the aid of biofeedback, which was provided with an interactive computer program that measured heart rate. Through biofeedback, Charlie was able to practise his newly acquired relaxation skills and see the physiological benefits in real time on a computer screen, which he thought was entertaining and which provided salient reinforcement of his skills. Finally, the connection of thoughts, feelings and behaviours was explored to illustrate how negative, 'what if'-style thinking promoted anxious feelings and produced symptoms. Charlie was taught how to 'reframe' his thoughts into positive, realistic, evidence-based thoughts that promoted more positive or neutral patterns of emotions and behaviours. Each week he was provided homework to practise his newly learned skills at home and chart his progress, with his family's support. By the end of the 6-week treatment, Charlie had not had any more CVS episodes and was confidently utilising his skills. Psychological treatment was discontinued because of his success; however, Charlie continued to be treated by his paediatric gastroenterologist, who informed the psychologist of his ongoing success.

EMPIRICAL REVIEW OF THE TEAM TREATMENT APPROACH

While it is common for integrated care models to be recommended in the healthcare literature, the efficacy of team approaches is understudied. Many authors conclude that patients would benefit from integrated care approaches that mirror the biopsychosocial model (*see* Chapter 7). This is often illustrated in discussion of treatment of functional gastrointestinal disorders. As Chiou and Nurko (2010) put it:

> The lack of a single, proven intervention highlights the complex interplay of biopsychosocial factors probably involved in the development of childhood functional abdominal pain and the need for a multidisciplinary, integrated approach. (p. 293)

The following section reviews what is known about the efficacy of the team approach in the paediatric literature, the efficacy of psychological interventions within the field of paediatric gastrointestinal psychology, and challenges to studying an integrated team care model.

Efficacy of the team approach

In 1976, Palmer and Thompson were among the first to describe an interdisciplinary approach in the paediatric health literature:

> The purpose of this paper is not to disseminate new findings or to review past research, but simply to state a progressive clinical philosophy in practical terms. Current emphasis on specialization and the simultaneous need for comprehensive health care seriously challenge the health professional's ability to provide adequate services without a well-integrated interdisciplinary approach. (p. 138)

Notably, the authors describe this approach as 'progressive' and note a number of benefits from the providers working together. Of particular interest is the population that the authors are referring to: children with nutritional problems. It is significant that one of the first articles highlighting the benefits of multidisciplinary treatments centred on the care of paediatric gastroenterology patients.

The terms 'multidisciplinary team' and 'multidisciplinary approach' started appearing regularly in the literature in the early 1980s. Another descriptive study published on multidisciplinary treatment, again in the field of paediatric gastroenterology, focused on team-based treatment of failure to thrive:

> A multidisciplinary team approach to treatment of failure to thrive in infancy and early childhood permits the simultaneous consideration of nutritional, medical, and psychosocial risk factors associated with this complex syndrome. The registered dietitian works with the physician, nurse, and social worker to provide an integrated evaluation of nutrition history, feeding patterns, medical status, social situation, developmental level, and interactional qualities of the child with failure to thrive … Long-term follow-up [occurs] at regular intervals in coordination with other members of the failure-to-thrive team. (Peterson *et al.*, 1984, p. 810)

In this way, many studies reiterate the benefit of a multidisciplinary approach without testing the approach itself. There are a few published studies designed to explicitly test the multidisciplinary approach. One study in paediatric gastroenterology examined inpatient multidisciplinary intervention for children with feeding disorders and found that 'results based on case studies and overall programme evaluation indicate that medically complicated, severe feeding disorders can be treated successfully in a few months with a multidisciplinary approach' (Babbit *et al.*, 1994, p. 278). Another study in the field of child protective services examined children evaluated in a multidisciplinary child protective services clinic and concluded that the multidisciplinary approach was more successful in eliciting the recommended follow-up services in a variety of disciplines than existing reports of abused and neglected children who did not have a multidisciplinary evaluation (Hochstadt and Harwicke, 1985). They concluded that a 'multidisciplinary team plays a central role in acquiring the services needed to reduce the deficits and sequelae suffered by victims of child abuse and neglect' (Hochstadt and Harwicke, 1985, p. 365).

Finally, other studies have focused on changes in treatment outcomes when multiple providers are involved. Finney and colleagues found that when psychologists collaborated with paediatricians in primary care, there was a higher level of problem resolution and lower healthcare utilisation in patients than in those who were not seen by the psychologist (Finney et al., 1991). Overall, there is some evidence for the positive benefits of multidisciplinary treatment for patients, providers, service coordination, symptom resolution and financial savings.

Efficacy of psychological intervention

As a branch of multidisciplinary treatment, there are many published treatment approached demonstrating the efficacy of psychological intervention specific to paediatric gastroenterology populations. For instance, randomised and control trial studies have shown efficacy for:

- cognitive behavioural therapy for treating functional abdominal pain (Robins et al., 2005)
- biofeedback therapy for decreasing pain-associated functional gastrointestinal disorders (Schurman et al., 2010)
- combination cognitive behavioural therapy, biofeedback and parental support for treating functional abdominal pain (Humphreys and Gevirtz, 2000)
- hypnotherapy for treating pain in irritable bowel syndrome (Vlieger et al., 2007)
- group therapy for improving fibre consumption, appropriate toileting and decreasing accidents in encopresis (McGrath et al., 2000; Stark et al., 1990)
- behaviour therapy for feeding disorders (Babbitt, et al., 1994; Bithoney et al., 1991; Fischer and Silverman, 2007).

In combination with the literature on empirically supported treatment in other major paediatric gastroenterology treatment areas (e.g. medicine, nutrition, speech and language pathology, nursing), providers as a whole are practising empirically supported treatment, even though the combined approach itself has not been widely validated.

Challenges to studying the team approach

There are a number of challenges to studying the multidisciplinary model that have likely contributed to a lack of empirical studies of this approach. From a study design standpoint, it is difficult to standardise each branch of treatment and carry it out uniformly across patients. In practice, many multidisciplinary interventions occur simultaneously, which adds to the complexity of understanding the additive effects of each branch of treatment. As such, studies tend to use a broad-outcome measure that provides information about the total intervention, as opposed to describing the relative benefits of each discipline's work. Finally, the biopsychosocial framework and corresponding multidisciplinary approach has now been so widely adopted, especially in the field of paediatric gastroenterology, that providers may feel that it is not ethical or necessary to have patients undergo an alternative treatment approach for research purposes.

Moving forward, it would be useful for future studies of the multidisciplinary treatment approach to look at the efficacy of individual treatment components, broaden illness groups, and conduct longitudinal follow-up assessments to measure treatment success over time. It also would be useful for studies of the multidisciplinary approach to identify what factors in individuals predict treatment success and examine those predictors of success across treatment components.

Strategies for building successful integrated teams

The most essential elements of building of integrated care clinics include:
- the combination of the personnel who have essential skills in each of the areas needed for care
- a well-developed organisational strategy including institutional support for the care clinic
- an infrastructure with designated support personnel to support the care model.

Without these elements, the clinic is likely to encounter obstacles that make the delivery of care overly complex or inefficient, increasing the likelihood of key players withdrawing support.

Key personnel

An integrated care team should consist of enthusiastic individuals who are willing to work closely together despite the likelihood of encountering a variety of logistical and philosophical challenges. Unfortunately, very few clinical training programmes include interdisciplinary training experiences. As a result, most professionals have their first interdisciplinary care experiences 'on the job'. Each team member should contribute unique knowledge and skills to the greater treatment team. It is particularly advantageous to have clinical staff members who recognise the unique contributions of other disciplines and enjoy the collaborative care process. Provided that there are relatively few additional clinical tasks and that the provision of care can be completed within the same workload expectation, clinicians are generally enthusiastic about the team process. As providers are able to learn from a variety of other disciplines and educate their professional colleagues about their roles, this leads many to greater job satisfaction.

Organisational strategy

Multidisciplinary and interdisciplinary programmes also need an organisational strategy, or clinical model of care, to ensure that the complexity of the care does not negatively affect service delivery efforts. Typically, this demands that the clinic adopts a singular philosophy of care and a plan for how clinicians communicate. Successful programmes generally develop the model of care before trying to implement any services to ensure a smooth programme launch. Relative advantages go to programmes that adopt a true interdisciplinary care model, especially if records and clinical services are offered out of the same system. Multidisciplinary programmes can overcome these relative disadvantages by using telehealth technologies to allow providers and patient families to share records or to have integrated care despite barriers associated with distance (e.g. videoconferencing or electronic medical records that offer shared access).

Infrastructure

Finally, the project will need infrastructure support including support staff, especially a clinical coordinator, to manage the daily operation of the project. To ensure the success of a multidisciplinary or interdisciplinary clinic, there should be a well-trained clinic coordinator and a scheduling assistant to ensure that clinics are well organised. Few things will undermine the best-intended efforts to develop an interdisciplinary clinic as the failures of logistical supports, including clinic coordination, scheduling and billing. The administrative support personnel will require many of the same skills as the clinical staff, including an ability to be flexible, have knowledge about the clinical practices of the various providers (as this will often need to be explained to families and other care partners), and these individuals will also need to be ambassadors to the administration to help them understand the added value to the hospital or care programme within which the clinic operates. Daily operations will include many of the traditional responsibilities of clinic coordination (e.g. scheduling patients, communication with families, ordering supplies for the clinic). Furthermore, if the project involves research, then the coordinator may also be asked to help with participant recruitment, data collection, tracking of patients and collecting longitudinal data. Without these core components, multidisciplinary care is difficult to utilise and may not be a viable option for care.

Service delivery plan

Prior to starting a multidisciplinary or interdisciplinary clinical programme, a plan for service delivery should be developed with a rationale for why multidisciplinary care is being considered. The programme plan should include the descriptions of the clinical population to receive services (diagnosis, medical needs), general treatment approach and protocols, a rationale for why multidisciplinary care would be advantageous over traditional services for the patient population (e.g. reduces barriers to care associated with complexity of underlying condition, improves clinical outcomes, reduces additional stressors on family associated with coordination of care). A detailed list of infrastructure needs should also be developed, including key personnel, a proposal for the model for care provision, and administrative supports needed. A plan for tracking progress should also be considered, which might include tracking of clinical outcomes, tracking patient and provider treatment satisfaction, frequency and ease of use of multidisciplinary visits, and economic benefits to families and the treatment facility.

If the providers plan to complete clinical research as part of their care a method should be developed a priori and all methods should be reviewed by the human subjects institutional review board before conducting any data collection.

TABLE 2.1 Integrated clinic start-up essentials

I.	*Administrative support and institutional vision*
	No integrated care clinic will be successful without the full support of the institution within which the clinic operates. The first step in developing an integrated care clinic is to identify key administrative personnel who support and are willing to become directly involved in the clinic. Typically, this requires a medical director, a hospital administrator and service line directors from each of the key disciplines involved in the clinic.
II.	*Staff selection and training*
	Staff selection will vary widely, dependent upon which disciplines are required to provide the clinical care. However, individual providers should be collaborative individuals who have a wide breadth of knowledge about the clinical problems seen within a clinical service. Clinicians will likely avoid integrated care until they feel adequately trained and comfortable with the care model. A special effort to invite personnel to observe integrated sessions, completing training sessions with trained staff and having professional colleagues who are well versed in integrated care available for consultation the first few clinics is advisable.
III.	*Scheduling and record keeping*
	As integrated care clinics are developed, confusion regarding responsibilities for scheduling and keeping patient records is common. A dedicated support person for the integrated clinic should reduce problems associated with logistics and record keeping. Prior to starting the clinical service, development of procedures for scheduling and documentation should also be established. In some integrated practice settings, treatment team assessment reports and notes are often generated.

SUMMARY

Integrated care models are increasingly becoming the gold standard of care delivery, particularly in paediatric healthcare. Utilisation of these practice models theoretically benefits patient families and providers alike. Many of the traditional barriers to optimal care are overcome by integrated models, including improved access to providers, ability to streamline care, cohesive treatment plans reducing confusion regarding treatment recommendations, and improved treatment satisfaction for families and providers alike. Unfortunately, these care models are more demanding on providers and the administrative system making these clinical services more difficult to offer for many systems. However, for those systems that have the vision and infrastructure to implement these models, all parties seem to benefit. While these models are well established and are largely considered to be the gold standard of care, there is still much work to be done from an investigational standpoint. Future research may want to focus on relative clinical outcome comparisons with traditional care, to study cost comparisons between models of care and to explore user satisfaction from provider, consumer and administrative standpoints.

REFERENCES

Armstrong FD. Individual and organizational collaborations: a roadmap for effective advocacy. In: Roberts MC, Steele RG, editors. *Handbook of Pediatric Psychology.* 4th ed. New York, NY: Guilford Press; 2009. pp. 774–84.

Armstrong FD, Drotar D. Multi-institutional and multi-disciplinary research collaboration: strategies and lessons from cooperative trials. In: Drotar D, editor. *Handbook of Research in Pediatric and Clinical Child Psychology: practical strategies and methods.* New York, NY: Kluwer Academic/Plenum Press; 2000. pp. 281–303.

Armstrong FD, Reaman GH. Psychological research in childhood cancer: the Children's Oncology Group perspective. *J Pediatr Psychol.* 2005; **30**(1): 89–97.

Babbitt RL, Hoch TA, Coe DA, *et al.* Behavioral assessment and treatment of pediatric feeding disorders. *Journal of Developmental and Behavioral Pediatrics.* 1994; **15**: 278–91.

Bithoney WG, McJunkin J, Michalek J, *et al.* The effect of a multidisciplinary team approach on weight gain in nonorganic failure-to-thrive children. *J Dev Behav Pediatr.* 1991; **12**(4): 254–8.

Buckloh LM, Greco P. Professional development, roles, and practice patterns. In: Roberts MC, Steele RG, editors. *Handbook of Pediatric Psychology.* 4th ed. New York, NY: Guilford Press; 2009. pp. 35–51.

Carter BD, Von Weiss RT. Inpatient pediatric consultation-liaison. In: Roberts M, Reis J, editors. *Handbook of Mental Health Services for Children and Adolescents.* New York, NY: Kluwer. 2004. pp. 63–83.

Chiou E, Nurko S. Management of functional abdominal pain and irritable bowel syndrome in children and adolescents. *Expert Rev Gastroenterol Hepatol.* 2010; **4**(3): 293–304.

Finney JW, Riley AW, Cataldo MF. Psychology in primary health care: effects of brief targeted therapy on children's medical care utilization. *J Pediatr Psychol.* 1991; **16**(4): 447–61.

Fischer E, Silverman A. Behavioral conceptualization, assessment, and treatment of pediatric feeding disorders. *Semin Speech Lang.* 2007; **28**(3): 223–31.

Froese AP, Kamin LE Levine CA. Teamwork: a multidisciplinary pediatric-liaison service. *Int J Psychiatry Med.* 1976–77; **7**(1): 47–56.

Guralnick MJ. Interdisciplinary assessment for young children. In: Guralnick MJ, editor. *Interdisciplinary Clinical Assessment of Young Children with Developmental Disabilities.* Baltimore, MD: Brookes; 2000. pp. 3–15.

Hochstadt NJ, Harwicke NJ. How effective is the multidisciplinary approach? A follow-up study. *Child Abuse Negl.* 1985; **9**(3): 365–72.

Humphreys PA, Gevirtz RN. Treatment of recurrent abdominal pain: components analysis of four treatment protocols. *J Pediatr Gastroenterol Nutr.* 2000; **31**(1): 47–51.

Kedesdy JH, Budd KS. Assessment of environmental factors in feeding: an overview. In: Kedesdy JH, Budd KS, editors. *Childhood Feeding Disorders: biobehavioral assessment and intervention.* Baltimore, MD: Brookes; 1998a. pp. 79–114.

Kedesdy JH, Budd KS. Introduction: feeding from a biobehavioral perspective. In: Kedesdy JH, Budd KS, editors. *Childhood Feeding Disorders: biobehavioral assessment and intervention.* Baltimore, MD: Brookes; 1998b. pp. 1–31.

Koocher GP, Keith-Spiegel P. *Ethics in Psychology and the Mental Health Professions: standards and cases.* 3rd ed. New York, NY: Oxford University Press; 2008.

Li BU, Balint JP. Cyclic vomiting syndrome: evolution in understanding of a brain-gut disorder. *Adv Pediatr.* 2000; **47**: 117–60.

McGrath ML, Mellon MW, Murphy L. Empirically supported treatments in pediatric psychology: constipation and encopresis. *J Pediatr Psychol.* 2000; **25**(4): 255–6.

Opipari-Arrigan L, Stark L, Drotar D. Benchmarks for work performance of pediatric psychologists. *J Pediatr Psychol.* 2006; **31**(6): 630–42.

Palmer S, Thompson RJ. Nutrition: an integral component in the health care of children. The interdisciplinary team in action. *J Am Diet Assoc.* 1976; **69**(2): 138–42.

Peterson KE, Washington J, Rathbun JM. Team management of failure to thrive. *J Am Diet Assoc.* 1984; **84**(7): 810–15.

Rae WA, Brunnquell D, Sullivan JR. Ethical and legal issues in pediatric psychology. In: Roberts MC, Steele RG. *Handbook of Pediatric Psychology.* 4th ed. New York, NY: Guilford Press; 2009. pp. 19–34.

Robins PM, Smith SM, Glutting JJ, Bishop CT. A randomized controlled trial of a cognitive-behavioral family intervention for pediatric recurrent abdominal pain. *J Pediatr Psychol.* 2005; **30**(5): 397–408.

Sampson P. Interdisciplinary teamwork. In: Kessler DB, Dawson P, editors. *Failure to Thrive and Pediatric Undernutrition: a transdisciplinary approach.* Baltimore, MD: Paul H Brookes; 1999. pp. 303–5.

Schurman JV, Wu YP, Grayson P, *et al.* A pilot study to assess the efficacy of biofeedback-assisted relaxation training as an adjunct treatment for pediatric functional dyspepsia associated with duodenal eosinophilia. *J Pediatr Psychol.* 2010; **35**(8): 837–47.

Stark LJ, Charlies-Stively J, Spirito A, *et al.* Group behavioral treatment of retentive encopresis. *J Pediatr Psychol.* 1990; **15**(5): 659–71.

Tarbell S, Li BU. Psychiatric symptoms in children and adolescents with cyclic vomiting syndrome and their parents. *Headache.* 2008; **48**(2): 259–66.

Vlieger A, Menko-Frankenhuis C, Wolfkamp S, *et al.* Hypnotherapy for children with functional abdominal pain or irritable bowel syndrome. *Gastroenterology.* 2007; **133**: 1430–6.

Walter RS. The multidisciplinary approach to management of swallowing disorders in the pediatric patient. In: Tuchman DN, Walters RS, editors. *Disorders of Feeding and Swallowing in Infants and Children.* San Diego, CA: Singular; 1994. pp. 251–7.

CHAPTER 3

Cognitive behavioural therapy for abdominal pain

Sara King, Jessica Boutilier and Christine T Chambers

INTRODUCTION

Various terms and definitions have been used to describe recurrent abdominal pain (RAP). Apley and Naish (1958) diagnose RAP as three episodes of abdominal pain that interfere with typical function and that last at least 3 months. Within this definition, typical functioning is defined as meeting academic standards based on grade level, participation in activities with peers in and outside of school, and functioning within the home environment with both siblings and parents on a daily basis (Cunningham and Banez, 2006). Although the term 'recurrent abdominal pain' is often used interchangeably with functional abdominal pain (or FAP), for the purposes of this chapter RAP is described as a dull, poorly localised pain that manifests in the abdominal area (Cunningham and Banez, 2006).

Given that a definable organic cause is typically not identified for children and adolescents who suffer from RAP (Levine and Rappaport, 1984; Cunningham and Banez, 2006), it is important to acknowledge that there are both physical and psychological components to chronic pain. It is generally accepted that RAP is an interaction of both biological (i.e. visceral hyperalgesia) and psychological factors (i.e. environmental stressors) (Chambers *et al.*, 2004). As such, it is important that both medical and psychological treatments are available for paediatric abdominal pain to appropriately address both the physical and psychological components of the condition (Barakat *et al.*, 2007).

With some studies suggesting prevalence rates as high as 44%, it is also important that children and adolescents with abdominal pain are treated in the most effective and efficient manner possible (King *et al.*, 2011). With such high numbers of children and adolescents suffering from RAP, there is an excessive burden being placed on the healthcare system. Frequent physician consultation, medication use and hospitalisation are just a few of the factors that appear to contribute to the burden that RAP places on healthcare resources (Chambers *et al.*, 2004). Adding to the overburdened healthcare system, patients with RAP also tend to be the most challenging patients for physicians to treat, as there is often no identified organic cause and very few empirically supported treatment and management strategies (Chambers *et al.*, 2004).

In this chapter we will look at the application of cognitive behavioural therapy (CBT) for RAP. A 'typical' case of an adolescent with presenting symptoms of abdominal pain can be followed in Part III, 3.4 (*FGID letter*).

EVIDENCE-BASED TREATMENTS

Evidence-based medications that target the physical symptomatology of RAP have been effective in the treatment and management of this state (Chambers *et al.*, 2004). However, many parents dislike the use of pharmaceuticals and often search for alternative treatment and management strategies. Alternative therapy and treatments can be costly and have questionable efficacy, especially for long-term use (Barry and Von Baeyer, 1997). With few empirically supported interventions targeting the physical symptomatology of RAP, psychological interventions are becoming increasingly popular as an evidence-based strategy to treat and manage RAP.

To date, RAP has not been linked to a specific organic cause. Standard paediatric practice is usually to reassure the child and his or her parent(s) that there is no serious disease present, that many children often 'grow out' of the pain, and that the child needs to learn how to cope with the pain (Sanders *et al.*, 1994). However, it has been noted that many children who experience RAP often lack coping strategies and do not believe they have any control over their symptoms (Sanders *et al.*, 1994). Teaching coping skills and relaxation strategies have been suggested as possible treatments for children with RAP. Operant and cognitive behavioural models of chronic pain posit that the family environment, specifically parental cues and attention to pain behaviour, also serve to reinforce the child's behaviour and maintain the pain (Sanders *et al.*, 1994). In effect, the interaction of the parent with the child may serve to increase or decrease the child's expression of pain. This would suggest that the behavioural expression of pain in children with RAP is not entirely under the control of the biological manifestations of the problem. Some authors have highlighted similarities between RAP and anxiety in children (Kendall and Chansky, 1991; Kendall *et al.*, 1992). This, in turn, has led to the belief that many features of CBT interventions for anxiety could be used to treat RAP (Sanders *et al.*, 1994).

COGNITIVE BEHAVIOURAL THERAPY

CBT is a psychological treatment modality that focuses on the interrelation between thoughts, feelings and behaviours in the development and maintenance of maladaptive behaviours. The treatment is delivered either individually or in group format over approximately eight sessions by a trained psychologist or other highly trained mental health professional (Chambers *et al.*, 2004). Using a 'collaborative empiricism' model, both the clinician and the client are active participants in the therapy process, as opposed to the patient following the instructions of the clinician. Therapy content is delivered both verbally and in writing and the patient is typically assigned 'homework' or 'practice' to complete between sessions. As is the case for most child-focused treatments, it is important to note that CBT for RAP will be most effective if both the child and the parent(s) participate actively in the programme (Chambers *et al.*, 2004). CBT has been shown to be an *effective* treatment for a variety of mental and physical health disorders in children, including anxiety and depression as well as chronic and recurrent pain conditions such as headache and RAP (Chambers *et al.*, 2004; Noel *et al.*, 2012).

Sanders *et al.* (1994) described the most widely used CBT treatment protocol for RAP. The goal of CBT for RAP is to provide children and parents with a range of coping strategies for pain and its associated functional impairment. Within the therapeutic sessions, environmental factors that reinforce and maintain the pain behaviour are uncovered and their function eliminated or controlled (Noel *et al.*, 2012). Specifically, maladaptive thoughts that serve to promote pain behaviour and maintain pain (e.g. 'If I go out with my friends my stomach will just start to hurt and I won't be able to do anything') are replaced with more adaptive or helpful thoughts (e.g. 'My stomach might start to hurt, but it won't stop me from having fun'). This will, in turn, lead to more adaptive behaviours that do not perpetuate pain. It is important to note that the goal of CBT for RAP is not to eliminate pain altogether but, rather, to improve daily functioning and to help the child reintegrate into activities such as school and extracurricular activities in spite of his or her pain. As a result of this focus on reintegration and functionality, the child and family are able to move towards acceptance of the pain and the child no longer avoids activities that may have been thought to exacerbate pain (e.g. attending school, playing sports). Similarly, parents no longer allow the child to avoid activities on account of his or her pain and learn to reinforce well behaviour rather than pain behaviour (Noel *et al.*, 2012; Chambers *et al.*, 2004).

Cognitive behavioural therapy for recurrent abdominal pain
Evidence supporting the use of cognitive behavioural therapy for recurrent abdominal pain

Recent Cochrane reviews of randomised controlled trials for chronic pain in children have found large positive effects for psychological interventions (i.e. behavioural relaxation-based programmes and CBT including cognitive coping, coping skills training and parent training) in reducing pain intensity when compared with no-treatment groups (Eccleston *et al.*, 2009; Palermo *et al.*, 2010). It is encouraging that these positive effects have been shown for headache and RAP – two of the most common types of pain in children (King *et al.*, 2011). The reported positive effects of CBT for RAP translate into clinically significant reductions in pain intensity (i.e. 50% reduction in pain). Children with pain were approximately four times more likely to have reduced pain than children who did not receive a CBT intervention. Web-based interventions for RAP have also been found to have similar effects to in-person interventions and are good alternatives for children and families who cannot access therapists face-to-face (Macea *et al.*, 2010).

Group-based cognitive behavioural therapy for recurrent abdominal pain

Recent studies have indicated that group-based CBT for children and families can also be an effective treatment for RAP. Specifically, our group, in partnership with the Paediatric Health Psychology Service at our local children's health centre, runs a CBT group for children and their parents based on the CBT principles (Noel *et al.*, 2012; Chambers *et al.*, 2004). The group is delivered to children between the ages of 8 and 12 years over the course of 6 weeks and consists of a 90-minute session for children and a concurrent 90-minute session for parents each week. Children and parents complete their sessions in separate rooms and then typically join one another for the last 10–15 minutes of the session to review the material that was covered in the child session. The group is developed and implemented by PhD students in clinical psychology under the supervision of a registered psychologist, as well as various pre-doctoral psychology residents and postdoctoral fellows; therefore, the specific content of the group varies from year to year, but the core components of CBT are always present.

Generally, the group begins with psychoeducation about pain and RAP and how the treatment will help children cope with their pain when it occurs. Children are also provided with pain diaries in the first session to monitor their symptoms throughout treatment. Following the psychoeducation component of treatment, children are introduced to relaxation strategies that can help them manage their pain and encouraged to practise at home with their parent(s). The CBT model of RAP (i.e. the thoughts, feelings and behaviours associated with RAP) is presented in the middle of the treatment, with the focus being placed on educating children how their thoughts, feelings and behaviours can exacerbate and maintain RAP. Children are taught to identify negative cognitions (or 'unhelpful thoughts') they have about their pain and to replace these thoughts with more helpful coping thoughts. Children are provided with a manual that they can complete during each session and also with homework sheets each week. Pain diaries and homework from the previous week are reviewed at the beginning of each session.

The concurrent parent group is similar to the child group, in that parents are provided with psychoeducation about RAP and are also introduced to the CBT model of RAP. Parents are encouraged to take on the role of 'coaches' for their children and are taught behavioural principles such as operant models of positive and negative reinforcement, differential attention, and modelling with respect to promoting well behaviour (e.g. reinforcing or praising children for attempting to cope positively with pain). Parents are taught that using these behavioural techniques does not imply that they are ignoring or invalidating their child's pain; parents are taught to allocate specific times to discuss pain briefly and to gradually decrease the amount of time spent attending to or discussing pain. During the final sessions of the parent group, parents are taught about relapse prevention and to develop a plan for coping with future instances of pain. Recommendations regarding sleep hygiene, school refusal behaviours and healthy lifestyle are provided. Preliminary results suggest that the child and parent CBT groups are effective in reducing pain duration and intensity (see Noel *et al.*, 2012). Children also reported that medication use had decreased significantly as a result of treatment, whereas parents reported significantly less encouragement of illness behaviour in their children.

COMPONENTS OF COGNITIVE BEHAVIOURAL THERAPY FOR RECURRENT ABDOMINAL PAIN

What distinguishes CBT from many other treatment modalities is that this type of treatment is typically delivered in a highly structured and manualised format and consists of several standardised components. With respect to RAP, a standard course of CBT would generally consist of the following elements (examples of each element can be found in Table 3.1).

Psychoeducation

It is important to distinguish formal psychoeducation from supportive advice. The psychoeducation component of any CBT protocol involves educating the child and his or her parents about the difficulty they face and how the psychologist will work with them to ameliorate it. With respect to RAP, the child and parent(s) are provided with information about the nature and prevalence of chronic and recurrent pain in children and also about the psychological factors that can exacerbate and maintain pain (e.g. the gate control theory of pain (Melzack and Wall, 1965) may be used to explain this). The role of cognitive behavioural pain management techniques is discussed with the child and parent(s) and they are given the message that the pain is real, despite the lack of organic cause.

Self-monitoring

Self-monitoring is especially important in the early phases of treatment, as the child and family are asked to record the intensity, frequency and duration of pain. Additionally, the child and parents are asked to record mood and behaviours around the time of the pain episode, as this allows for the identification of possible pain triggers and, therefore, allows the child and parent(s) to learn to manage the behavioural antecedents and consequences of pain.

Coping skills

At this stage of treatment, children are taught a variety of developmentally appropriate coping strategies to help them manage their pain; children practise these techniques in the session with the psychologist but are also strongly encouraged to practise them at home with their parent(s). As already noted, 'homework' or 'practice' is usually an expectation of children taking part in CBT; as such, practising their coping skills outside of the session often forms part of their homework assignment. Skills that are typically taught as part of a CBT treatment protocol include relaxation strategies (e.g. deep breathing, progressive muscle relaxation, guided imagery), recognising negative thoughts about pain (e.g. 'Going to school will make my stomach hurt'), replacement of negative thoughts with more positive, helpful thoughts (e.g. 'My stomach might hurt when I'm at school but I can get through it and still have a good day'), and rewarding oneself for making the effort to cope with the pain in an appropriate and helpful way (e.g. extra television time, choosing a special treat).

Parent training

As with many psychological treatments for children, parents play an essential role in delivering CBT for RAP (Chambers *et al.*, 2004; Noel *et al.*, 2012). Parents are encouraged to play the role of 'coach' to their child and to support the child in practising and applying the psychological techniques that are part of the CBT programme. Sanders *et al.* (1994) specifies that parents should reinforce well behaviour, respond to pain complaints by encouraging the child to engage in an alternate activity, ignore non-verbal pain behaviour, avoid modelling pain behaviour, and learn to distinguish between RAP and a physical complaint that may require medical intervention.

Relapse prevention

A key feature of CBT for RAP is to provide children and parents with the tools they need to manage future occurrences of pain, as well as anxiety-provoking situations (e.g. starting a new school year, trying a new activity, being away from home).

Homework

As noted, assigning the child 'homework' or 'practice' to complete between sessions is an essential component of any CBT programme. The homework assignments are typically short and easy to complete; however, they allow for the generalisation of skills to real-life situations outside of the clinician's office.

TABLE 3.1 Examples of cognitive behavioural therapy (CBT) elements for recurrent abdominal pain (RAP)

Element	Examples
Psychoeducation	• This is not simply giving the child and family advice
	• Information provided regarding the nature and prevalence of chronic and recurrent pain (i.e. by explaining gate control theory of pain)
	• Overview of pain management techniques that will be covered in sessions
	• Parents and children assured that the pain is real, despite the lack of organic cause
Self-monitoring	• Parents and children asked to monitor intensity, frequency and duration of pain (important in initial phases of treatment)
	• Parents and children asked to record disruption to daily functioning as a result of pain
	• Parents and children encouraged to record events happening before and after the pain episode (to identify possible triggers)
Coping skills	• Deep breathing exercises: children taught diaphragmatic breathing techniques (e.g. pretending to blow up and deflate a balloon in their stomachs)
	• Progressive muscle relaxation: children taught to relax and tense various groups of muscles. Developmentally appropriate examples given to assist children with this task (e.g. children told to pretend to be a 'robot' and a 'rag doll' or 'uncooked spaghetti' and 'cooked spaghetti')
	• Guided imagery: the therapist assists the child in imagining a relaxing scene (e.g. being at the beach) and to focus on each element of this scene. The therapist can record the narration so that the child can practise at home
	• Positive self-talk (coping thoughts): children are taught to replace negative self-talk or unhelpful thoughts (e.g. 'my pain will never go away') with positive self-talk or coping thoughts (e.g. 'I am the boss of my pain and I can handle this')
	• Distraction techniques: children come up with a list of activities they can do that will focus their attention away from the pain
	• Self-reinforcement: children are taught to praise themselves or give themselves a 'pat on the back' for coping with their pain successfully
Parent training	Parents taught to be 'coaches' in helping their children manage RAP using strategies such as:
	• Limiting or removing attention from pain: when the child complains of pain, the parent can acknowledge it, but should keep discussion to a minimum and shift attention to other activities (e.g. play or homework)

(*continued*)

Element	Examples
Parent training (*cont.*)	• Reinforcing well behaviour: parents are taught to provide attention and special privileges on days when the child does not complain of pain. This encourages the child to keep up with daily activities and takes attention away from pain
	• School attendance: parent is encouraged to send child to school every day, even if pain is present. Discussion of pain should be limited in the morning before school and if child complains of pain at school, he or she should be allowed to rest briefly at school and should not be sent home unless signs and symptoms of illness (e.g. fever) are present
	• Limiting activities on days when child complains of pain: if the child is too sick to attend school, then he or she is too sick to participate in activities in the home (e.g. playing on the computer, talking with friends, watching television)
	• Identifying stress: the parent can help the child identify stress at home or at school and develop a plan to cope with the stress
	• Encouraging use of coping skills: the parent should encourage the child to engage in strategies that have been taught as part of CBT (e.g. breathing/relaxation techniques)
Relapse prevention	• During the course of CBT for RAP, the child and parent(s) are taught to develop a plan for how to cope with pain in the future
	• The child is encouraged to continue practising relaxation strategies and developing coping thoughts to deal with future episodes of pain
Homework	• The therapist typically prepares worksheets and short homework assignments to be completed between sessions
	• It is important to hold the child accountable for homework completion – if the child arrives at a session without his or her homework completed, the therapist should assist the child in completing the homework for 10 minutes at the beginning of the session

Note: adapted from Chambers *et al.*, 2004

In addition to the components of parent training mentioned in Table 3.1, parents are also taught to liaise appropriately with school officials to ensure that the child receives consistent messages about pain management across settings.

COGNITIVE BEHAVIOURAL THERAPY AT SCHOOLS

Children spend a large portion of their time in school. Therefore, it is important to involve school personnel in the treatment of RAP. School personnel do not require a special skill set or knowledge of CBT principles to implement CBT-based accommodations and modifications in the classroom; rather, management of RAP in the classroom requires good communication between parents and teachers. Some frequently recommended accommodations are presented in this chapter (*see* Box 3.1); these accommodations are based on several of the key concepts of CBT and include reinforcing behaviour unrelated

---

BOX 3.1 Classroom accommodations for children with recurrent abdominal pain

- Provide two sets of books for children so that they can keep one set at home and are not forced to carry their books to and from school
- Allow the student to get up from the desk and stretch his or her legs periodically so as not to force the student to sit for long periods of time
- If the student suffers from stomach problems and requires frequent trips to the bathroom, allow the student to sit close to the exit and do not require the student to raise his or her hand when he or she needs to leave the classroom to go to the bathroom
- If there are policies that prohibit students from participating in extracurricular activities because of frequent absences, revisit this policy in order to ensure that the student is not being excluded from these activities unfairly
- Provide special attention to the student when he or she is having a day without pain
- Avoid concentrating on or discussing the student's pain, so as to avoid dwelling on the occurrence
- Refocus the student's attention when he or she begins discussing pain
- Identify a safe space within the school for the student to go for a short break when he or she begins to feel overwhelmed by the pain
- Try to avoid having the student call home when he or she begins experiencing pain – try to implement some of the strategies already listed to avoid further absenteeism
- Assign a classmate as a 'buddy' to collect homework and work on projects together

---

to illness through contingent social attention, responding to verbal complaints with distracting activities and ignoring non-verbal pain behaviours (Cunningham and Banez, 2006). Common accommodations implemented in the classroom are based on natural reinforcement schedule practices rather than implementing a focused reinforcement schedule. These, in some instances, may distract the teacher from his or her primary task of teaching the class and improving the academic success of the child with RAP. Common school practices include sending students home when they are in pain or giving them extensions for work they failed to complete. This accommodation allows the student to fall further behind in his or her coursework (Logan *et al.*, 2008). These types of accommodation simply reinforce the escape behaviour and perpetuate the cycle of absenteeism and poor academic performance often observed in students with RAP and other recurrent pain conditions. For children with RAP, it is essential that they are encouraged to manage their pain at school. It is important that teachers understand and adhere to the CBT approach to ensure treatment efficacy and consistency. With the support of parents and mental health professionals, school personnel can implement small adjustments in the school environment to ensure that students with chronic pain are receiving in-school support in conjunction with the treatment they are receiving outside of the school system. It is important that healthcare professionals consistently relay the message that school personnel are capable of implementing small changes in the school system that have the potential to create larger, long-term changes for students with RAP.

SUMMARY

The current chapter has detailed the use of CBT for families with children suffering from RAP. Evidence-based interventions for these children are still in their infancy, therefore there is a limited amount of data to definitively suggest what are and are not effective approaches to adopt to aid children with RAP in coping with their condition. CBT has received some initial support for helping children with RAP. This form of psychological therapy can be delivered through individual or group-based sessions, as long as they contain psychoeducation, self-monitoring, teaching of coping strategies and parental training as central tenets to the intervention. When employing CBT techniques, the clinician should be mindful of incorporating methods to limit relapse and provide the family with targets to achieve outside of the therapeutic session. To maximise success, incorporation of the child's school will aid in generalising the new coping strategies into all of the important environments of the child's daily life. The current chapter offers a method to implement a CBT intervention for children with RAP. If the intervention is implemented correctly by a suitably qualified professional, the initial evidence suggests that the child will achieve clinically significant reductions in pain and that this will help the child to achieve better grades at school.

REFERENCES

Apley J, Naish N. Recurrent abdominal pains: a field survey of 1,000 school children. *Arch Dis Child.* 1958; **33**(168): 165–70.

Barakat LP, Gonzalez ER, Weinberfer BS. Using cognitive-behaviour group therapy with chronic mental illness. In: Christner RW, Stewart J, Freeman A, editors. *Handbook of Cognitive Behaviour Group Therapy with Children and Adolescents: specific settings and presenting problems.* New York, NY: Routledge; 2007. pp. 427–46.

Barry J, Von Baeyer CL. Brief cognitive-behavioral group treatment for children's headache. *Clin J Pain.* 1997; **13**(3): 215–20.

Chambers CT, Holly C, Eakins D. Cognitive-behavioural treatment of recurrent abdominal pain in children: a primer for paediatricians. *Paediatr Child Health.* 2004; **9**(10): 705–8.

Cunningham CL, Banez GA. Recurrent abdominal pain. In: Cunningham CL, Banez GA. *Pediatric Gastrointestinal Disorders: biopsychosocial assessment and treatment.* New York, NY: Springer; 2006. pp. 93–111.

Eccleston C, Palermo TM, Williams AC, *et al.* Psychological therapies for the management of chronic and recurrent pain in children and adolescents. *Cochrane Database Syst Rev.* 2009; (2): CD003968.

Kendall PC, Chansky TE. Considering cognition in anxiety-disordered children. *J Anxiety Disord.* 1991; 5: 167–85.

Kendall PC, Kortlander E, Chansky TE, *et al.* Comorbidity of anxiety and depression in youth: treatment implications. *J Consult Clin Psychol.* 1992; 60(6): 869–80.

King S, Chambers CT, Huguet A, *et al.* The epidemiology of chronic pain in children and adolescents revisited: a systematic review. *Pain.* 2011; 152(12): 21–9.

Levine MD, Rappaport LA. Recurrent abdominal pain in school children: the loneliness of the long-distance physician. *Pediatr Clin North Am.* 1984; 31(5): 969–91.

Logan DE, Simons LE, Stein MJ, *et al.* School impairment in adolescents with chronic pain. *J Pain.* 2008; 9(5): 407–16.

Macea DD, Gajos K, Calil YAD, Fregni F. The efficacy of Web-Based Cognitive Behavioral Interventions fro Chronic Pain: A Systematic Review. *J Pain.* 2010; 11(10): 917–29.

Melzack R, Wall PD. Pain mechanisms: a new theory. *Science.* 1965; 150(3699): 971–9.

Noel M, Petter M, Parker JA, *et al.* Cognitive behavioural therapy for pediatric chronic pain: the problem, research, and practice. *J Cogn Psychother.* 2012; 26(2): 143–56.

Palermo TM, Eccleston C, Lewandowski AS, *et al.* Randomized controlled trials of psychological therapies for management of chronic pain in children and adolescents: an updated meta-analytic review. *Pain.* 2010; 148(3): 387–97.

Sanders MR, Shepherd RW, Cleghorn G, *et al.* The treatment of recurrent abdominal pain in children: a controlled comparison of cognitive-behavioral family intervention and standard pediatric care. *J Consult Clin Psychol.* 1994; 62(2): 306–14.

CHAPTER 4

Children with FGIDs: considerations of family factors (a social learning perspective)

Jennifer V Schurman and Amanda D Deacy

INTRODUCTION

The prevailing biopsychosocial model of functional gastrointestinal disorders (FGIDs) (described in Chapter 7) suggests that chronic abdominal pain and other gastrointestinal symptoms in children occur as a result of varying contributions from, and dynamic interactions among, biological, psychological and social factors. Equally important to understand, however, is that biopsychosocial factors are situated within a larger ecological context that includes the family. Several theoretical models have been put forth to account for the 'ecology' in which a child with chronic health concerns finds him- or herself. One such model, the Social-Ecological Model of Health, fits particularly well with the biopsychosocial model of FGIDs in proposing that individual health is influenced by biological and genetic functioning, environmental contingencies and social and familial relationships, as well as by broader social and economic trends (Smedley and Syme, 2001). Family factors clearly intersect with all of these components in one way or another, and yet have remained relatively neglected in discussion of pediatric FGIDs.

This chapter presents the current empirical evidence for familial contribution to each component outlined in the Social-Ecological Model of Health as it relates to pediatric FGIDs, as well as the assessment and treatment implications for clinical practice. A thorough assessment of potential familial contributions may help better define the generating and maintaining factors for an individual child's symptoms, as well as guide creation of a targeted and effective treatment plan that minimises family-based risk factors and enhances family strengths. Specific assessment strategies, and relevant parent- or family-level interventions (when applicable), are highlighted in brief following each discussion section.

A more broad discussion of treatment approaches in paediatric FGIDs can be found elsewhere in this book. Finally, a case study is serialised throughout the chapter to illustrate how specific family factors may present in clinical practice

BIOLOGICAL AND GENETIC FUNCTIONING

Case Study: Ryan

Ryan, a 10-year-old boy, gets a 'stomach bug', along with the rest of his family. Although the symptoms last for only a few days for his other family members, Ryan's abdominal pain and nausea persist. He also continues to have some loose bowel movements.

Ryan's father has had problems with occasional cramping and diarrhoea since his own childhood. He remembers being embarrassed by a bowel accident that occurred in class at school one day when a teacher asked him to wait until the end of the lesson to visit the bathroom. He has never been treated for this issue, since it only interferes with his life on rare occasions. Most of the time, Ryan's dad feels fine. On bad days, he just stays home where he can be close to the bathroom, 'just in case'.

Human biology (*see* 'the development of the digestive system' in Part III, 3.0) may be considered to 'set the stage' for the development of many chronic health conditions. The genes that a child inherits from his or her parents may individually, or in combination, place that child at risk for a specific constellation of symptoms. Although genetic research in FGIDs is relatively new and is far from complete, early data suggest that familial inheritance may contribute to the development of FGIDs in children by two pathways:
1. Direct – via genes controlling gastroenterological function
2. Indirect – via genes controlling stress and anxiety pathways.

Inheritance of gastrointestinal issues
Genetic associations have been demonstrated for both of the two most common FGIDs related to abdominal pain – irritable bowel syndrome (IBS) and functional dyspepsia (FD). Data on genetic associations for other FGIDs associated with pain (e.g. functional abdominal pain syndrome, abdominal migraine) are not currently available in the literature. IBS has been shown to aggregate in families and affect multiple generations. Specifically, first-degree relatives of patients with IBS are two to three times more likely to have IBS than the general population (Saito *et al.*, 2010). This symptom clustering within families may be explained in part by genetic predisposition. Candidate genes suggested for IBS generally have been related to specific pathways operating within the gastrointestinal tract, including serotonin, G-protein receptors and inflammation. Serotonin pathways have received particular attention in the

research literature, as serotonin is known to be involved in motility and has a key role in modulating sensitivity (Saito, 2011). To date, IBS has been associated with polymorphisms of genes encoding for specific serotonin receptors (e.g. HTR2A and HTR3E), as well as the serotonin transporter protein (Saito, 2011; Markoutsaki *et al.*, 2011). IBS also has been associated with polymorphisms related to pro- and anti-inflammatory cytokines (e.g. IL6 and IL10), as well as genes encoding for G-protein coupling receptors that may be involved in motility (e.g. GNB3) (Saito, 2011; Markoutsaki *et al.*, 2011).

FD also has been associated with genetic polymorphisms related to serotonin metabolism, including specific receptors (i.e. 5HTR3A) and a promoter region for the serotonin transporter gene (i.e. 5HTTLPR) (Mujakovic *et al.*, 2011; Toyoshima *et al.*, 2011). Similar to IBS, FD is associated with polymorphisms in the GNB3 gene described earlier, but the specific allele is different than that associated with IBS (Oshima *et al.*, 2010). These genetic associations provide reason to believe that a similar symptom clustering within families may be observed, although specific rates of family risk in FD have not yet been established.

While there are genes associated with specific FGIDs, it should be noted that their presence alone does not appear to be sufficient to generate the specific FGID. In the case of IBS, for example, estimations of the proportion of phenotypic variation that is inherited through genetic factors have varied from 0% to 57% (Saito, 2011). Clearly, while familial inheritance of specific genes involved in gastroenterological function may impart heightened risk for an individual child, the actual development of an FGID occurs via a more complex pathway. Still, for the child presenting with gastroenterological symptoms, assessment of the child's genetic risk for a specific FGID may help to guide the diagnostic process and is easily accomplished as part of the standard medical history-taking.

BOX 4.1 Inheritance of gastrointestinal problems

Assessment strategies

Include items in medical history that ask about gastroenterological symptoms or conditions in first-degree relatives.

Inherited vulnerability towards anxiety

The contribution of familial genetic factors may extend beyond the gastrointestinal system in FGIDs. Children also may inherit a tendency towards a heightened sensitivity to stress and/or anxiety that predisposes them to the development of FGIDs. Stress in various forms predisposes adults to develop IBS and has been found to increase symptoms in children with FGIDs (Katiraei and Bultron, 2011; Walker *et al.*, 2011). Further, early temperament markers of anxiety may predict a relative increased risk for the development of FGIDs in early school age (Ramchandani *et al.*, 2006). Clearly, then, familial inheritance of anxiety warrants some consideration.

Similar to IBS, genetic heritability estimates for anxiety has ranged from 0% to 59% (Middeldorp *et al.*, 2005; Thapar and McGuffin, 1995). However, single candidate genes have not been identified. Instead, recent large-scale genomic studies have suggested the anxiety susceptibility is polygenic, with many loci each contributing a small amount to the overall effect (Demirkan *et al.*, 2011). Genotype also appears to function as a moderator of the relationship between environment and phenotypic expression of anxiety. In other words, genes may make some individuals more susceptible to developing problems with anxiety than others when exposed to the same environmental events or adversities (Franić *et al.*, 2010). In the case of FGIDs, pain may function as the event that triggers the onset of problems with anxiety, with anxiety then contributing to the further maintenance of that pain.

Again, the presence of anxiety does not appear to be sufficient, on its own, to generate a specific FGID. Many children experiencing anxiety do not have corresponding gastrointestinal symptoms. In the end, it is likely that FGIDs are multifactorial, resulting from a polygenic predisposition interacting with biologic factors, the patient's psychosocial milieu and the broader social environment. Although the end result (i.e. abdominal pain) may be the same, the relative contribution of genes and environment is likely to be different for each individual child. Identifying genetic risk for anxiety issues represents one potentially important piece of the overall clinical picture.

BOX 4.2 Inherited vulnerability towards anxiety

Assessment strategies

Include items in the medical history that ask about anxiety issues in first-degree relatives.

ENVIRONMENTAL CONTINGENCIES

Ryan: what happened next?

At first, Ryan's parents keep him home from school, believing that Ryan will recover with just a little more time. His mother takes some time off from work to care for him at home. His father, appreciating first-hand how uncomfortable he is, brings home special treats to help lift his spirits and asks his little sister to be especially nice to him right now. After a few more days, Ryan's parents call the school and make arrangements for work to be sent home, where they can help him get caught up on what he is missing during those times when he feels up to it.

Parents of children with FGIDs may react to their children's pain episodes in a variety of ways. Some of these reactions may be beneficial and help children to increase their use of positive coping skills. Other reactions, however well intended, may be detrimental and result in symptoms increasing in intensity, occurring more frequently or being maintained over time.

Social learning mechanisms

Social learning theory has been suggested as a context for understanding the association between parental behaviours and child outcomes, both positive (e.g. effective coping) and negative (e.g. increased somatic complaints), in FGIDs (Levy, *et al.*, 2007). This theory would suggest that children learn how to behave in response to pain by attending to, remembering and imitating the reactions of their family members. Further, the child's imitation of this observed behaviour must be reinforced in some way. Parents of patients with FGIDs do tend to have more physical complaints, as well as more symptoms of anxiety and depression, leading to speculation that these parents model more illness behaviour for their child and provide more attention to their child's own physical symptoms (Di Lorenzo *et al.*, 2005).

BOX 4.3 Social learning mechanisms

Assessment strategies

- Include items in the medical history that ask about parent illness and/or disability
- Behavioural observation during evaluation and subsequent clinic visits

Parent-level interventions

Recommend that parents (and other caregivers) avoid modelling pain or disability behaviour, for example:

- attend school, work or other daily commitments as scheduled, regardless of symptoms
- seek own individual psychotherapy to address disability and/or symptoms of anxiety and depression.

Coach parents to provide positive modelling of coping skills (and model this behaviour during visits), for example:

- maintain behavioural expectations for the child's participation in school and other activities
- demonstrate good emotional self-regulation in front of the child
- freely discuss strategies used to manage own symptoms and/or stressors effectively throughout the day
- focus attention on the child's successes and progress
- use neutral language when discussing pain within the family.

Although data are limited in children, modelling and reinforcement of behaviour consistent with the sick role by family members has been associated with more chronic illness-related behaviour in adults. In one study (Whitehead *et al.*, 1986), individuals whose mothers had modelled and encouraged behaviour consistent with the sick role during their childhood were found to report more menstrual symptoms, clinic visits and disability days as adults. A similar pattern of modelling and reinforcement of the sick role emerged in a study of adults with FGIDs (Whitehead *et al.*, 1994). This type of social learning of illness behaviour is argued to begin in childhood and continue throughout the lifespan (Walker and Zeman, 1992).

Assessing and addressing these issues as part of the treatment for a child with an FGID can be critical. Inclusion of a few key questions about the parents' own history of illness or disability in the medical history-taking can be very helpful in identifying potential problems related to modelling of behaviour consistent with the sick role, as well as potential opportunities for modelling of positive coping skills. Additional information can be gleaned from observing family members during the clinical evaluation and subsequent follow-up visits. For example, families will often share information during conversation (e.g. 'I can remind her to take her morning medications – I am home on disability right now, anyway') or through their actions (e.g. repeatedly cancelling appointments because of illness) that may be valuable to consider in the development of the child's treatment plan.

Parental reinforcement

While reinforcement may come from a variety of sources – including extended family, peers, school staff and even strangers – parents are especially powerful sources of reinforcement for children. Parental behaviours that serve to reinforce the sick role may involve social rewards (e.g. more time with parents or special attention), material gain (e.g. increased provision of treats or privileges), removal of a noxious stimulus (e.g. protection from being bothered by siblings) and/or avoidance of undesirable responsibilities (e.g. school attendance or completion of chores). These parental behaviours have been found to predict prolonged illness, symptom reoccurrence and increased disability in children with chronic medical conditions, including FGIDs (Walker and Zeman, 1992; Brace *et al.*, 2000). Even under carefully controlled, experimental conditions, parental attention to the child's abdominal pain has been shown to increase verbal complaints in response to a water load task (see explanation added later in the chapter to explain the cold presser task) as compared with parental distraction; these behavioural changes were found despite children reporting similar levels of experienced pain across conditions (Walker *et al.*, 2006). In one recent study (Kessler *et al.*, 2012), greater report of parental engagement in negatively reinforcing behaviours (i.e. allowing the child to stay home from school and leave chores or homework uncompleted) was found to predict lower functioning in children with FGIDs, whether or not parents reported providing any other type of reinforcement. This effect was particularly strong for adolescents in terms of predicting psychosocial (i.e. emotional, social and school) functioning. However, combining high levels of negative and positive reinforcement (e.g. providing the child with special attention or treats) appeared to be the most problematic, as this combination was associated with the lowest levels of child functioning across both physical and psychosocial domains.

BOX 4.4 Parental reinforcement

Assessment strategies

- Illness Behavior Encouragement Scale
- Adult Responses to Childhood Symptoms
- Include items in the medical history asking about the number of full or partial days absent from school, extracurricular activities missed and social activities missed with family and friends in the past month
- Behavioural observation during evaluation and subsequent clinic visits

Parent-level interventions

Coach parents on the appropriate use of reinforcement (and model this behaviour during visits), for example:
- differentially reinforce 'well' rather than 'sick' behaviors
- reward child's effort to use positive coping strategies and/or engage in normal daily activities (e.g. schoolwork, chores, activities with friends)
- set the bar low to ensure success and gradually increase expectations.

Coach parents to encourage increased focus on functioning (and model this behaviour during visits), for example:
- avoid asking the child about pain or other symptoms
- briefly acknowledge and redirect the child's attention when reports are made about bodily symptoms and sensations
- join in with the child when involved in appropriate activities
- encourage the parent to work with the child and school personnel on a graduated school re-entry plan (as needed)
- ask the school to reduce the volume of make-up work in a thoughtful way to preserve learning
- discuss other accommodations (e.g. bathroom access) that may be needed with school personnel
- commit to a small amount of time that the child will attend school daily regardless of symptoms
- gradually add time to the school day as tolerated
- use home study sparingly, as a support to catch-up prior to adding each class to the child's in-school schedule
- recommend family therapy (including Parent-Child Interaction Therapy, as appropriate) to provide ongoing support for parents enacting the behavioural coaching recommendations listed here.

Several brief questionnaires exist to aid in the assessment of parental behaviour in response to their child with an FGID. The Illness Behaviour Encouragement Scale (Walker and Zeman, 1992) is a 12-item parent self-report measure assessing provision of parental attention, special privileges and relief from normal responsibility during a child's abdominal pain episodes. A parallel child proxy-report form is also available. The Adult Responses to Childhood Symptoms (Van Slyke and Walker, 2006) is a 29-item parent self-report measure assessing parents' responses to their children's pain. The Adult Responses to Childhood Symptoms contains three subscales: (1) Parent Protectiveness, (2) Minimisation of Pain and (3) Encouraging and Monitoring Responses. Alternatively, much information can be gained from close observation of the interaction between a child and parent during evaluation and subsequent treatment visits. Important information can also be gained from including questions on the medical history that ask about the specific number of school days and other activities missed recently. This will more directly get at the issue of negative reinforcement, or parental willingness to release the child from his or her daily responsibilities in response to FGID symptoms, and determine whether specific intervention is needed to help parents return the child to school.

Parental beliefs

Parental behaviour often is underscored by a set of beliefs regarding the child's pain and other symptoms. Several studies of chronic pain conditions in childhood have found associations between parental beliefs and thoughts, parental behaviour and child disability. Parental belief that symptoms are 'real' and not being used for attention seeking has been found to differentiate between families seeking medical treatment and those who do not in response to a child's abdominal pain (Van Tilburg et al., 2009). Catastrophic thinking in parents has been associated with illness-related parenting stress, parental depression and anxiety, and the child's disability – including school attendance – beyond the child's reported pain intensity (Goubert et al., 2006). Parental worries about both physical and emotional or behavioural health have been positively associated with parents' use of behaviours known to promote pain behaviour and reinforce the sick role, including granting permission to stay home from school, allowing homework or regular chores to go uncompleted, and providing special privileges or extra attention to the adolescent (Guite et al., 2009). In terms of outcomes, parental worry about the child's physical health has also been positively associated with child disability (Guite et al., 2009). This finding is consistent with the fear-avoidance model, which asserts that fear of pain, or the belief that pain is harmful, is associated with fear and avoidance of physical activity, which can in turn lead to deconditioning and the maintenance of pain and disability (Waddell et al., 1993). Interestingly, current evidence suggests that children whose parents accept a biopsychosocial, as opposed to a purely biological or psychological, conceptualisation of abdominal pain and its treatment are more likely to experience symptom improvement and, thus, are less likely to experience long-term disability (Scholl and Allen, 2007).

Evaluation of parental beliefs may include both formal and informal assessment. The Pain Catastrophising Scale (Goubert *et al.*, 2006) is a questionnaire consisting of 13 items that describe different thoughts and feelings parents may have when their child is experiencing pain. Each item is rated on a 5-point scale (0 = 'not at all', 4 = 'extremely'). The Pain Catastrophising Scale yields three subscale scores: (1) Rumination, (2) Magnification and (3) Helplessness. The Worries and Beliefs about Abdominal Pain questionnaire (Van Tilburg *et al.*, 2009) is another alternative. The Worries and Beliefs about Abdominal Pain is a 31-item parent-report questionnaire comprised of four subscales that assess (1) the parental beliefs about the child's pain, (2) need for diagnosis and frustration with physician care, (3) difficulties in coping with the child's abdominal pain and (4) recognition of the role of stress and heredity on the child's symptoms. Paying close attention to the thoughts and beliefs informally espoused by parents about their child's FGID symptoms during evaluation and subsequent clinic visits (e.g. 'Are you sure we aren't missing something?') can help to supplement formal questionnaire data.

BOX 4.5 Parental beliefs

Assessment strategies

- Pain Catastrophising Scale
- Worries and Beliefs about Abdominal Pain
- Behavioural observation during evaluation and subsequent clinic visits

Parent-level interventions

- Educate parents regarding the biopsychosocial model and its application to FGIDs on an as-needed basis throughout treatment
- Ensure that all members of the child's treatment team (e.g. nursing, physical therapy, psychology, nutrition) clearly and consistently communicate a biopsychosocial conceptualisation
- Recommend that parents avoid dichotomising their child's pain and symptoms as *either* biological *or* psychological
- Assure parents that symptom flares likely are temporary and that paced, moderate activity is beneficial, not at all harmful, to their child

---

SOCIAL AND FAMILIAL RELATIONSHIPS

Ryan: what happened next?

After missing more than a week of school, Ryan starts to fall behind in his classes. His pile of makeup work grows taller on the kitchen table and he begins to feel overwhelmed and worried about not being able to catch up. Thinking about the work makes him feel worse. Feeling worse keeps him from working on the pile. Ryan's mother begins to think that staying home is not helping him and that he just needs to get back to school, but Ryan resists her encouragement each morning. Ryan's father, on the other hand, believes that Ryan's pain is 'real' and worries about the potential embarrassment Ryan might face with peers if he returns to school while continuing to have problems with loose bowel movements and nausea. He tells Ryan's mother that she just does not understand. In the meantime, Ryan's parents are watching him carefully for any signs of improvement or deterioration that might help them decide what direction to take. The whole family stays closer to home than usual. Most recently, Ryan's little sister even had to miss a friend's birthday party because Ryan's mother did not feel comfortable leaving him alone for the few hours it would require.

Naturally, just as children with FGIDs are affected by their families, so too are families affected by the chronic nature of a child's FGID. For example, it is reasonable to assume that problems with family functioning, parenting stress and conflicting views of the child's symptoms may be a logical outgrowth of a family system taxed by a high level of child symptoms and associated distress and impairment. In turn, these stressors may play a reciprocal role in further exacerbating and/or maintaining gastrointestinal symptoms (O'Malley *et al.*, 2011).

Family functioning

Paediatric chronic pain has been shown to have a deleterious effect on family functioning in a variety of ways. Mothers of adolescents with chronic pain, including those with abdominal pain, report restrictions in the social life of the family, as well as problems dealing with the stress of the adolescents' pain; further, greater pain intensity is associated with more problems in these areas (Hunfeld *et al.*, 2001). In turn, family conflict and enmeshment predict functional disability in children with chronic abdominal pain over and above reported pain intensity (Logan and Schraff, 2005). Siblings of children with FGIDs also have been found to report higher levels of emotional or behavioural symptoms than peers (Guite *et al.*, 2007). In sum, family dynamics appear to influence, and are influenced by, the functional status of the child with an FGID.

Given the potential negative and reciprocal impact of a child's FGID symptoms on family functioning, formal and/or informal assessment of overall family health and relationship dynamics is strongly encouraged. The Family

Environment Scale (Moos and Moos, 1986) is a 90-item parent self-report questionnaire that provides one formal option for measuring family functioning, particularly in the areas of interpersonal relationships, personal growth and family structure or organisation. Alternatively, the McMaster Family Assessment Device (Miller *et al.*, 1985) is slightly shorter, with 60 items assessing seven dimensions of family functioning: (1) problem-solving, (2) communication, (3) roles, (4) affective responsiveness, (5) affective involvement, (6) behavioural control and (7) general functioning. The McMaster Family Assessment Device has the advantage of established cut-offs that categorise families as demonstrating healthy versus unhealthy functioning. In addition to obtaining this broad look at family functioning, inserting specific questions into the medical history-taking to assess family restrictions on social activity secondary to the child's FGID can be helpful in identifying potentially important targets of treatment. Behavioural observations, including careful attention to language used in interaction among family members, also may provide insight into family dynamics during the evaluation and follow-up process.

BOX 4.6 Family functioning

Assessment strategies

- Family Environment Scale
- Family Assessment Device
- Include items in the medical history asking about restrictions on parent and sibling activities secondary to the patient's FGID
- Behavioural observations during evaluation and subsequent clinic visits

Family-level interventions

- Educate families about the ways that their relational patterns may influence child functioning and treatment outcomes
- Refer for traditional systems-based family therapy to address disruptions in family functioning, daily routines, relationships, and so forth
- Refer for individual evaluation of sibling(s) of FGID patients, as needed

---

Parenting and family stress

A seminal paper published in 1984 (Hodges *et al.*, 1984) compared stressful life events in a sample of children with recurrent abdominal pain against children with behaviour disorders and healthy children. Parents of the children identified the presence of certain life events, as well as the readjustment required and stress associated with the events. Children in the abdominal pain and behaviour disorders groups experienced significantly more critical life events and more stress associated with them than children in the healthy comparison group. The children in the abdominal pain and behaviour disorders groups differed in terms of the types of life events endorsed, with children in the former being more likely to have experienced illness, hospitalisation and death. The limitations of this study notwithstanding (e.g. correlational design, lack of use of current FGID symptom criteria), results suggest that children with chronic abdominal pain experience stress at a level likely greater than that of their well peers.

Several measures are available to assess parenting and family stress. Some evaluate stress in the context of a family struggling with a child's illness. Others are not specific to families with an ill child and, instead, focus on family stress more broadly. As an example of the former, the Pediatric Inventory for Parents (Streisand *et al.*, 2001) contains a list of 42 difficult events frequently faced by parents of children with a chronic illness. Parents are asked to rate, on a 5-point scale, the frequency of each event in the past 7 days, as well as the difficulty associated with it. Frequency and difficulty scores are summed for each of four domains – (1) communication, (2) emotional functioning, (3) medical care and (4) role function – with higher scores indicating greater frequency and difficulty. A more general measure of parenting stress, the Parenting Stress Index-Short Form (Abidin, 1990), assesses the quality of the parent–child relationship, as well as specific child (e.g. adaptability and mood) and parent (e.g. competence, isolation and health) characteristics, via 36 items rated on a 5-point scale. In contrast, the Social Readjustment Rating Scale (Holmes and Rahe, 1967) evaluates the occurrence and impact of stressful life events by asking individuals to identify which of 43 stressful life events they have encountered in the previous 12 months. Each of the events is assigned a number of 'life change units' to reflect the presumed magnitude of impact of the specific stressor; these are summed to produce a total Social Readjustment Rating Scale score. In addition to these standardised measures, it can be helpful to include questions in the medical history that ask about the parent or family's current level of stress, as well as the presence of past or upcoming stressful life events.

BOX 4.7 Parenting and family stress

Assessment strategies
- Pediatric Inventory for Parents
- Parenting Stress Index-Short Form
- Social Readjustment Rating Scale
- Include items in the medical history asking about past or recent occurrence of stressful life events

Family-level interventions
Refer for traditional systems-based family therapy to provide support and problem-solving related to parent and family stressors.

Symptom disagreement

To the extent that involved family members hold different beliefs and, thus, disagree about the causes and/or best practices for managing children's symptoms, the risk for family conflict and thereby stress is increased. This risk is further enhanced as attempts to manage symptoms fail and children become more and more disabled. Although there are no existing data that clearly address the relationship between family members' disagreement regarding symptoms and resulting family stress, the empirical literature has confirmed that lack of agreement, itself, among family members is not at all uncommon. One study evaluated the concordance between parental and child reports regarding pain intensity in a sample of paediatric patients with juvenile idiopathic arthritis. Results indicated that there was only a moderate level of agreement between parents and their children (Garcia-Munitis *et al.*, 2006). In another study of healthy children undergoing an ethical experimental pain assessment through the cold presser task, agreement between children and their mothers was classified as poor (Moon *et al.*, 2008). This phenomenon is less well studied for paediatric FGIDs; however, the existing data are comparable with those described earlier regarding agreement on general pain symptoms. Agreement between parents and children about irritable bowel symptoms, for example, has ranged from poor (or uncorrelated; Czyzewski *et al.*, 2011) to fair (Schurman *et al.*, 2005).

BOX 4.8 Symptom disagreement

Assessment strategies
- Straightforward numerical or visual analogue rating scales
- Abdominal Pain Index
- Questionnaire on Gastrointestinal Symptoms in Children and Adolescents

Family-level interventions
- Refer for traditional systems-based family therapy to provide education and communication training
- Recommend that caregivers (parents, grandparents, teachers, and so forth) discuss disagreements regarding symptoms and expectations in private, and present a unified front when in the child's presence

---

To help assess the frequency, intensity and duration of gastrointestinal symptoms, as well as to determine the extent to which there is agreement among family members regarding the prominence of these symptoms, providers often obtain some kind of pain or symptom rating. Straightforward numerical or visual analogue rating scales that are completed by parents and/or children and assess symptoms on a continuum of severity (e.g. from 1 to 10) are quite efficient. The Abdominal Pain Index (Walker *et al.*, 1997), another assessment methodology, is a five-item child self-report scale used to assess the frequency, duration and intensity of abdominal pain episodes occurring over the previous 2-week period. Similarly, the Questionnaire on Paediatric Gastrointestinal Symptoms (Walker *et al.*, 2000) contains items designed to measure the frequency (i.e. never to everyday) and duration (i.e. less than an hour to all day) of abdominal pain and associated symptoms occurring in a child during the past 2 weeks. Items are based on the paediatric Rome II diagnostic criteria for FGIDs (Rasquin-Weber *et al.*, 1999), and both a child self-report and a parent proxy-report are available.

SOCIAL AND ECONOMIC TRENDS

Ryan: what happened next?

Several months after the initial onset of his symptoms, Ryan continues to have abdominal pain, nausea and loose bowel movements. Over time, the cramping has actually gotten worse and Ryan occasionally vomits now as well. Ryan's mother and father have been sharing the burden of staying at home to care for Ryan, but now Ryan's mother is beginning to get pressure from her supervisor at work regarding the number of days she has been absent or requested to work from home recently. The family needs both incomes to keep up with their monthly bills, so one parent quitting or even cutting back to part-time is not an option. To further complicate matters, when Ryan's parents took him to the doctor for evaluation last month, they did not really understand the explanation they were given about his symptoms and left the office somewhat confused about how to proceed. At this point, they are unsure how to implement the recommendations given and where to turn for further help or advice.

Depending on the type and number of socio-economic barriers present, families' abilities to understand their child's condition and execute the recommended treatment plan can be significantly compromised. Certain social and economic issues can be particularly problematic, as they intersect with the requirements for treatment of the child's FGID, such as low education and/or health literacy; poor or absent health insurance, including prescription coverage; parental un- or underemployment; parental job inflexibility; inadequate housing; unreliable transportation; custody issues; and so forth. Although these factors have not been studied exclusively in FGIDs, insurance coverage, education and income have all been shown to influence individuals' abilities to effectively access quality healthcare in general and, in turn, to follow through on provider recommendations (Schwartz *et al.*, 2011). A Swedish study recently investigated the relationship between household socio-economic conditions and psychosomatic complaints in children aged 10–18 years (Ostberg *et al.*, 2006). Although FGIDs are not considered 'psychosomatic' conditions in the way these authors defined them, their findings are notable nonetheless. Economic stress in the household was associated with headache, recurrent abdominal pain and difficulties falling asleep. Children in single-parent families also reported significantly more symptoms than children in two-parent families. In contrast, there was no consistent relationship found between parental employment status or social class, determined by parental occupation, and children's symptoms.

The potential specific impact of the aforementioned factors on the treatment course of paediatric FGIDs cannot be understated. Without sufficient socio-economic resources and social support, key treatment plan components that could be especially difficult to enact include enforcing a set of structured daily activities to promote functioning, supporting good-quality sleep hygiene practices, regular monitoring of stools to avoid constipation and/or accessing appropriate school-related activities. It is quite reasonable to assume, for instance, that in a single-parent home where the custodial parent must work in order to provide for his or her family, it will be difficult for that parent to monitor the implementation of a daily schedule for a youngster with an FGID who has become quite disabled and is not attending school. Similarly, 'flexible' transportation to and from school, as would be required by a graduated school re-entry programme, would be extraordinarily difficult for a family without reliable personal transportation facilities. In such cases, providers will need to be adaptable and creative in their approaches to treatment recommendations.

The initial assessment of important potential socio-economic barriers to care easily can be done as part of the routine workup for a child presenting with an FGID. Questions may be posed in the form of a semi-structured interview as part of the medical history-taking or via a psychosocial screener developed for a specific provider's practice. Questions may be tailored based on the general socio-economic status of that provider's patient population and the resources available in the local community. However, as social and economic forces are dynamic, with family circumstances changing rapidly at times, assessment in this area will need to be ongoing. Regardless of the format for collecting this information, a clear understanding of the specific social and economic burdens currently affecting the family is needed to support adherence to the prescribed treatment plan and promote recovery of the child with an FGID.

SUMMARY

Family factors play an understudied yet unique, important and complex role in the aetiology and maintenance of paediatric FGIDs. Factors warranting consideration include a child's biological and genetic predisposition (both to FGIDs and to anxiety), environmental contingencies to which a child's illness-related behaviours are subject, social and family relationships and the socio-economic culture of a child's family. While these factors have been relatively neglected in the empirical literature, familiarity with them is critical for a paediatric provider caring for children with FGIDs and their families. A thorough assessment of potential familial contributions may help to define the biopsychosocial, as well as ecological, factors relevant to an individual child's symptoms. Ultimately, consideration of familial factors may help guide creation of a targeted and effective treatment plan that minimises family-based risk factors and enhances family strengths.

REFERENCES

Abidin R. *Parenting Stress Index.* Odessa, FL: Psychological Assessment Resources; 1990.

Brace MJ, Smith MS, McCauley E, *et al.* Family reinforcement of illness behavior: a comparison of adolescents with chronic fatigue syndrome, juvenile arthritis, and healthy controls. *J Dev Behav Pediatr.* 2000; **21**(5): 332–9.

Czyzewski DI, Lane MM, Weidler EM, *et al.* The interpretation of Rome III criteria and method of assessment affect the irritable bowel syndrome classification of children. *Ailment Pharmacol Ther.* 2011; **33**(3): 403–11.

Demirkan A, Penninx BW, Hek K, *et al.* Genetic risk profiles for depression and anxiety in adult and elderly cohorts. *Mol Psychiatry.* 2011; **16**(7): 773–83.

Di Lorenzo C, Colletti RB, Lehmann HP, *et al.* Chronic abdominal pain in children: a technical report of the American Academy of Pediatrics and the North American Society for Pediatric Gastroenterology, Hepatology, and Nutrition. *J Pediatr Gastroenterol Nutr.* 2005; **40**(3): 249–61.

Franić S, Middeldorp CM, Dolan CV, *et al.* Childhood and adolscent anxiety and depression: beyond heritability. *J Am Acad Child Adolesc Psychiatry.* 2010; **49**(8): 820–9.

Garcia-Munitis P, Bandeira M, Pistorio A, *et al.* Level of agreement between children, parents, and physicians in rating pain intensity in juvenile idiopathic arthritis. *Arthritis Rheum.* 2006; **55**(2): 177–83.

Goubert L, Eccleston C, Vervoort T, *et al.* Parental catastrophizing about their child's pain. The parent version of the Pain Catastrophizing Scale (PCS-P): a preliminary validation. *Pain.* 2006; **123**(3): 254–63.

Guite JW, Lobato DJ, Shalon L, *et al.* Pain, disability, and symptoms among siblings of children with functional abdominal pain. *J Dev Behav Pediatr.* 2007; **28**(1): 2–8.

Guite JW, Logan DE, McCue R, *et al.* Parental beliefs and worries regarding adolescent chronic pain. *Clin J Pain.* 2009; **25**(3): 223–32.

Hodges K, Kline JJ, Barbero G, *et al.* Life events occurring in families of children with recurrent abdominal pain. *J Psychosom Res.* 1984; **28**(3): 185–8.

Holmes TH, Rahe RH. The Social Readjustment Rating Scale. *J Psychosom Res.* 1967; **11**(2): 213–18.

Hunfeld JA, Perquin CW, Duivenvoorden HJ, *et al.* Chronic pain and its impact on quality of life in adolescents and their families. *J Pediatr Psychol.* 2001; **26**(3): 145–53.

Katiraei P, Bultron G. Need for a comprehensive medical approach to the neuro-immuno-gastroenterology of irritable bowel syndrome. *World J Gastroenterol.* 2011; **17**(23): 2791–800.

Kessler ED, Roberts MR, Schurman JV. *Parental Influences on Children's Chronic Abdominal Pain Experiences: exploring the relationship between parental protective behaviors and child quality of life.* Poster presented at the Midwest Regional Conference on Pediatric Psychology, Milwaukee, WI; April 2012.

Levy RL, Langer SL, Whitehead WE. Social learning contributions to the etiology and treatment of functional abdominal pain and inflammatory bowel disease in children and adults. *World J Gastroenterol.* 2007; **13**(17): 2397–403.

Logan DE, Schraff L. Relationships between family and parent characteristics and functional abilities in children with recurrent pain syndromes: an investigation of moderating effects on the pathway from pain to disability. *J Pediatr Psychol.* 2005; **30**(8): 698–707.

Markoutsaki T, Karantanos T, Gazouli M, *et al.* Serotonin transporter and G protein beta 3 subunit gene polymorphisms in Greeks with irritable bowel syndrome. *Dig Dis Sci.* 2011; **56**(11): 3276–80.

Middeldorp CM, Birley AJ, Cath DC, *et al.* Familial clustering of major depression and anxiety disorders in Australian and Dutch twins and siblings. *Twin Res Hum Genet.* 2005; **8**(6): 609–15.

Miller IW, Epstein NB, Bishop DS, *et al.* The McMaster Family Assessment Device: reliability and validity. *J Marital Fam Ther.* 1985; **11**(4): 345–56.

Moon EC, Chambers CT, Larochette AC, *et al.* Sex differences in parent and child pain ratings during an experimental child pain task. *Pain Res Manag.* 2008; **13**(3): 225–30.

Moos R, Moos B. *Family Environment Scale Manual.* 2nd ed. Palo Alto, CA: Consulting Psychologists Press; 1986.

Mujakovic S, ter Linde J, de Wit N, *et al.* Serotonin receptor 3A polymorphism c.-42C>T is associated with severe dyspepsia. *BMC Med Genet.* 2011; **12**: 140.

O'Malley D, Quigley EM, Dinan TG, *et al.* Do interactions between stress and immune responses lead to symptom exacerbations in irritable bowel syndrome? *Brain Behav Immun.* 2011; **25**(7): 1333–41.

Oshima T, Nakajima S, Yokoyama T, *et al.* The G-protein β3 subunit 825 TT genotype is associated with epigastric pain syndrome-like dyspepsia. *BMC Med Genet.* 2010; **11**: 13.

Ostberg V, Alfven G, Hjern A. Living conditions and psychosomatic complaints in Swedish schoolchildren. *Acta Paediatr.* 2006; **95**(8): 929–34.

Ramchandani PG, Stein A, Hotopf M, *et al.* Early parental and child predictors of recurrent abdominal pain at school age: results of a large population-based study. *J Am Acad Child Adolesc Psychiatry.* 2006; **45**(6): 729–36.

Rasquin-Weber A, Hyman PE, Cucchiara S, *et al.* Childhood functional gastrointestinal disorders. *Gut.* 1999; **45**(Suppl. 2): 60–8.

Saito YA. The role of genetics in IBS. *Gastroenterol Clin North Am.* 2011; **40**(1): 45–67.

Saito YA, Petersen GM, Larson JJ, *et al.* Familial aggregation of irritable bowel syndrome: a family case-control study. *Am J Gastroenterol.* 2010; **105**(4): 833–41.

Scholl J, Allen P. A primary care approach to functional abdominal pain. *Pediatr Nurs.* 2007; **33**(3): 247–59.

Schurman JV, Friesen CA, Danda CE, *et al.* Diagnosing functional abdominal pain with the Rome II criteria: parent, child, and clinician agreement. *J Pediatr Gastroenterol Nutr.* 2005; **41**(3): 291–5.

Schwartz L, Tuchman L, Hobbie W, *et al.* A socio-ecological model of readiness for transition to adult-oriented care for adolescents and young adults with chronic health conditions. *Child Care Health Dev.* 2011; **37**(6): 883–95.

Smedley B, Syme S. Promoting health: intervention strategies from social and behavioral research. *Am J Health Promot.* 2001; **15**(3): 149–66.

Streisand R, Braniecki S, Tercyak KP, *et al.* Kazak AE. Childhood illness-related parenting stress: the pediatric inventory for parents. *J Pediatr Psychol.* 2001; **26**(3): 155–62.

Thapar A, McGuffin P. Are anxiety symptoms in childhood heritable? *J Child Psychol Psychiatry.* 1995; **36**(3): 439–47.

Toyoshima F, Oshima T, Nakajima S, *et al.* Serotonin transporter gene polymorphism may be associated with functional dyspepsia in a Japanese population. *BMC Med Genet.* 2011; **12**: 88.

Van Slyke DA, Walker LS. Mothers' responses to children's pain. *Clin J Pain.* 2006; **22**(4): 387–91.

Van Tilburg MA, Chitkara DK, Palsson OS, *et al.* Parental worries and beliefs about abdominal pain. *J Pediatr Gastorenterol Nutr.* 2009; **48**(3): 311–17.

Waddell G, Newton M, Henderson I, *et al.* A fear-avoidance beliefs questionnaire (FABQ) and the role of fear-avoidance beliefs in chronic low back pain and disability. *Pain.* 1993; **52**(2): 157–68.

Walker LS, Caplan-Dover A, Rasquin-Weber A. *Manual for the Questionnaire on Pediatric Gastrointestinal Disorder.* Nashville, TN: Department of Pediatrics, Vanderbilt University School of Medicine; 2000.

Walker LS, Smith CA, Garber J, *et al.* Development and validation of the Pain Response Inventory for children. *Psychol Assessment.* 1997; **9**: 392–405.

Walker LS, Williams SE, Smith CA, *et al.* Parent attention versus distraction: impact on symptom complaints by children with and without chronic functional abdominal pain. *Pain.* 2006; **122**(1–2): 43–52.

Walker LS, Zeman JL. Parental response to child illness behavior. *J Pediatr Psychol.* 1992; **17**(1): 49–71.

Walker MM, Warwick A, Ung C, *et al.* The role of eosinophils and mast cells in intestinal functional disease. *Curr Gastroenterol Rep.* 2011; **13**(4): 323–30.

Whitehead WE, Busch CM, Heller BR, *et al.* Social learning influences on menstrual symptoms and illness behavior. *Health Psychol.* 1986; **5**(1): 13–23.

Whitehead WE, Crowell MD, Heller BR, *et al.* Modeling and reinforcement of the sick role during childhood predicts adult illness behavior. *Psychosom Med.* 1994; **56**(6): 541–50.

CHAPTER 5

Adherence, concordance, compliance and barriers to gastrointestinal treatments in children

Kevin A Hommel and Wendy N Gray

INTRODUCTION

Adherence, defined as 'the extent to which a person's behaviour coincides with medical or health advice' (Modi *et al.*, 2012), is a significant issue in paediatric chronic illness. Medical or health advice can refer to specific medications, medical procedures or overall health lifestyle habits (e.g. diet, exercise, avoiding alcohol consumption or tobacco use). While some recommendations are easily adhered to, others are much more difficult to follow because of financial limitations, time constraints or other barriers.

Overall, non-adherence to medical treatment is common, particularly among paediatric populations. Across all paediatric chronic conditions, non-adherence prevalence is estimated to be 50% (Rapoff, 2010) among children and 65%–88% in adolescents (Hommel *et al.*, 2009; Logan *et al.*, 2003; Rapoff and Barnard, 1991), with particularly high rates of non-adherence reported in paediatric inflammatory bowel disease (IBD) and liver transplant. For example, in IBD, non-adherence prevalence rates are as high as 88% (Hommel *et al.*, 2009). In liver transplant, non-adherence prevalence is as high as 76% (Fredericks *et al.*, 2008). These rates are alarming, given the severe and potentially irreversible consequences of non-adherence. In IBD, non-adherence is associated with increased disease severity (Greenley *et al.*, 2012; Reed-Knight *et al.*, 2010), poorer quality of life (Hommel *et al.*, 2008a), increased healthcare costs (Higgins *et al.*, 2009) and increased risk of disease recurrence (Kane *et al.*, 2003). In liver transplant, increased healthcare utilisation (e.g. frequency and duration of hospital stay) (Fredericks *et al.*, 2007), lower quality of life

(Fredericks *et al.*, 2007), treatment resistance, greater medical complications, graft rejection (Berquist *et al.*, 2006; Fredericks *et al.*, 2007; Molmenti *et al.*, 1999; Shemesh *et al.*, 2004), re-transplantation (Berquist *et al.*, 2006), and death have been reported. These severe outcomes may have been prevented with better adherence.

The current chapter reviews and summarises the literature on adherence in paediatric IBD and liver transplant. Following a discussion of factors that influence adherence in these populations, we will discuss strategies for identifying and addressing non-adherence, both in clinical practice and in the context of research trials. The chapter will conclude with a discussion of current challenges in adherence research and new directions.

FACTORS INFLUENCING ADHERENCE TO GASTROINTESTINAL TREATMENT

The extent to which a patient adheres to medical advice is influenced by numerous disease, individual and family factors. The following provides a brief summary of the existing literature on factors influencing adherence in paediatric IBD and liver transplant. Although similarities exist across paediatric conditions with regard to factors influencing adherence, there are unique differences between IBD and liver transplant, and the research literatures in each area have developed independently of each other. Therefore, for the purpose of clarity, each condition is discussed separately.

Inflammatory bowel disease
Disease and regimen-specific factors
Crohn's disease, ulcerative colitis and indeterminate colitis, collectively known as IBD, are characterised by unpredictable periods of gastrointestinal inflammation and symptom remission. Symptoms of IBD include diarrhoea, fatigue, delayed puberty, growth failure and abdominal pain. Although treatment varies by patient, IBD is primarily managed with oral medications (e.g. systemic corticosteroids, immunosuppressants, over-the-counter medications), dietary modifications, routine clinical appointments and, in some cases, surgery.

Adherence is generally best when treatment is time-limited, provides immediate benefit and is minimally burdensome (Osterberg and Blaschke, 2005; Rapoff, 2010; Riekert and Drotar, 2002). Unfortunately, few, if any, of these characteristics describe the IBD regimen. Lifelong adherence to a complex treatment regimen, often involving multiple medication doses per day, is required. Treatment fatigue is common, with newly diagnosed patients more adherent than those with a greater time since diagnosis (Reed-Knight *et al.*, 2010). Although patients are more likely to engage in health behaviours when they are associated with immediate benefits (Becker, 1974), the benefits of adhering to IBD treatment are not always apparent. Some medications must be taken for up to 16 weeks before demonstrating therapeutic effect (Verhave *et al.*, 1990) and the unpredictable waxing and waning course of IBD symptoms may make it difficult to observe a direct connection between adherence behaviour and general well-being. This may cause patients who do not see an immediate benefit to their adherence to erroneously conclude their medications are not working (Greenley *et al.*, 2010) and discontinue treatment. In addition, adherence may be lower for patients burdened by a higher number of medications or doses prescribed per day (Greenley *et al.*, 2010; Oliva-Hemker *et al.*, 2007), those whose treatment interferes with activities (Gray *et al.*, 2012; Ingerski *et al.*, 2010) and those experiencing the unpleasant and potentially embarrassing side effects (Ingerski *et al.*, 2010) associated with systemic corticosteroid and immunosuppressant medication (e.g. weight gain, acne, cushingoid appearance, immune suppression, inflammation, excess facial hair) (CCFA, 2009).

Individual and family factors

(For individual and family factors, *see* also Chapter 4.) Children and adolescents comprise 25% of IBD diagnoses and many patients with IBD are diagnosed during the adolescent years (mean age at diagnosis = 15 years) (Auvin *et al.*, 2005). This developmental period, characterised by rapid cognitive, emotional and physical development (Holmbeck, 2002), is known for high rates of non-adherence. Increases in academic, family and social demands during adolescence contribute to non-adherence. Commonly reported barriers to adherence, such as forgetting, interference with an activity and being away from home (Ingerski *et al.*, 2010), reflect the difficulties paediatric patients experience in incorporating their treatment regimen into their busy lives. Social concerns may also affect adherence. Patients may intentionally skip prescribed treatments to avoid teasing or feeling different from peers (Janicke *et al.*, 2009). Social concerns may be particularly salient when adhering to treatment causes embarrassing and socially stigmatising symptoms (e.g. weight gain, acne, facial hair). Poor emotional or behavioural functioning and coping may also affect adherence (Mackner and Crandall, 2005). Youth with IBD are at increased risk for anxiety and depression (Burke *et al.*, 1989; Szigethy *et al.*, 2004). These emotional difficulties may amplify pre-existing barriers to adherence (Gray *et al.*, 2012) and interfere with a patient's ability to access support from family and friends.

Families play a critical role in promoting adherence, with higher family functioning and more parent involvement predicting greater adherence (Mackner and Crandall 2005). However, as children grow into adolescence, responsibility for the treatment regimen is often transferred from parent to adolescent and parents become less involved in their child's day-to-day medication management (Greenley *et al.*, 2010). This can have significant ramifications on adherence, as adolescents often lack the self-management skills to manage their health independently. Thus, it is important for parents to continue to be involved in their child's care.

Liver transplant
Disease and regimen-specific factors
Numerous diagnoses can lead to end-stage liver disease and subsequent need for liver transplant (e.g. extrahepatic biliary atresia, hepatitis, metabolic disorder). Many patients awaiting a liver transplant look towards the procedure as a turning point from a life filled with anxiety and fears of death to one of prolonged life, renewed hope and freedom (Olausson *et al.*, 2006). While liver transplants provide patients with a second chance at life, the surgical procedure is not an end point or cure. Following transplant, patients must take multiple prescription (e.g. immunosuppressant) and over-the-counter medications, each with a different dosing schedule and number of pills. This may be an abrupt change from the pre-transplant regimen and the limited amount of time between notification of an available organ and actual transplantation provides little time for families to adjust to increased treatment demands. Not surprisingly, non-adherence is more prevalent following transplant.

By its nature, the post-transplant treatment regimen is designed to prevent symptom recurrence, rather than alleviate acute symptoms. In the absence of immediate observable benefits (i.e. symptom relief), patients may not recognise the value of remaining adherent, and adherence tends to decline the further a patient is removed from their date of transplant (Berquist *et al.*, 2008). Patients experiencing medication side effects may also be less adherent. Consequences of immunosuppressant medication include weight gain, depression, agitation, hirsutism and short stature (Griffin and Elkin, 2001). Certain side effects may be particularly troublesome for adolescent females (i.e. weight gain, hirsutism) or males (i.e. short stature) because of their social implications. When faced with such symptoms, patients may intentionally skip prescribed doses or only adhere to certain medications.

Individual and family factors
Several developmental factors affect adherence. As children age, they are more likely to be non-adherent to prescribed medications and clinic appointments (Fredericks *et al.*, 2010). Alarmingly, for every year of child age, the odds of non-adherence increase by 26% (Berquist *et al.*, 2008). This may be due to decreased parent involvement and the transfer of responsibility for the treatment regimen that naturally occurs as children age (Fredericks *et al.*, 2010). Transferring responsibility for the treatment regimen from the parent to the child or adolescent patient is challenging. For most families, the transfer of responsibility is an informal process and there is no explicit discussion about division of responsibility (Pai *et al.*, 2011). In liver transplant, this transfer begins in childhood. Findings from a recent study indicate that children as young as 9 years of age are primarily responsible for taking their medications and the average age at which parents transfer responsibility for the treatment regimen to the child is 12 (Shemesh *et al.*, 2004). This transition occurs at the beginning of a developmental period in which increased competing academic

and social demands already place adolescents at higher risk for non-adherence. Although the impact of emotional factors on adherence has been understudied, one study has linked depression with poorer adherence in children and adolescents with liver transplant (Maikranz *et al.*, 2007).

Family and environmental factors also affect adherence. Adherence is lower in children whose families exhibit lower cohesion and poorer problem-solving skills (Fredericks *et al.*, 2007). These factors may make it difficult for family members to work together to overcome barriers to adherence. Adherence is also lower for children whose parents report greater illness-related parenting stress and greater presence of post-traumatic stress disorder symptoms or psychopathology (Fredericks *et al.*, 2007; Shemesh *et al.*, 2000). Finally, adherence is lower in children from single-parent households and among those receiving public assistance or from low-socio-economic status backgrounds (Berquist *et al.*, 2008). These findings highlight the importance of the family system in maintaining adherence in children and adolescents with liver transplant.

IDENTIFYING AND ADDRESSING NON-ADHERENCE (PAEDIATRIC INFLAMMATORY BOWEL DISEASE AND LIVER TRANSPLANT)
Conceptualisation of adherence

Patients are often classified as either 'adherent' or 'non-adherent' based on predetermined but arbitrary cut-off values (e.g. 80%). This approach is becoming less popular because of several limitations. First, creating artificial dichotomies impedes comparison of results across studies, as the cut-off values used vary across studies. Second, dichotomising patients truncates the natural variability in adherence and results in the potential grouping of very dissimilar patients into the same category (i.e. patients demonstrating 0% and 79% adherence are both labelled 'non-adherent'). This has significant clinical implications, as the approach one might take for a patient who misses 20% of his or her doses because of organisational barriers differs significantly from the approach one might take when working with a patient who is completely non-adherent because of beliefs about treatment efficacy. Finally, the percentage of adherence that results in treatment efficacy varies across treatments; thus, applying an 80% cut-off point for two different medications to determine adherence can result in misclassification of adherence behaviour. Given these shortcomings, it is becoming common practice to treat adherence as a continuous variable with capped values ranging from 0% to 100%. In this system, patients can be completely non-adherent (0%) to perfectly adherent (100%). Those in between these numbers represent varying degrees of adherence or non-adherence. Although rarely discussed in the literature, some patients may be over 100% adherent. This overadherence is clinically relevant, as it can cause health concerns (e.g. overdosing, drug toxicity). Because adherence is defined as the extent to which a person's behaviour coincides with medical or health advice, and patients who take over 100% of their prescribed medications are not following medical advice, overmedicating is also considered a non-adherent behaviour.

TABLE 5.1 Overview of strengths and weaknesses of methods for assessing adherence

Method	Advantages	Disadvantages
Self-report or parent proxy report	Easy and inexpensive to obtain Can provide qualitative information to guide intervention	Overestimates adherence Subject to social desirability bias
Clinician estimate	Easy to obtain Clinician has intimate knowledge of patient's medical history	Unreliable Easily influenced by knowledge of patient's health status, patient or parent report of adherence or history of non-adherence
Direct observation	High accuracy Can confirm ingestion of medication	Resource-intensive Limited feasibility in research and clinical settings
Pill count	Reliable Inexpensive to obtain	May be cumbersome and time-consuming Can be positively or negatively manipulated
Pharmacy refill records	Accurate record of refill history Can be obtained for multiple medications	May be difficult to obtain because of privacy regulations May cost money to obtain Cannot confirm refilled medications were ingested
Bioassays	Measures concentration of medication in blood stream Can facilitate treatment decision-making	Costly Easily influenced by most recent medication-taking behaviour and pharmacokinetic factors Not available for all medications
Electronic monitoring	Reliable Can provide information on patterns of adherence to guide intervention	Costly May not be accepted by patients or families Equipment may fail or malfunction

Note: objective methods are shaded in grey.

It is important to recognise that adherence is not a static concept, but rather a constantly changing, multidimensional construct. Adherence can vary across situation (e.g. home vs. school), time (e.g. weekday vs. weekend), development (e.g. childhood vs. adolescence) and behaviour (e.g. oral medications vs. dietary recommendations). In IBD and liver transplant, where youth are prescribed multiple medications and instructed to adhere to different dietary and lifestyle habits, it is possible to obtain multiple calculations of adherence. Each numerical representation of adherence is specific to a particular medication, treatment or recommendation, and adherence behaviours can vary within the same individual (e.g. greater adherence to oral medications than dietary recommendations). Given the variable, multidimensional nature of adherence, it is not surprising that multiple methods exist for assessing adherence. Furthermore, there is no consensus on the best way to assess adherence. The following section provides an overview of the different methods of assessing adherence in paediatric populations. Strengths and weaknesses for each method are discussed in the context of the existing literature in IBD and liver transplant. For a brief overview, *see* Table 5.1. When considering an assessment method, clinicians and researchers should consider the strengths and weaknesses of each approach, and, if needed, consider using multiple assessment methods.

Subjective assessment strategies

Adherence assessment strategies are broadly categorised as subjective or objective. While either subjective or objective assessment categories can be used in clinical practice and research, the low cost and minimal burden of subjective methods make them particularly appealing in clinical settings. Subjective methods include patient self-report, parent proxy-report and clinician or provider estimates.

PATIENT AND PARENT REPORT

Self-report or parent proxy report of adherence is the most common method of assessing adherence and comes in many different forms (e.g. verbal report, questionnaires or diaries, and structured interviews). In addition to being easy and inexpensive to obtain, self-report and parent proxy report allow for the assessment of behaviours that more objective measures, such as pill count, are unable to assess, such as dietary recommendations. Self-report and parent proxy reports also allow patients to provide additional information regarding the challenges they've experienced adhering to their regimen, potentially guiding the delivery of targeted intervention.

Despite these benefits, there is significant concern regarding the validity of self-report and parent proxy report data. Patients or parents may be reluctant to disclose non-adherence because of social desirability bias or may not accurately recall episodes of non-adherence. As a result, self-report and parent proxy report generally overestimate adherence. For example, when self-report or parent proxy report of adherence is used, non-adherence prevalence rates in IBD are 10% for 6-MP/azathioprine and 2% for 5-aminosalicylates. However, when objective methods (e.g. pill counts) are used, non-adherence prevalence rates jump to 64% for 6-MP/azathioprine and 88% for 5-aminosalicylates (Hommel *et al.*, 2009). In a study with paediatric liver transplant patients, mean self-reported adherence was 97.5%. Using electronic monitors, however, mean adherence was estimated at 69.1% (Maikranz *et al.*, 2007). Furthermore, patient and parent report of adherence were not associated with any health outcome variable (i.e. number of biopsies and rejection episodes, number of hospital admissions or inpatient stays) (Shemesh *et al.*, 2004), limiting their clinical utility.

Although concerns exist regarding the validity of self-report or parent proxy report, recent efforts to improve the accuracy of this method hold promise. Normalising non-adherence, asking about non-adherence in a non-judgemental manner, and limiting the time frame in which patients and parents are asked to recall adherence information may yield more accurate self-report estimates (Mackner and Crandall, 2005). In addition, structured interviews, such as the Medication Adherence Measure (Zelikovsky and Schast, 2008), may yield more accurate self-reporting.

CLINICIAN ESTIMATE

Clinician estimate of adherence is another common method for assessing adherence. Clinicians are uniquely positioned to assess adherence, as they often have provided medical care for their patients over a long period of time and are intimately familiar with their medical history. Clinician estimates are easy to obtain and, compared with patient or parent report, may be less susceptible to social desirability (Hommel *et al.*, 2008b). However, there are significant concerns regarding the reliability and validity of provider estimates of adherence (La Greca and Bearman, 2003). They are generally poor at identifying non-adherence, underestimate adherence and are not associated with health outcome (Finney *et al.*, 1993; Shemesh *et al.*, 2004). The limited reliability of clinician estimates may be in part because clinician estimates are partially based on unreliable factors such as the patient's self-report, current health status and past history of non-adherence. As mentioned earlier, patients often under-report non-adherence. Health status is not a good proxy for adherence, as many factors (e.g. medication resistance, sub-therapeutic medication dosing, illness) may also affect a patient's overall health. Finally, clinician ratings may be influenced by their knowledge of the patient's past non-adherence. Because of the numerous shortcomings of clinician estimate of adherence, this method of adherence assessment is not commonly used in research studies involving patients with paediatric IBD or liver transplant.

Objective assessment strategies

Numerous methods for objectively assessing adherence have been reported in the paediatric IBD and liver transplant literature. Objective methods of assessing adherence include health status, direct observation, pill count, pharmacy refill records, bioassays and electronic monitoring. With the exception of direct observation and bioassays, these methods are considered *indirect* adherence estimators because they cannot confirm whether medication was actually ingested by the patient. With subjective measures, one should consider the strengths and weaknesses associated with each objective method prior to implementing adherence assessment in clinical practice or research.

HEALTH STATUS

Health status is often used as a proxy measure of adherence, as it is generally believed that patients who take their medications consistently are more likely to benefit from treatment and thus have better health and symptom control. While it is generally true that greater adherence is associated with better health status in paediatric IBD and liver transplant, this relationship is imperfect. Numerous factors can affect health status, such as the presence of co-morbid conditions, common illnesses and disease recurrence (Shemesh *et al.*, 2004). Furthermore, if patients have developed resistance to their medications, if they are undermedicated (i.e. insufficient dosing or pharmacokinetic and pharmacodynamic factors) or if their disease has progressed because of past non-adherence, health status may not reflect their current adherence behaviours.

DIRECT OBSERVATION

Direct observation of adherence involves the patient taking his or her medication in the presence of observers. This is typically done in a setting where the patient's actions can be highly monitored, such as an inpatient hospital or in the presence of a family member (e.g. parent). Advantages of this method include a high level of accuracy in adherence assessment and the ability to confirm that the patient ingests the medication. However, because of the resource-intensive nature of this assessment method (e.g. need for hospitalisation, presence of an observer), the feasibility of using this approach in clinical and research settings is limited (Hommel *et al.*, 2008b).

PILL COUNT

Pill counts generate an estimate of adherence by comparing the number of pills remaining and the number of pills expected to have been consumed over a set period of time. Pill counts are considered more accurate than self-report of adherence (Hommel *et al.*, 2009) and their low cost makes them appealing in both research and clinical practice (Hommel *et al.*, 2008b). These advantages notwithstanding, pill counts may be cumbersome and time-consuming, particularly if a patient has more than one prescribed medication. Also, pill counts can be positively or negatively manipulated as a result of combining old and new medication bottles or discarding medication. Because pill counts depend on patients remembering to bring their medication with them to appointments, missing data is also a possibility. Furthermore, in the absence of complementary data (i.e. pharmacy refill data), unusual pill count data (i.e. increasing rather than decreasing number of pills) may be difficult to interpret.

PHARMACY REFILL RECORDS

Rather than directly assessing medication consumption, pharmacy records assess *refill behaviours*. Inherent in the use of pharmacy refills as a proxy of adherence is the belief that the extent to which a patient refills medications on time corresponds to how well the patient takes his or her prescribed medications. While this relationship has been demonstrated in other chronic illness populations, there are currently no data examining the accuracy of pharmacy refill records in estimating adherence in paediatric IBD or liver transplant. Comparison of refill records with other adherence assessment methods (e.g. electronic monitoring, bioassays) is needed in these populations. Additionally, access to pharmacy refill data may be limited by privacy regulations, and some pharmacies may charge a fee prior to releasing refill records.

BIOASSAYS

Bioassays are considered to be a direct measure of adherence, as they measure the concentration of a particular medication in a person's body using a small sample of his or her blood. A benefit is that bioassay data can confirm ingestion of medication. Additionally, assay data may help with treatment decision-making. Providers may change medication dosing to ensure that assay values fall within a specific therapeutic range and patients are not over- or under-medicated. In spite of these benefits, bioassays have several limitations. While bioassays can confirm that medication has been ingested, it cannot confirm how much has been taken. In addition, bioassays are costly and not all medications have established therapeutic levels to assist with bioassay interpretation. Other factors, such as pharmacokinetic variations in drug absorption, metabolism and excretion (Lakatos, 2009) and white coat compliance (Cramer *et al.*, 1990) may also affect assay levels. As bioassays are highly influenced by the patient's most recent medication-taking behaviour, patients who are generally non-adherent but take their medication prior to an upcoming medical appointment (i.e. white coat compliance) will likely appear more adherent. With the exception of extreme cases of non-adherence, bioassays do not strongly correspond with objective measures of adherence (e.g. pill count) in IBD (Hommel *et al.*, 2009). In transplant, bioassays are used somewhat differently. Rather than relying on one assay value, several blood levels of a target medication (e.g. tacrolimus) are collected across time and the *variability* (i.e. standard deviation, or SD) in these blood levels is used. This approach better reflects how consistently a patient is taking his or her medication (Venkat *et al.*, 2008). Higher SD values suggest inconsistent adherence and patients whose SD of tacrolimus blood levels exceed established cut-off values (2.5–3.0 ng/mL) undergo more biopsies and are at greater risk for rejection episodes (Stuber *et al.*, 2008).

ELECTRONIC MONITORING

Numerous companies have marketed electronic monitors to measure adherence. (For a review of existing technologies, please see Ingerski *et al.*, 2011.) Although the manner in which an electronic monitor measures adherence varies by manufacturer, they generally work by comparing the patient's actual medication-taking behaviour (i.e. the time and date that a medication was removed from its container) and the prescribed regimen via recordings of container openings using a microchip embedded in the container. Information from the microchip is then downloaded onto a computer to obtain various adherence data. In addition to providing an overall estimate of adherence, electronic monitors can also provide information on patterns of adherence that would otherwise be unknown. This information may be helpful in identifying specific barriers to adherence (i.e. weekend doses missed most often) and aid in the subsequent delivery of targeted interventions. Because of the wealth of information provided by electronic monitors, it is not surprising that they are increasingly used in research. The advantages of electronic monitors, however, must be weighed against the weaknesses of these devices. High cost is a major barrier to their widespread use, and given that patients with IBD and liver transplant are often prescribed multiple medications, it may not be financially possible to measure all medications electronically. Furthermore, in order to track adherence, patients must be willing to transfer their medication into a specially designed container (i.e. medication bottle or pill box with an embedded microchip). These containers may be bulky and difficult to transport, they may interfere with current adherence routines and they may not accommodate all forms of medication (e.g. those in liquid form). Finally, electronic monitors may misestimate adherence because of malfunctioning equipment, user error or other unknown factors (Ingerski et al., 2011).

INTERVENTIONS TO IMPROVE ADHERENCE IN PAEDIATRIC IRRITABLE BOWEL DISEASE AND LIVER TRANSPLANT

It is important to intervene with patients who have been identified as non-adherent in order to avoid negative health consequences. Improving adherence in paediatric populations can be challenging and, as previously discussed, patients experience numerous barriers to adhering to their prescribed treatment regimen. Unfortunately, there are few published adherence promotion interventions in paediatric IBD and liver transplant. The following section provides a summary of the published research on interventions to improve adherence in these populations. Interventions are broadly grouped into clinic-based, multicomponent and technological interventions. Ongoing research is also summarised to illustrate current trends in adherence interventions.

Clinic-based

Clinic-based approaches involve the delivery of adherence interventions within the context of routine clinical care. Only one such intervention has been reported in the liver literature and no studies have been reported in IBD. Shemesh and colleagues (Shemesh et al., 2008) reported outcomes of 23 paediatric liver transplant patients following implementation of a clinic-based adherence intervention protocol. As part of this clinic-based approach, adherence was assessed at each appointment via three methods: (1) tacrolimus blood level, (2) SD of tacrolimus and (3) patient report of adherence. The intervention was applied any time a patient reported non-adherence or by examining tacrolimus blood levels. As part of the clinic-based adherence protocol, non-adherent patients participated in an intensified clinic visit schedule and received more frequent blood monitoring. They were also provided with feedback on their SD of tacrolimus blood levels and were educated on the importance of taking their medication. Finally, clinic staff analysed the family's current medication management plan and provided recommendations to improve their adherence. Key outcomes were measured and compared with clinic data collected prior to the implementation of the protocol. Following 2 years of implementation, the number of patients with high alanine aminotransferase levels (100 and above) decreased. Improvements in SD of tacrolimus and number of rejection episodes were also observed. Moreover, the intervention did not increase health system costs. Strengths of this clinic-based approach include long duration of follow-up (1 year) after implementation of the protocol, multi-method assessment of adherence and integration within the clinical setting. Limitations of the study include small sample size, lack of a control group and potential selection bias due to study inclusion criteria.

Multicomponent behavioural interventions

Multicomponent behavioural interventions focus on helping patients and their families develop the skills to successfully manage their health and overcome barriers to adherence. As their name implies, these interventions target multiple skills and behaviours that either support or hinder adherence. Three such interventions have been reported in the literature, all of which are in paediatric IBD.

Increasing dietary calcium intake in paediatric inflammatory bowel disease

Stark and colleagues conducted a randomised clinical trial to improve calcium intake in 32 children (aged 5–12 years) with IBD (Stark *et al.*, 2005). A three-session nutritional counselling intervention was compared with a six-session behavioural intervention (i.e. nutritional education, goal setting, child behaviour management, contingency management) and adherence to calcium was measured via parent-completed food diaries. Following the intervention, participants in the behavioural treatment demonstrated a greater mean increase in dietary calcium (M = 948 mg) than those in the nutritional counselling group (M = 274 mg). Additionally, 81% of those in the behavioural intervention achieved their recommended daily calcium intake, compared with 19% in the nutritional counselling group. Strengths of this study include a randomised clinical trial design and adaptation of a behavioural intervention with previously demonstrated efficacy (Stark *et al.*, 2006). Limitations include uneven number of contacts with the healthcare team across treatment groups, use of a subjective measure of adherence and potential selection bias (43% recruitment rate).

Individually tailored treatment of medication non-adherence in paediatric irritable bowel disease

Hommel and colleagues (Hommel *et al.*, 2011) reported findings from a randomised clinical trial comparing an individualised behavioural treatment and a wait-list control for 14 adolescents (aged 11–18) with IBD and their parents. Each adolescent in the behavioural condition and his or her parent met together with a study interventionist for four sessions focused on IBD education, behaviour modification principles, problem-solving skills, and family functioning and communication. Adherence was measured via pill count.

Following receipt of treatment, participants demonstrated an average increase in mesalamine adherence of 25%. Strengths of this study include use of an objective measure of adherence, randomisation to treatment, 0% attrition, and assessment of treatment feasibility and acceptability. Limitations include small sample size and lack of long-term follow-up.

Group-treatment of medication non–adherence in paediatric irritable bowel disease

In this randomised clinical trial, Hommel and colleagues (Hommel *et al.*, 2012) compared a group-based behavioural intervention to promote adherence and usual care. The participants were 40 adolescents (aged 11–18) with IBD and their parents. Adolescents and parents in the behavioural treatment met in separate but simultaneous groups three times, and once jointly. The behavioural condition emphasised IBD education, problem-solving skills to overcome barriers to adherence, behavioural contracting and principles of behaviour modification. In addition, a multi-method adherence assessment method was used (i.e. electronic monitoring caps, pill count and self-report). Although participants in the behavioural treatment reported significant improvements in mesalamine adherence, there were no differences in adherence according to electronic monitoring, pill count or caregiver report. Strengths of this study include larger sample size, multi-method adherence assessment, inclusion of a control group, randomisation to treatment and a 99% session attendance rate. As with all existing interventions in IBD, lack of diversity in participant socio-economic and ethnic background limits study generalisability. Additionally, the high baseline levels of adherence at pre-intervention may have limited the extent to which significant improvements in adherence could be detected.

Technological interventions

Technological interventions broadly include any work that utilises some form of technology (e.g. phone, video conferencing, Internet) to deliver an intervention to promote adherence. To date, only one intervention utilising technology has been published. Miloh and colleagues (2009) used text messaging to improve adherence and health outcomes in paediatric liver transplant recipients. Forty-one patients (aged 1–27 years) were enrolled in the study. For each participant, text message reminders were sent to the primary medication administrator (patient or parent). As part of the intervention, participants were required to respond to each text and indicate whether or not the medication was taken. These text responses were used as the measure of adherence. Significant improvements were seen in both adherence and health outcome following the intervention. On average, SD of tacrolimus and SD of sirolimus blood levels decreased post intervention and there was a significant decrease in the number of biopsy-proven rejection episodes (i.e. from 12 to 2). Higher rates of adherence were observed for participants who completed the study (69% adherence) than for those who dropped out (48% adherence). Strengths of this study include multi-method measurement of adherence (self-report, bioassays), use of a low-cost intervention and assessment of health outcome. Limitations include high attrition (58.5% completion rate), lack of a control group and selection bias. As only those who had text-capable cell phones were able to participate in the study, patients from lower socio-economic backgrounds may have been excluded.

Ongoing interventions

As of the date of this book's publication, there are several ongoing interventions utilising technology to improve adherence in paediatric IBD and liver transplant. Building upon prior work, Hommel and colleagues (2012) are currently testing three different adherence interventions among adolescents with IBD: (1) a small telehealth (i.e. web-based video conferencing) individualised behavioural intervention, (2) comparison of group-based behavioural intervention to a group intervention enhanced by individualised telehealth sessions and (3) a large-scale, multisite telehealth randomised controlled trial.[5] Also in IBD, Greenley and colleagues (2012) are collecting preliminary efficacy data of an adherence intervention delivered entirely via telephone.[6] In liver transplant, Fredericks is developing and testing an adherence intervention that is delivered entirely via text message and web-based modules.[7] These interventions represent the cutting edge of adherence research in IBD and liver transplant and will have a profound effect on the future delivery of care in these populations.

CHALLENGES IN ADHERENCE RESEARCH
Paediatric irritable bowel disease and liver transplant

Adherence research in paediatric IBD and liver transplant is a developing and rapidly changing field. Advances in medical treatment have made it possible for patients to achieve better disease management, improved quality of life and increased longevity. However, the extent to which patients benefit from treatment and achieve these outcomes depends in part on how well they adhere to treatment. Numerous challenges, including transition to adult care and the need to optimise interventions, disseminate findings and integrate comparative effectiveness and quality improvement (QI) research, must be considered in order to advance practice in this field.

Transition to adult care

As advances in medical treatment have led to increased patient longevity, we now find ourselves struggling with how to maintain adherence over time, particularly as patients transition from paediatric to adult care. Transition, defined as 'the purposeful, planned movement of adolescents and young adults with chronic physical conditions from child-centred to adult-oriented healthcare

---

5   K Hommel, personal communication.
6   R Greenley, personal communication.
7   E Fredericks, personal communication.

systems' (Blum *et al.*, 1993), is a critical issue affecting care in paediatric IBD and liver transplant. Although transition to adult care plays an essential role in ensuring patients receive developmentally appropriate care, transition is also associated with declines in medication adherence, clinic attendance and other important medical care (Pai and Ostendorf, 2011). Differences in expectations between paediatric and adult care settings (Escher, 2009) very likely contribute to the challenges patients experience. Adult care providers expect patients to be fully responsible for the management of their disease. However, in paediatrics, responsibility for the treatment regimen is often shared between parent and adolescent. Existing transition programmes, which are largely focused on *transfer* of care (e.g. the logistical aspects of moving to adult care, such as transferring medical records and identifying an adult provider), do not adequately prepare patients for adult care. Few, if any, are focused on the *process of transition* (e.g. gradually helping adolescent patients develop the skills necessary to effectively manage their health independently). These skills, collectively known as self-management, play a central role in successful transition to adult care and the lifelong management of IBD and liver transplant. It is essential that transition programmes place a greater emphasis on self-management. Although transition to adult care poses a significant challenge to adherence, if properly managed we can avoid negative outcomes and achieve optimal health management.

Optimising interventions

It has become increasingly important to demonstrate treatment efficacy and optimise interventions to ensure that patients receive only those components that have been empirically validated. This is a significant challenge to the field of adherence intervention as much of the published work in IBD and liver transplant is in its infancy. Only a few interventions have demonstrated preliminary efficacy and large-scale testing of these interventions is needed to replicate findings and demonstrate their generalisability to diverse populations. Moreover, as many of the published interventions have multiple components, it is difficult to isolate the active ingredients or mechanisms of change in such interventions. This prevents us from dismantling treatment components and only offering the most effective interventions.

Although additional research on adherence interventions in paediatric IBD and liver transplant is generally needed, there is a particular need for interventions to expand their focus on oral medications to include adherence to other important aspects of the treatment regimen (e.g. dietary adherence, tube-feedings, exercise). Despite suboptimal rates of adherence to oral medications, there is evidence to suggest that adherence to other aspects of treatment, such as those already mentioned, is even lower (Rapoff, 2010). Unfortunately, many of the adherence assessment strategies discussed in this chapter are tailored to oral medications, making assessment of adherence to other treatment recommendations challenging. Self-report methods (e.g. exercise diaries and 24-hour diet recall) may be used in such cases. However, their validity and reliability in IBD and transplant is unknown. It is important that we overcome the challenge of measuring adherence to other aspects of treatment, as these treatment components also contribute to promoting the overall health of youth with IBD and liver transplant.

Another challenge in the optimisation of adherence interventions is our ability to deliver services in a minimally burdensome way and target those families in greatest need of intervention. As many interventions require families to make additional trips to a treatment facility, it is likely that only those who have the time and material resources to meet these demands are receiving treatment. At our treatment facility located in a major metropolitan area, 52% of those approached to participate in our adherence intervention studies live more than 32 km from the hospital (M = 49.76 km; Range = 1.61–500.51 km) and 45% live over a half-hour drive away. Inability to commit to the time or travel required for adherence interventions is a primary reason for study refusal. As a result, many families are not receiving needed services. In order to reach underserved families, researchers and clinicians must overcome the challenges posed by such barriers and adapt treatments to ensure they are acceptable and feasible for families. Delivery of interventions via telehealth may enable a larger number of patients to receive treatment and, as previously mentioned, several interventions utilising telehealth and other technology are currently under way in IBD[8,9] and liver transplant.[10]

Comparative effectiveness research and quality improvement

Treatments that have been developed in a research setting need to be compared in clinical samples via comparative effectiveness research. Establishing treatment efficacy is an important but not a final step in improving adherence to paediatric IBD and liver transplant regimens. It is critical that efficacious treatments be tested in clinical practice to determine their generalisability. Unfortunately, few interventions that have been determined as efficacious in research have been successfully translated into real-world settings (Glasgow *et al.*, 2004). This is because certain characteristics of efficacy trials are not reflective of real-world practice. Efficacy trials generally have homogeneous and highly motivated participants without significant co-morbidities. They usually have secured funding and a highly trained and dedicated research team deliver the treatment. In contrast, patients in real-world settings are often heterogeneous, with varying levels of motivation and other comorbidities. Funding for such programmes may be questionable or unavailable and staff delivering the intervention may have varying skill sets and other demands on their time. Although numerous models for bridging the gap between efficacy trials to real-world practice have been proposed to overcome barriers to the translation and dissemination of research trials (Glasgow *et al.*, 2004; Klesges *et al.*, 2005;

---

8   K Hommel, personal communication.
9   R Greenley, personal communication.
10 E Fredericks, personal communication.

Nathan *et al.*, 2000), we have yet to apply these models to improve adherence in paediatric IBD and liver transplant because of the nascence of the field.

QI methods may facilitate the transition of efficacy trials to clinical practice. QI in healthcare is focused on improving processes and procedures to result in better health outcomes and higher satisfaction (Plsek, 1999). By applying QI models and methods, clinicians can optimise and tailor the most effective interventions to their unique clinical context. This is particularly helpful in settings where limited resources and provider expertise mean it would be difficult to implement an intervention as it was originally designed in a research setting.

Dissemination and implementation of research findings

Interventions proven effective in clinical settings must be disseminated to and implemented in other patient populations and clinics in order to have widespread impact. Interventions in IBD and liver transplant are in the beginning stages of development and efficacy testing. However, in order to move the literature forwards and improve adherence and health outcomes in these populations, researchers and clinicians must work collaboratively to design, test, implement and disseminate findings. Given the small number of patients with IBD or liver transplant at any given treatment facility, multisite collaborations that harness the collective expertise of researchers and health providers throughout the world will likely become more common. Although improving adherence in IBD and liver transplant is a challenging task, the promise of better disease control, quality of life and patient longevity warrant continued dedication to this area.

REFERENCES

Auvin S, Molinie F, Gower-Rousseau C, *et al.* Incidence, clinical presentation and location at diagnosis of pediatric inflammatory bowel disease: a prospective population-based study in northern France (1988–1999). *J Pediatr Gastroenterol Nutr.* 2005; **41**(1): 49–55.

Becker MH. The health belief model and personal health behavior. *Health Educ Monogr.* 1974; **2**: 324–508.

Berquist RK, Berquist WE, Esquivel CO, *et al.* Adolescent non-adherence: prevalence and consequences in liver transplant recipients. *Pediatr Transplant.* 2006; **10**(3): 304–10.

Berquist RK, Berquist WE, Esquivel CO, *et al.* Non-adherence to post-transplant care: prevalence, risk factors and outcomes in adolescent liver transplant recipients. *Pediatr Transplant.* 2008; **12**(2): 194–200.

Blum RW, Garell D, Hodgman CH, *et al.* Transition from child-centered to adult healthcare systems for adolescents with chronic conditions. A position paper of the Society for Adolescent Medicine. *J Adolesc Health.* 1993; **14**(7): 570–6.

Burke P, Meyer V, Kocoshis S, *et al.* Depression and anxiety in pediatric inflammatory bowel disease and cystic fibrosis. *J Am Acad Child Adolesc Psychiatry.* 1989; **28**(6): 948–51.

Cramer JA, Scheyer RD, Mattson RH. Compliance declines between clinic visits. *Arch Intern Med.* 1990; **150**(7): 1509–10.

Crohn's and Colitis Foundation of America (CCFA). *Treating Children and Adolescents.* New York, NY: CCFA; 2009. Available at: www.ccfa.org/info/treatment/kidsmeds (accessed 6 April 2009).

Escher JC. Transition from pediatric to adult health care in inflammatory bowel disease. *Dig Dis.* 2009; **27**(3): 382–6.

Finney JW, Hook RJ, Friman PC, *et al.* The overestimation of adherence to pediatric medical regimens. *Child Health Care.* 1993; **22**(4): 297–304.

Fredericks EM, Dore-Stites D, Well A, *et al.* Assessment of transition readiness skills and adherence in pediatric liver transplant recipients. *Pediatr Transplant.* 2010; **14**(8): 944–53.

Fredericks EM, Lopez MJ, Magee JC, *et al.* Psychological functioning, nonadherence and health outcomes after pediatric liver transplantation. *Am J Transplant.* 2007; **7**(8): 1974–83.

Fredericks EM, Magee JC, Opipari-Arrigan L, *et al.* Adherence and health-related quality of life in adolescent liver transplant recipients. *Pediatr Transplant.* 2008; **12**(3): 289–99.

Glasgow RE, Goldstein MG, Ockene JK, *et al.* Translating what we have learned into practice: principles and hypotheses for interventions addressing multiple behaviours in primary care. *Am J Prev Med.* 2004; **27**(2 Suppl.): 88–101.

Gray WN, Denson LA, Baldassano RN, *et al.* Treatment adherence in adolescents with inflammatory bowel disease: the collective impact of barriers to adherence and anxiety/depressive symptoms. *J Pediatr Pscyhol.* 2012; **37**(3): 282–91.

Greenley RN, Stephens M, Doughty A, *et al.* Barriers to adherence among adolescents with inflammatory bowel disease. *Inflamm Bowel Dis.* 2010; **16**(1): 36–41.

Greenley RN, Kunz JH, Biank V, *et al.* Identifying youth nonadherence in clinical settings: data-based recommendations for children and adolescents with inflammatory bowel disease. *Inflamm Bowel Dis.* 2012; **18**(7): 1254–9.

Griffin KJ, Elkin TD. Non-adherence in pediatric transplantation: a review of the existing literature. *Pediatr Transplant.* 2001; **5**(4): 246–9.

Higgins PDR, Rubin DT, Kaulback K, *et al.* Systematic review: impact of non-adherence to 5-aminosalyciclic acid products on the frequency and costs of ulcerative colitis flares. *Aliment Pharmacol Ther.* 2009; **29**(3): 247–57.

Holmbeck GN. A developmental perspective on adolescent health and illness: an introduction to the special issues. *J Pediatr Psychol.* 2002; **27**(5): 409–16.

Hommel KA, Davis CM, Baldassano RN. Medication adherence and quality of life in pediatric inflammatory bowel disease. *J Pediatr Psychol.* 2008a; **33**(8): 867–74.

Hommel KA, Davis CM, Baldassano RN. Objective versus subjective assessment of oral medication adherence in pediatric inflammatory bowel disease. *Inflamm Bowel Dis.* 2009; **15**(4): 589–93.

Hommel KA, Hente EA, Odell S, *et al.* Evaluation of a group-based behavioural intervention to promote adherence in adolescents with inflammatory bowel disease. *Eur J Gastroenterol Hepatol.* 2012; **24**(1): 64–9.

Hommel KA, Herzer M, Ingerski LM, *et al.* Individually tailored treatment of medication nonadherence. *J Pediatr Gastroenterol Nutr.* 2011; **53**(4): 435–9.

Hommel KA, Mackner LM, Denson LA, *et al.* Treatment regimen adherence in pediatric gastroenterology. *J Pediatr Gastroeneterol Nutr.* 2008b; **47**(5): 526–43.

Ingerski LM, Baldassano RN, Denson LA, *et al.* Barriers to oral medication adherence for adolescents with inflammatory bowel disease. *J Pediatr Psychol.* 2010; **35**(6): 683–91.

Ingerski LM, Hente EA, Modi A, *et al.* Electronic measurement of medication adherence in pediatric chronic illness: a review of measures. *J Pediatr.* 2011; **159**(4): 528–34.

Janicke DM, Gray WN, Kahhan NA, *et al.* Brief report: the association between peer victimization, prosocial support, and treatment adherence in children and adolescents with inflammatory bowel disease. *J Pediatr Psychol.* 2009; **34**(7): 769–73.

Kane S, Huo D, Aikens J, *et al.* Medication nonadherence and the outcomes of patients with quiescent ulcerative colitis. *Am J Med.* 2003; **114**(1): 39–43.

Klesges LM, Estabrooks PA, Dzewaltowski DA, *et al.* Beginning with the application in mind: designing and planning health behavior change intervention to enhance dissemination. *Ann Behav Med.* 2005; **29**(2): 66–75.

La Greca AM, Bearman KJ. Adherence to prescribed medical regimens. In: Roberts MC, editor. *Handbook of Pediatric Psychology.* New York, NY: Guilford Press; 2003. pp. 119–40.

Lakatos PL. Prevalence, predictors and clinical consequences of medical adherence in IBD. How to improve it? *World J Gastroenterol.* 2009; **15**(34): 4234–9.

Logan D, Zelikovsky N, Labay L, *et al.* The Illness Management Survey: identifying adolescents' perceptions of barriers to adherence. *J Pediatr Psycho.* 2003; **28**(6): 383–92.

Mackner LM, Crandall WV. Oral medication adherence in pediatric inflammatory bowel disease. *Inflamm Bowel Dis.* 2005; **11**(11): 1006–12.

Maikranz JM, Steele RG, Dreyer ML, *et al.* The relationship of hope and illness-related uncertainty to emotional adjustment and adherence among pediatric renal and liver transplant recipients. *J Pediatr Psychol.* 2007; **32**(5): 571–81.

Miloh T, Annunziato R, Arnon R, *et al.* Improved adherence and outcomes for pediatric liver transplant recipients by using text messaging. *Pediatrics.* 2009; **124**(5): e844–50.

Modi AC, Pai AL, Hommel KA, *et al.* Pediatric self-management: a framework for research, practice, and policy. *Pediatrics.* 2012; **129**(2): e473–85.

Molmenti E, Mazariegos G, Bueno J, *et al.* Noncompliance after pediatric liver transplantation. *Transplant Proc.* 1999; **31**(1–2): 408.

Nathan PE, Stuart SP, Dolan SL. Research on psychotherapy efficacy and effectiveness: between Scylla and Charybdis? *Psychol Bull.* 2000; **126**(6): 964–81.

Olausson B, Utbult Y, Hansson S, *et al.* Transplanted children's experiences of daily living: children's narratives about their lives following transplantation. *Pediatr Transplant.* 2006; **10**(5): 575–85.

Oliva-Hemker MM, Abadom V, Cuffari C, *et al.* Nonadherence with thiopurine immunomodulator and mesalamine medications in children with Crohn disease. *J Pediatr Gastroenterol Nutr.* 2007; **44**(2): 180–4.

Osterberg L, Blaschke T. Adherence to medication. *N Engl J Med.* 2005; **353**(5): 487–97.

Pai ALH, Ingerski LM, Perazzo L, *et al.* Preparing for transition? The allocation of oral medication regimen tasks in adolescents with renal transplants. *Pediatr Transplant.* 2011; **15**(1): 9–16.

Pai ALH, Ostendorf HM. Treatment adherence in adolescents and young adults affected by chronic illness during the health care transition from pediatric to adult health care: a literature review. *Childrens Health Care.* 2011; **40**(1): 16–33.

Plsek PE. Quality improvement methods in clinical medicine. *Pediatrics.* 1999; **103**(1 Suppl. E): 203–14.

Rapoff MA. *Adherence to Pediatric Medical Regimens.* New York, NY: Springer; 2010.

Rapoff MA, Barnard MU. Compliance with pediatric medical regimens. In: Cramer JA, Spilker B, editors. *Patient Compliance in Medical Practice and Clinical Trials.* New York, NY: Raven Press; 1991. pp. 73–98.

Reed-Knight B, Lewis JD, Blount RL. Association of disease, adolescent, and family factors with medication adherence in pediatric inflammatory bowel disease. *J Pediatr Psychol.* 2010; **36**(3): 308–17.

Riekert KA, Drotar D. The beliefs about medication scale: development, reliability and validity. *J Clin Psychol Med Settings.* 2002; **9**(2): 177–84.

Shemesh E, Annunziato RA, Shneider BL, *et al.* Improving adherence to medications in pediatric liver transplant recipients. *Pediatr Transplant.* 2008; **12**(3): 316–23.

Shemesh E, Lurie S, Stuber ML, *et al.* A pilot study of posttraumatic stress and nonadherence in pediatric liver transplant recipients. *Pediatrics.* 2000; **105**(2): E29.

Shemesh E, Shneider BL, Savitzky JK, *et al.* Medication adherence in pediatric and adolescent liver transplant recipients. *Pediatrics.* 2004; **113**(4): 825–32.

Stark LJ, Davis AM, Janicke DM, *et al.* A randomized clinical trial of dietary calcium to improve bone accretion in children with juvenile rheumatoid arthritis. *J Pediatr.* 2006; **148**(4): 501–7.

Stark LJ, Hommel KA, Mackner LM, *et al.* Randomized trial comparing two methods of increasing dietary calcium intake in children with inflammatory bowel disease. *J Pediatr Gastroenterol Nutr.* 2005; **40**(4): 501–7.

Stuber ML, Shemesh E, Seacord D, *et al.* Evaluating non-adherence to immunosuppressant medications in paediatric liver transplant recipients. *Pediatr Transplant.* 2008; **12**(3): 284–8.

Szigethy E, Levy-Warren A, Whitton S, *et al.* Depressive symptoms and inflammatory bowel disease in children and adolescents: a cross-sectional study. *J Pediatr Gastroeneterol Nutr.* 2004; **39**(4): 395–403.

Venkat VL, Nick TG, Wang Y, *et al.* An objective measure to identify pediatric liver transplant recipients at risk for late allograft rejection related to non-adherence. *Pediatr Transplant.* 2008; **12**(1): 67–72.

Verhave M, Winter HS, Grand RJ. Azathiorpine in the treatment of children with inflammatory bowel disease. *J Pediatr.* 1990; **117**(5): 809–14.

Zelikovsky N, Schast AP. Eliciting accurate reports of adherence in a clinical interview: development of the medical adherence measure. *Pediatr Nurs.* 2008; **34**(2): 141–6.

CHAPTER 6

Young people with gastrointestinal conditions on home parenteral nutrition and their transition to adult services

Sue Protheroe

INTRODUCTION

Developments in home care have transformed the management of chronic illnesses so that children with a continuing need for parenteral nutrition (PN) as treatment for intestinal failure are discharged home and survive through adolescence into adulthood. Children receiving PN for primary digestive disorders – for example, short bowel syndrome and Crohn's disease – expect a better probability of survival and weaning off PN than adults on PN and benefit from early home discharge on home PN.

Although PN is a life-saving intervention, it is time-consuming therapy that requires technical competencies and adherence to daily routines (*see* also Chapter 13). Home PN is cost-effective and reduces the risks of infection compared with hospital PN; home PN also encourages normal development and participation in family activities. Having a child at home on home PN places an immense responsibility on families and is associated with physical and psychological stresses. High-quality, well-planned transition from hospital to home for children and young people with complex health needs is an important part of enabling children and their families to enjoy as good a quality of life as possible. This involves not only addressing the child's physical needs but also the multidisciplinary team must identify social, emotional, spiritual and education needs of the whole family, helping families to achieve a life that allows educational and work achievements, participation in social activities and a sense of belonging and self-worth. Arranging transition for young people on home PN to the adult health sector is one of the greatest challenges for health services that care for young people. Both areas of transition to home care and to the adult health services are multidimensional processes covering psychosocial, educational and vocational aspects and are key quality issues for health services.

CONDITIONS REQUIRING HOME PARENTERAL NUTRITION

Intestinal failure is diagnosed when intestinal function becomes insufficient to allow adequate absorption of fluid, electrolyte or nutrient requirements (Puntis, 1995). Home PN is instituted when intestinal failure is expected to last for 3 months or more resulting from a variety of different gastrointestinal diseases. Short bowel syndrome is the most common reason for intestinal failure. Short bowel syndrome is acquired as a result of extensive bowel resection, usually in the neonatal period, but it may be due to Crohn's disease in children. Permanent intestinal failure may result from inherited conditions diagnosed in the neonatal period, which include:

- severe motility disorders such as chronic intestinal pseudo-obstruction where children have recurrent symptoms suggesting bowel obstructions in the absence of an obstructing lesion or long-segment Hirschsprung's disease
- congenital enteropathies, such as microvillus inclusion disease and tufting enteropathy.

The ability to successfully wean from home PN is greater in those with short bowel syndrome or Crohn's disease. Approximately 75% of these children would be expected to wean off PN, but this may take many years.

Home PN is a safe treatment with high probability of long-term patient survival; however, patients may have an increased risk of death because of factors related to home PN or the underlying disease. There is a risk of catheter-related blood stream infection when strict aseptic techniques are not adhered to. Recurrent infections with late presentation are a risk factor for intestinal failure–associated liver disease.

How common is home parenteral nutrition in children and young people?

The point prevalence of paediatric home PN is estimated to be 13.7 patients per million in 2011, a fourfold increase since 1993. Short bowel syndrome accounted for 63% of cases (Beath *et al.*, 2011). It is estimated that in the United Kingdom up to 30 adolescents on home PN are poised to transfer to adult services over the next 5 years (BANS, 2007). Many of these adolescents will have been dependent on PN since early infancy. Of this cohort, 40% have short bowel syndrome secondary to neonatal causes, 30% have congenital enteropathy and a smaller number (15%) have severe motility problems.

'ADOLESCENT MEDICINE' AND TRANSITION TO ADULT SERVICES

Adolescence includes young people aged 10–20 years (UNICEF, 2011) and the Department of Health recognises that health services for young people cover those individuals aged 16–19 years (Department of Health, 2009). Young people are new users of health services and have specific requirements. Provision of confidential healthcare that allows engagement with young people and promotes disease self-management behaviour (e.g. central venous line care) and successful engagement with the new home PN team is pivotal (Johnson and Sexton, 2006).

Screening for health risk behaviours (mental health, diet, exercise, cardiovascular risk and smoking) is as important in adolescents on home PN as in other young people in the population (Sawyer and Aroni, 2005). Opportunities exist for health promotion, disease knowledge and prevention (e.g. osteoporosis). There is growing evidence that skills training for young people with chronic illness can be associated with positive outcomes (e.g. improved information seeking, social competence and behaviour), which can maximise functioning and potential (McDonagh *et al.*, 2006a; Viner, 2008). There have been several reports of increased unemployment in young adults that is not always related to their disability or educational achievement. Young adult clinics or wards covering those aged 18–24 years may help an adolescent's complete transition, are associated with improved quality of care and may cost no more to implement than an ad hoc approach (Kennedy and Sawyer, 2008; Rosen *et al.*, 2003).

PSYCHOSOCIAL SEQUEL OF CHRONIC INTESTINAL FAILURE AND LONG-TERM HOME PARENTERAL NUTRITION

Costs to the family

The carers of the patient who is discharged home on PN have to provide care of a highly technical and intensive nature that in the past would have been the domain of professionals. Repeat hospitalisation for complications has a serious impact on quality of life for the children and their families and on healthcare costs. Home PN poses significant safety challenges and requires coordination of care between several healthcare disciplines within and outside hospital.

We assume that 'being home is good' but there are challenges in achieving ordinary lives, and home PN is not the same as 'hospital at home'. Parents struggle with the emotional strain and physical tiredness from the burden of care (Holden, 2001). While the majority of parents successfully provide long-term care at home with excellent outcomes, over prolonged periods, with competing demands, strict adherence to routines may break down. Recurrent catheter-related blood stream infections have been attributed to fabricated or induced illness, which resolved with a change of carer (Frederick *et al.*, 1990; Wu *et al.*, 2006).

The British Artificial Nutrition Survey collected questionnaire data from families of 81 children receiving home PN between 1996 and 1999. Most of the burden of care fell on the families, as many of the children were under the age of 1 year and time spent in hospital was less than 2%. Sleep disturbance was common, with deterioration in their family life, poor social life activities and reduced quality of life. Ethnicity, family structure, coping strategies, educational ability, housing and geographical location varied between families.

Sexton *et al.* (2005) explored the needs of families and their views about nursing home care packages. Families felt that nursing their child at home was a major advantage but three themes that families face emerged: (1) physical burden, (2) psychosocial and emotional stress due to social isolation in light of their child's medical needs and (3) feelings of guilt and financial burden because of job loss.

Physical burden

Parents struggled with the emotional strain, physical tiredness and the burden of care, living with the threat of complications. Children may need gastrostomy feeding, ileostomy care, administration of medications, management of vomiting, frequent stool output or urinary bladder catheterisation, and the overall care of the child may take several hours per day with disturbance overnight responding to infusion pump alarms. In addition to the overall care of the child, parent–child conflict or sibling rivalry may be observed.

Psychosocial and emotional stress due to social isolation in light of their child's medical needs

Neither the extended family nor the medical system can support families' respite needs, since arranging for baby-sitting is virtually impossible. Respite by community hospices is generally designed for children with life-limiting conditions and may not be able to support these families' respite needs. Parents have difficulties in taking holidays and admit to feeling frustrated, annoyed, stressed and having problems sleeping. Tensions arise between 'parenting and nursing' (Kirk *et al.*, 2005).

Feelings of guilt and financial burden because of job loss

A national multicentre study of 72 patients, 67 fathers and 69 mothers showed that quality of life was significantly impaired in parents, especially in mothers, who showed lower levels of satisfaction than did fathers for items related to work, inner life and freedom (Gottrand *et al.*, 2005). A further study showed that 7 out of 11 families exceeded the threshold for psychiatric morbidity measured by the General Health Questionnaire (Wong *et al.*, 2000). In contrast, a high level of family functioning was seen in a UK study (Emedo *et al.*, 2010), which is encouraging, as is associated with good psychosocial outcome and emotional well-being in children with chronic illness (Michaud *et al.*, 2004).

Other factors

WHEN CARE AT HOME MAY BREAK DOWN IN CHILDREN ON HOME PARENTERAL NUTRITION: FABRICATED OR INDUCED ILLNESS?

Concerns of suspected fabricated or induced illness have been previously reported in children on home PN when recurrent central venous access line infections have occurred more commonly than would have been expected (Frederick *et al.*, 1990; Menahem and Halasz, 2000). It is difficult to prove if complications were caused intentionally, but they seem likely to have arisen because of lack of adherence to routines by parents. When the infant was placed with foster parents, the complications were reversible with a change of carer (Wu *et al.*, 2006). Parents may not be able to meet their child's physical needs if they are unable to cope emotionally with the stresses surrounding long-term home treatment and may find it difficult to admit feeling under stress through fear, or guilt or from losing the child (Menahem and Halasz, 2000). At times, the burden of responsibility in addition to other family pressures may result in inability to maintain complex care routines, despite the technical competence of carers.

WHEN PARENTERAL NUTRITION HAS REACHED ITS LIMITS: INTESTINAL TRANSPLANTATION

Intestinal transplantation may be offered when PN has reached its limits because of life-threatening complications – for example, recurrent line infections, loss of venous access or intestinal failure–associated liver disease. Overall survival rates in a large cohort after intestinal transplantation (n = 814) were 73% at 1 year, 61% at 3 years and 55% at 5 years (Lao *et al.*, 2010).

The parents of the child recipients of intestinal transplantation reported significant limitations in the physical and psychosocial well-being of their children compared with that of normal school children. In contrast, the intestinal transplant recipients themselves reported a quality of life similar to normal school children. This discrepancy could be explained by the fact that the children grow accustomed to differences in life relative to their peers and their parents may have had a stronger recollection of the pre-transplant status and had lingering concern over their child's overall well-being (Sudan *et al.*, 2002).

THE EFFECTS OF LIVING AT HOME WITH PARENTERAL NUTRITION: QUALITY-OF-LIFE STUDIES

Published studies typically involved parents' ratings of their child's quality of life or have studied only the impact of the therapy on parents' lives. Three recently published studies (Emedo *et al.*, 2010; Engström *et al.*, 2003; Gottrand *et al.*, 2005) have attempted to evaluate the quality of life of children on home PN and show differing conclusions regarding the impact of the therapy on quality of life.

France

The first study was a national multicentre study of 72 French patients that reported that the quality of life of home PN-dependent children and siblings was not different from that of healthy children. Children may use effective coping strategies (Gottrand *et al.*, 2005). Lower scores were recorded when children younger than 11 years of age were questioned about health-related subjects, obligations and 'thinking about being a grown-up'. Presence of an ileostomy was the only factor that influenced quality of life, especially adolescents. In contrast to their children, the quality of life of parents of home PN–dependent children was low, especially in mothers who showed a lower level of satisfaction than fathers for items related to work, inner life and freedom.

Sweden

A national questionnaire-based study showed that children on home PN in Sweden score similarly to children with inflammatory bowel disease, but significantly lower than children with diabetes (Engström *et al.*, 2003). Commercial home care companies were not available in Sweden and families exclusively managed their children's home PN. The study raised questions about whether the psychological distress in families could be reduced. The major factor seems to be reducing the worry about complication associated with the treatment. The authors concluded that a multi-professional team input (Puntis *et al.*, 1991) could reduce complications.

United Kingdom

The third study (Emedo *et al.*, 2010) interviewed seven children in the United Kingdom about their lifestyle and health. Children coped well but were troubled when complications of the underlying condition disease persisted (e.g. abdominal pain, stool frequency). Children were aware of life restrictions – for example, fewer sleepovers with friends and fewer late nights. Despite the problems, patients developed a level of resilience, maintained a positive outlook, and coped well with illness-related demands. Coping strategies and support perceived to help the children were identified as
- parental support
- good understanding of illness and treatment
- good peer relationships
- emotional support from siblings
- participation in usual childhood activities
- household pets.

UNDERSTANDING OF CHRONIC ILLNESS BY YOUNG PEOPLE

Accurate understanding of their chronic illness has been found to be related to a sound emotional state and good overall health-related quality of life in children (Garrison and McCuiston, 1989). Children can play a part in their treatment and cooperate with management tasks such as helping with the aseptic technique when accessing a central line. Portable infusion pumps can allow mobility around the home in the evenings and social activities such as sleepovers are possible if home PN infusions are reduced to 6 or fewer nights per week. The ability to cope so well may be related to their lack of experience with any other way of life, because this group of children has had virtually lifelong treatment.

Relationships

Social support can buffer the effects of stress on well-being and enhance adaptive coping (Cohen and Wills, 1985). Children were also enabled to cope by support from parents, siblings, friends and household pets. The relative importance of a good relationship with peers increases during childhood and is known to peak in adolescence. Challenges conforming to peers, making decisions about disclosure, dealing with missing school, attending hospital and coming to terms with living with the illness are pertinent issues in the lives of these young people.

Education

School is an important area for child socialisation and missing school can impede individualisation from the family and establishment of an independent identify (Geist *et al.*, 2003). Frequent and extended absences from school are experienced because of illness and hospital visits.

Eating

While studies have shown intellectual and motor skills to be near normal limits in most children on long-term home PN (Ament and O'Conner, 1984), many children experience problems with normal eating behaviour including failure of weaning, oral hypersensitivity and food refusal. Eating is invariably restricted and there may be limitations on types of foods, frequency of meals or amount of food per meal. Children who miss out on development of oral feeding skills in the first year of life, or if food has been associated with negative consequences such as nausea and discomfort, may experience persistent eating problems that continue as young adults. Enteral calorie intake may be reliant on gastrostomies or feeding tubes because of tolerability of specialised liquid feeds, which may be given nocturnally for convenience and to avoid daytime satiety, as well as problems with appetite, ability and willingness to eat.

SUPPORTING FAMILIES

Supporting young people and families for discharge home on parenteral nutrition: assessment of the needs of the child and family

Establishing core responsibilities for parent and professionals

Parents accept that they have no real choice in taking on the care of their child who is discharged home with complex medical needs, as the only other alternative for their child is prolonged hospitalisation. It is important to achieve a common understanding so that parents appreciate they have core responsibility as the primary caregivers, as they may have unrealistic expectations about the assistance that is available. Service provision will only supplement parental care at home, particularly as funding for provision is increasingly stretched. Resources that professionals offer must be achievable and tailored to family's needs and priorities.

Psychological transitions for parents

Professionals should enable parents to be supported in maintaining their role as the child's primary carers, with professional input supportive of, but not intrusive on, this role. Parents must also be prepared for the shifting of roles and responsibility from professionals. At home, parents will rapidly become more experienced, become experts in their child's health-related care and will face a significant workload over and above the usual requirements of childcare. Confidence in parenting may change to concerns about managing aspects of their child's care at home, with worry about the complexity of tasks faced alongside their emotional attachment to their child. Mothers particularly face a transition in their personal identity as their previous work role outside the home shifts to that of being only their child's unpaid carer. Conflict may arise with other home commitments, and families require support in accommodating the emotional workload of caring for their child at home and parenting other siblings, for example.

Detecting the burden on parents

How far parents' emotional and social needs are met may affect the whole family's quality of life. If these needs are not met, it may reduce the parents' ability to meet their child's needs. It may be difficult to assess the effectiveness of coping strategies informally, so it is important to explore parental adaption to their child's needs and consider the positive impact that meeting these will have on the family. Formal evaluation, using standardised, validated instruments may identify if the burden on parents is becoming problematic. Factors associated with adverse outcome may be identified – for example, parental separation, lack of extended family support, change in employment networks, financial difficulties or depression. Parental perceptions of caring for children receiving family-centred rehabilitation or disability services have been evaluated using Measures of Processes of Care (Dickens *et al.*, 2010), a 20-item questionnaire encompassing five domains: (1) Enabling and Partnership, (2) Providing General Information, (3) Providing Specific Information about the Child, (4) Co-ordinated and Comprehensive Care for the Family and Child and (5) Respectful and Supportive Care. Although the focus of provision is on the child, preparing for the child's transition home should be conducted within the context of the needs of the whole family, especially the child's siblings. As far as is possible, support should be organised in a way that maintains the siblings' quality of life as well as that of the child on home PN.

Integration between health and social care

Obtaining appropriate and coordinated home support services, particularly respite, can be problematic. Parents have reported that individualised home care
packages developed in response to family needs are essential and help counter
the significant distress endured. The presence of a 24-hour on-call service with
expert paediatric nursing staff was a key factor for families to feel secure and
prevent readmission to hospital (Sexton *et al.*, 2005). This service is an expensive resource and is not universally available.

Multi-agency working and integration within children's services is set out in
Every Child Matters: Change for Children (DfES, 2004) and the *National Service
Framework for Children, Young People and Maternity Services* (DoH, 2004). A
Common Assessment Framework (CWDC, 2007) is a needs-led plan for as
many disciplines as possible to use one system of assessment and documentation. If it works well, it can involve families in decision-making, provide
early intervention with a key worker to coordinate support, and advocate for
families (CWDC, 2007). A Common Assessment Framework does not provide
additional services but it should identify needs, ensure that families are heard,
review progress and escalate concerns to safeguarding.

BOX 6.1 Planning requirements for arranging for home parenteral nutrition

- Education from nutrition nurse specialist – possession of a good
  understanding of their illness and training for children in practical skills to
  assume more responsibility for their own care
- Discharge planning meeting for family and professionals led by key worker
  – nursing support to facilitate the discharge home and to provide ongoing
  support for families
- A named keyworker acts as a central point of contact and coordination for
  all the parties involved in providing the child's support
- Improving infection control and reducing catheter-related complications to
  reduce the burden of disease and hospital admissions
- A Common Assessment Framework asserts the need for appropriate
  community support services for families
- Signposting to options beyond statutory services, such as charities and
  voluntary organisations
- Contact with other parents and patient support networks, e.g. PINNT, a
  support group for people receiving artificial nutrition (www.pinnt.com)
- Practical support from specialist home care companies used to deliver
  disposable equipment and parenteral nutrition to the child's home

---

BOX 6.2 Recommendations for coordinated multidisciplinary input for emotional support for families of children on home parenteral nutrition

- Strategies to help children coming to terms with living with chronic illness
- Supportive counselling for children and families to encourage coping mechanisms
- Encouragement to participate in normal childhood activities, academic and extracurricular activities, extra help at school, sport, holidays, conforming to peers, and dealing with missing school
- Professionals to explore parents' adaptation to their child's needs and changes to social and employment networks; detection of possible breakdown of coping strategies should prompt close liaison with Social Care; respite care to be offered if possible
- Standardised Outcome Measures may detect factors associated with adverse outcome – for example, parental separation, single-parent families, lack of extended family support or employment outside the home
- Speech and language therapy and dietitian – eating behaviour – encouraging meals and avoiding dietary restrictions where possible
- Home care services aimed at supporting children and families at home should be tailored to, and sensitive to, the individual needs of each family; siblings to continue their school routines, extracurricular activities, social events and maintain friendships
- Liaison with school health services
- Transition – as these children move into adulthood, it is important to plan transition to adult services carefully and reassess young people's coping strategies as they take over responsibility for their care

BOX 6.3 Services and individuals who may be involved in supporting children or young people on home parenteral nutrition

Nutritional support team at regional centre of paediatric gastroenterology	Specialist paediatric nutrition nurse
	Consultant paediatric gastroenterologist
	Specialist paediatric pharmacist
	Specialist paediatric dietitian
	Paediatric clinical psychologist
	Speech and language therapist
	Paediatric surgeon
	Paediatric stoma nurse
	Venous access team
Local primary care centre	General practitioner
	Health visitor
	Transport

Local provider trust	Paediatrician
	Occupational therapist
	Dietitian
	Physiotherapist
	Clinical psychologist
	Speech and language therapist
Local community services	Community paediatrician
	Community children's nurses
	Community pharmacist
	Portage worker
Education services	School nurses
	Teaching staff
Commercial home care company	Home nursing staff
	Delivery staff
Social care	Social worker

TRANSITION OF YOUNG PEOPLE (YP) ON HOME PARENTERAL NUTRITION TO ADULT SERVICES

Definition of transition

The standard definition of transition is:

> a purposeful, planned process that addresses the medical, psychosocial and edu-
> cational/vocational needs of adolescents and young adults with chronic physical
> and medical conditions as they move from child-centred to adult-orientated
> health care systems. (DoH, 2006, p 14, Box 2)

Why is the planned transfer of healthcare so important?

Preparing patients for transition involves more than simply describing future
events and raising awareness of transfer (Protheroe, 2009). Paediatric care is
family-centred, focusing as much on the parents as on the children, but this
approach provides poor preparation for moving to the adult sector. Adult
health services assume that patients have an extent of autonomy and have the
capacity to negotiate the healthcare system. Shift from parent-managed to self-
managed care is required (McDonagh, 2007).

Effective transition is important not only in terms of the potential benefits
to patients from increased satisfaction and decreased morbidity, but also in
terms of the cost savings to enhance participation in society when the transition teams 'get it right' (Last et al., 2007). At worst, if it is not handled well,
failure to engage with adult tertiary services makes routine clinic attendance
less likely and quality of care may decline (Dobbels et al., 2005; Watson, 2000).
Young people, who have experienced skills training in transition programmes

and who secure a strong relationship with the new healthcare team have better adherence to follow-up, improved disease control and quality of life (McDonagh *et al.*, 2005).

Poorly planned transition results in difficulties when young people access adult specialist services. As a consequence, there may be increased risk of non-adherence or lack of follow-up, which carries dangers of morbidity and mortality as well as poor social and educational outcomes. Transition does not end at the exit from the paediatric clinic, but continues into the adult sector, which needs to provide developmentally appropriate clinical care. Department of Health initiatives are aimed at ensuring that young people do not miss out on healthcare during the transfer between paediatric and adult services. Transfer can be a major, often daunting, event for young people. Parents may also fear transfer and need to learn to 'let go' of some control, which may be particularly difficult.

Timing of transition to adult services

Flexibility in timing of transfer will ensure that the needs of individual young people are met. Generally the Department of Health recognises that health services for young people cover those individuals aged 16–19 years (Michaud *et al.*, 2004). Professionals and young people choose to plan transfer to the adult sector when patients are clinically stable, growth and puberty is complete, avoiding major life events such as school examinations, or starting college.

BOX 6.4 Key features of transition

Key features of transition

- An active period of preparation, which occurs before and after the event of transfer
- Adapted to the young person's needs and views
- Is not distinct from the principles and practice of adolescent healthcare
- Starts early, approximately the age of 12 years
- Continues into adulthood

Requirements for transition

- A shared written policy between adult and paediatric providers, which has the young person's wider needs for the future at the centre
- An individual transition plan with education programme and goals to be reached by certain dates (*see* Box 6.5)
- A nominated key worker, often a nurse specialist to involve the young individual in the planning process
- Independent visits; the importance of consulting with the young person alone, without their accompanying parents, is an important step towards building autonomy in healthcare and is one of main methods of demonstrating transition. An opportunity should be provided for self-

confidence to navigate and negotiate services previously accessed by parents on their behalf, and for self-advocacy.
● Opportunity to meet the adult physician before transfer
● Transfer to adult healthcare to be determined by the readiness of the young person and is usually after they have finished growth, puberty and school
● Transfer includes a comprehensive transfer of health information

Note: based on Viner (2008) and McDonagh *et al.* (2006b).

The challenges of transitioning to adult services
Challenges for young people

While the young person with a chronic medical condition may have outgrown the paediatric healthcare environment, they may have delayed psychosocial milestones, reduced independence, social isolation and increased educational and vocational difficulties (Stam *et al.*, 2006). Management tasks may present greater obstacles and be more problematic in young people. Children who miss out on development of oral feeding skills in the first year of life may have persistent eating problems that continue as young adults. Enteral intake may be reliant on gastrostomies or feeding tubes.

Skill acquisition – for example, setting up their own home PN – is variable and can be delayed in the context of chronic illness and be more problematic in young people, as psychosocial milestones such as cognitive maturity and autonomy have not yet been achieved (Sawyer *et al.*, 2007). Adolescents might reject medical care as part of separation from parental control. They may be more prone to risk-taking (Bolton-Maggs, 2007; Sawyer *et al.*, 2007) or overwhelmed by the burden of healthcare issues and inappropriate expectations of clinicians.

Depression and anxiety are common problems in the daily life of adults on home PN (who commence home PN in adulthood) and these difficulties may arise as a result of lack of freedom, limitations in social life and being dependent. Somatic problems such as fatigue and sleep disturbance impact on economic dependency (Huisman-de Waal *et al.*, 2007). Quality of life of adults on home PN is reduced in the presence of depression and narcotic dependency (Winkler, 2005). These findings are in contrast to young people who have been on home PN since infancy. In a supportive environment, young people may develop a sense of well-being, personal identity and worth because of their experiences, their coping strategies and their ability to adapt well, compared with adults, to the medical routines. Home PN teams should be aware of the problems that adults face and facilitate psychosocial support and/or cognitive training for young people to avoid a negative psychological transition and enable the young person to strive to achieve independence at home as well in their chosen vocation.

Challenges for parents and families

Families of young people on home PN may be overprotective and have difficulties with transition (CWDC, 2007) particularly if care appears discontinuous or they feel excluded. Demonstration that young people have developed independence in healthcare as well as other aspects of their lives allows parents (and their doctors) to 'let go'. Having a child on home PN is associated with physical and social stresses, social isolation, loneliness and depression in parents (Johnson and Sexton, 2006; Wong *et al.*, 2000) and parents may require support in re-establishing personal identity issues and having time to consider taking on work roles outside the home that may have been impossible prior.

Young people and their families may be concerned about a reduction in services following transfer and a lack of preparation for such differences. Home care services may be negotiated to support children and their families with nursing support (Sexton *et al.*, 2005), and families may face a change of services with a change of provider as well as a new adult nutritional care team.

TRANSITION: HOW TO DO IT

There have been a number of publications on how to provide quality services for adolescents during transition, including the *National Service Framework for Children, Young People and Maternity Services* (DoH, 2004) and the guidelines from the Royal College of Paediatrics and Child Health (Intercollegiate Working Party on Adolescent Health, 2003) and the Royal College of Nursing (RCN, 2004). They have been reviewed in the Department of Health's recent guidance in *Transition: Getting it Right for Young People. Improving the Transition of Young People with Long Term Conditions from Children's to Adult Health Services* (DoH, 2006).

Focus groups of adolescents have been helpful in developing models of care in rheumatology (Shaw *et al.*, 2004), with common themes emerging, for example:

- need for multidisciplinary team
- continuity and good coordination between professionals
- clear sources of information
- care that minimises the impact of the medical condition on their life
- a less-formal environment
- a need for information, and websites devoted to health issues for adolescents (McDonagh *et al.*, 2006a).

Planning transition to adult services

Important factors have been identified to help with both the successful transition and the recognition of potential barriers for enterally fed adolescents moving to adult services. These factors can be applied to adolescents on PN and highlight the need for flexibility to ensure the needs of individual children are met.

Health transitions are one part of the wider set of educational, family and social transitions that young people make. These transitions are outlined in Box 6.5.

BOX 6.5 Transitions undergone by the young person on home parenteral nutrition (PN) moving to adult healthcare services

- Health transitions – independent visits and phone calls, contacting the new team, self-care of the central venous line and techniques for independent setting up of PN
- New PN prescription
- New contacts, e.g. pharmacy, supplier or home care company may change
- Dry goods and pumps
- Stoma care
- Generic health issues, health and lifestyle, exercise, understanding of adult-onset diseases (e.g. osteoporosis), sexual health
- Smoking, alcohol, narcotics and illegal drugs, self-esteem and body image
- Home and psychosocial transitions
- Self-advocacy, knowledge of benefits, sources of support, peer support groups, e.g. PINNT (a charitable body that supports patients on intravenous and nasogastric nutrition)
- Educational transitions – examinations, work experience, moving away to college or university, career advice and plans
- Vocational transitions – career choice, moving away from home, financial planning, impact of disclosure of condition at college or workplace

---

SUMMARY

Planning the transition from hospital to home for a child with complex and continuing health needs on PN involves a range of services to ensure that care provision meets their health, social and educational needs, and that the needs of the family as a whole are met. A key worker, usually a children's nutrition nurse works with the child and the family and provides the link between hospital and community settings. A package of support should enable parents to be supported in maintaining their role as the child's primary carers, with professional input supporting but not intrusive on the parents' role. The requirements of families will differ and home-care services should be tailored to, and sensitive to, the individual needs of each family.

Transition to adult health services is a key quality issue for the National Health Service. It is vital that both paediatric and adult centres address the challenge to ensure transition is a well-managed active process that starts early and proceeds in a planned and purposeful way. Securing relationships for the young person with a new healthcare team can enhance his or her self-reliance and medical and vocational outcomes while at the same time continuing good medical care (McDonagh *et al.*, 2006b).

Despite initiatives and evidence, progress in developing transition programmes in some medical specialities has been slow. A concerted effort is required to put recommendations into practice and for commissioning bodies to consider the resource implications for development of transition policies. Knowledge and skills in adolescent medicine and transition should become more firmly incorporated into training programmes for healthcare professionals. Services need to work in partnership with families and with each other at both strategic and operational levels, to develop integrated and coordinated services that can meet the needs of this group of families (Hewitt-Taylor, 2012). The large overall increase in numbers of home PN patients suggests that a national strategy to integrate health and social care needs to be developed for their management.

Key messages and aims for future arrangements

- Improved outcomes for children with intestinal failure have led to more care at home and transfer of care to families. This may come at a cost to family functioning.
- Integration and continuum of care from hospital team and social care is necessary to supplement family care.
- Parental and young person's involvement and choice is vital at the outset and during transition to adult services.
- Standardised measures to determine the level of burden, ability to cope, and specific costs to family (such as loss of employment outside the home) should be developed to detect strain on the family and tailor home care packages and services to requirements.
- Professionals should consider supplementing home care by parents with realistic offers of respite from social care or charitable bodies and consider new ways of home support and follow-up.

REFERENCES

Ament ME, O'Connor MJ. Long-term cognitive development of children on home total parenteral nutrition (HTPN) for 42 to 96 months. *Pediatr Res.* 1984; 18: 100A.

Beath SV, Gowen H, Puntis JW. Trends in paediatric home parenteral nutrition and implications for service development. *Clin Nutr.* 2011; 30(4): 499–502.

Bolton-Maggs PH. Transition of care from paediatric services in haematology. *Arch Dis Child.* 2007; 92(9): 797–801.

British Artificial Nutrition Survey Committee (BANS). *Annual BANS Report, 2007: artificial nutrition support in the UK 2000–2006.* Redditch, Worcestershire: BAPEN; 2007. Available at: www.bapen.org.uk/pdfs/bans_reports/bans_report_07.pdf

Children's Workforce Development Council (CWDC). *Common Assessment Framework for Children and Young People: practitioners' guide. Integrated working to improve outcomes for children and young people.* Leeds: CWDC; 2007.

Cohen S, Wills TA. Stress, social support, and the buffering hypothesis. *Psychol Bull.* 1985; 98(2): 310–57.

Department for Education and Skills (DfES). *Every Child Matters: change for children.* London: Department for Education and Skills; 2004. Available at: http://webarchive.

nationalarchives.gov.uk/20130401151715/https://www.education.gov.uk/publications/eOrderingDownload/DFES10812004.pdf

Department of Health (DoH). *National Service Framework for Children, Young People and Maternity Services*. London: DoH; 2004.

Department of Health (DoH). *Healthy Lives, Brighter Futures – The Strategy for Children and Young People's Health*. London: DoH; 2009. Available at: www.fatherhoodinstitute.org/uploads/publications/409.pdf

Department of Health, Child Health and Maternity Services Branch (DoH). *Transition: getting it right for young people. Improving the transition of young people with long term conditions from children's to adult health services*. London: DoH; 2006. Available at: www.bspar.org.uk/DocStore/FileLibrary/PDFs/Transition-%20getting%20it%20right%20for%20young%20people%20-%2023rd%20March%202006.pdf

Dickens K, Matthews LR, Thompson J. Parent and service providers' perceptions regarding the delivery of family-centred paediatric rehabilitation services in a children's hospital. *Child Care Health Dev*. 2010; **37**(1): 64–73.

Dobbels F, Van Damme-Lombaert R, Vanhaecke J, *et al*. Growing pains: non-adherence with the immunosuppressive regimen in adolescent transplant recipients. *Pediatr Transplant*. 2005; **9**(3): 381–90.

Emedo MJ, Godfrey El, Hill SM. A qualitative study of the quality of life of children receiving intravenous nutrition at home. *J Pediatr Gastroenterol Nutr*. 2010; **50**(4): 431–40.

Engström I, Björnestam B, Finkel Y. Psychological distress associated with home parenteral nutrition in Swedish children, adolescents, and their parents: preliminary results. *J Pediatr Gastroenterol Nutr*. 2003; **37**(3): 246–50.

Frederick V, Luedtke GS, Barrett FF. Munchausen syndrome by proxy: recurrent central catheter sepsis. *Pediatr Infect Dis J*. 1990; **9**(6): 440–2.

Garrison W, McCuiston S. *Chronic Illness during Childhood and Adolescence*. London: Sage publications; 1989.

Geist R, Grdisa V, Otley A. Psychosocial issues in the child with chronic conditions. *Best Pract Res Clin Gastroenterol*. 2003; **17**(2): 141–2.

Gottrand F, Staszewski P, Colomb V, *et al*. Satisfaction in different life domains in children receiving home parenteral nutrition and their families. *J Pediatr*. 2005; **146**(6): 793–7.

Hewitt-Taylor J. Planning the transition of children with complex needs from hospital to home. *Nurs Child Young People*. 2012; **24**(10); 28–35.

Holden C. Review of home paediatric parenteral nutrition in the UK. *Br J Nurs*. 2001; **10**(12): 782–8.

Huisman-de Waal G, Schoonhoven L, Janeen J, *et al*. The impact of home parenteral nutrition on daily life: a review. *Clin Nutr*. 2007; **26**(3): 275–88.

Intercollegiate Working Party on Adolescent Health. *Bridging the Gap: healthcare for adolescents. Report of the Joint Working Party on Adolescent Health of the Royal Medical and Nursing Colleges of the UK*. London: Royal College of Paediatrics and Child Health; 2003.

Johnson T, Sexton E. Managing children and adolescents on parenteral nutrition: challenges for the nutritional support team. *Proc Nutr Soc*. 2006; **65**(3): 217–21.

Kennedy A, Sawyer S. Transition from pediatric to adult services: are we getting it right? *Curr Opin Pediatr*. 2008; **20**(4): 403–9.

Kirk S, Glendinning C, Callery P. Parent or nurse? The experience of being the parent of a technology-dependent child. *J Advanced Nurs*. 2005; **51**(5): 456–64.

Lao OB, Healey PJ, Perkins JD *et al*. Outcomes in children after intestinal transplant. *Pediatrics*. 2010; **125**(3): e550–8.

Last BF, Stam H, Onland-van Nieuwenhuizen AM, *et al*. Positive effects of a psycho-educational group intervention for children with a chronic disease: first results. *Patient Educ Couns*. 2007: **65**(1): 101–12.

McDonagh JE. Transition of care from paediatric to adult rheumatology. *Arch Dis Child*. 2007; **92**(9): 802–7.

McDonagh JE, Minnaar G, Kelly K, *et al.* Unmet education and training needs in adolescent health of health professionals in a UK children's hospital. *Acta Paediatr.* 2006a; **95**(6): 715–19.

McDonagh JE, Shaw KL, Southwood TR. Growing up and moving on in rheumatology: development and preliminary evaluation of a transitional care programme for a multicentre cohort of adolescents with juvenile idiopathic arthritis. *J Child Health.* 2006b; **10**(1): 22–42.

McDonagh JE, Southwood TR, Shaw KL. Growing up and moving on in rheumatology: disease knowledge in a multicentre cohort of adolescents with juvenile idiopathic arthritis. *Arch Dis Child.* 2005; **90**: G123.

Menahem S, Halasz G. Parental non-compliance: a paediatric dilemma. A medical and psychodynamic perspective. *Child Care Health Dev.* 2000; **26**(1): 61–72.

Michaud PA, Suris JC, Viner R. The adolescent with a chronic condition. Part II: healthcare provision. *Arch Dis Child.* 2004; **89**(10): 943–9.

Protheroe S. Young people artificial nutrition and transitional care: transition in young people on home parenteral nutrition. *Proc Nutr Soc.* 2009: **68**(4): 1–5.

Puntis JW. Home parenteral nutrition. *Arch Dis Child.* 1995; **72**: 186–90.

Puntis JW, Holden CE, Smallman S, *et al.* Staff training: a key factor in reducing intravascular cather sepsis. *Arch Dis Child.* 1991; **66**(3): 335–7.

Rosen DS, Blum RW, Britto M, *et al.* Transition to adult health care for adolescents and young adults with chronic conditions: position paper for the Society for Adolescent Medicine. *J Adolesc Health.* 2003: **33**(4): 309–11.

Royal College of Nursing (RCN). *Adolescent Transition Care: guidance for nursing staff.* London: RCN; 2004.

Sawyer S, Aroni R. Self-management in adolescents with chronic illness. What does it mean and how can it be achieved? *Med J Aust.* 2005; **183**(8): 405–9.

Sawyer S, Drew S, Yeo M, *et al.* Adolescents with a chronic condition: challenges living, challenges treating. *Lancet.* 2007; **369**(9571): 1481–9.

Sexton E, Coad J, Holden C. Review of home care packages for paediatric HPN patients. *Br J Nurs.* 2005; **14**(20): 1080–5.

Shaw KL, Southwood TR, McDonagh JE. User perspectives of transitional care for adolescents with juvenile idiopathic arthritis. *Rheumatology (Oxford).* 2004; **43**(6): 770–8.

Stam H, Hartman E, Deurloo J, *et al.* Young adult patients with a history of paediatric disease: impact on course of life and transition in adulthood. *J Adolesc Health.* 2006; **39**(1): 4–13.

Sudan D, Iyer K, Horslen S, *et al.* Assessment of quality of life after paediatric intestinal transplantation by parents and paediatric recipients using the child health questionnaire. *Transplant Proc.* 2002; **34**(3): 963–4.

UNICEF. United Nations Children's Fund. The State of the World's Children: Adolescence, An Age of Oportunity. 2011. www.unicef.org/sowc2011/pdfs/SOWC-2011-Main-Report_EN_02092011.pdf (accessed 14 January 2014).

Viner R. Transition of care from paediatric to adult services: one part of improved health services for adolescents. *Arch Dis Child.* 2008; **93**(2): 160–3.

Watson AR. Non-compliance and transfer from paediatric to adult transplant unit. *Pediatr Nephrol.* 2000; **14**(6): 469–72.

Winkler MF. Quality of life in adult home parenteral nutrition patients. *JPEN J Parenter Enteral Nutr.* 2005; **29**(3): 162–70.

Wong C, Akobeng AK, Miller V, *et al.* Quality of life of parents of children on home parenteral nutrition. *Gut.* 2000; **46**(2): 294–5.

Wu PA, Kerner JA, Berquist WE. Parenteral nutrition-associated cholestasis related to parental care. *Nutr Clin Pract.* 2006; **21**(3): 291–5.

CHAPTER 7

A biopsychosocial framework to understand children and young people with gastrointestinal problems

Terence Dovey

INTRODUCTION

There are many theories that explain human behaviour. Every undergraduate psychologist is exposed to the traditional core areas of social, cognitive and developmental psychology. The student may briefly cover other perspectives, before going on to his or her postgraduate training, but, even than, few will understand the sheer number of theoretical explanations for human behaviour that have been operationalised and implemented in clinical practice. At last count, the number was in excess of 400 (Corsini and Wedding, 2008). Other less well-covered approaches include the applied behavioural, biological/neural and affective models, as well as 'offshoots' and 'combined' approaches. In an attempt to provide a definitive measure of human experience, philosophers, psychologists and medics have attempted to bring the various strands of human existence into a single unified theory. One such attempt was put forward by Engel (1977) and was termed the biopsychosocial model. Since its inception, the biopsychosocial model has received wide theoretical acceptance by multidisciplinary teams and has, indeed, already been referenced by a number of authors thus far in this text. This chapter seems therefore well placed, coming as it does at the end of Part I, to present a critique of the impact of this model in practice.

Psychologists working as part of a multidisciplinary team can easily be seduced by a unified theory. By its very nature, a unified theory provides, and allegedly designates, a role for every professional in the process. Wide acceptance would assign roles to specific professional groups and eliminate potential conflict over culpability and ownership of treatment. However, vigilance is recommended. Acceptance of any perspective without fully understanding its underpinnings is never recommended. Indeed, any psychologist who suggests he or she adheres to the biopsychosocial model may actually misunderstand the fundamentals of this theory, as it was never intended or designed to include in the healing processes any other professionals beyond trained medical staff. It was a framework for medical practice, not a process for the inclusion of professionals outside of medicine. It was intended to 'bring home' psychiatry, not to 'bring in' psychology or any other applied health professional.

This chapter will focus on the biopsychosocial model and its purported impact on managing paediatric gastroenterological conditions. In order to fully comprehend the model four key aspects must be acknowledged.

1. An interpretation of the original author's intentions is necessary.
2. Irrespective of intention, subsequent interpretation and applications must be understood before it can be fully accepted and adopted.
3. Highlighting some of the shortcomings and the difficulties in implementation require consideration in order to understand the potential for this model.
4. The application of the model to gastroenterology and how a psychologist fits into the biopsychosocial model is necessary to fully understand the framework of multidisciplinary teams working with individuals with chronic medical conditions.

These four components form the structure of the current chapter.

THE ORIGINAL BIOPSYCHOSOCIAL MODEL

The seminal paper on the biopsychosocial model was that of Engel (1977). Published in the journal *Science*, Engel contends with the subject of the inclusion of psychiatry as a medical discipline. The historical context to the article was that psychiatry was undergoing an identity crisis. Prior to the crisis, medicine had been dependent on two forms of information, data gathered from observation and information gathered from discussion. In effect, medicine relied on a mixed measures approach, incorporating both qualitative and quantitative methods. In any given examination, and irrespective of sub-discipline, the medic would take a series of measurements, as well as talk to the patient about their general social and psychological wellbeing. On the basis of this collated information, the medic would make a diagnosis and recommend a treatment. Engel then argues that the various technological advances in molecular biology allowed medics to engage with illness in some cases prior to the onset of observable symptoms (Engel, 1997). Medicine quickly became reliant on measureable data rather than the impact of a perceived symptom. Engel refers to this as the 'dogma' of medicine. 'Dogma' in this instance was based on the medics' resistance to accept that information in the form of verbal markers had an impact on the underlying 'medical' problem. Instead, the medic looked at the data from the biological tests and told the patient whether they were 'sick' or not. In effect, the medic was operating on a process of 'fixing' biological problems. However, what they failed to understand was that the problems they were often fixing had developed as a consequence of problematic living. This narrow view of *'broken' biology* (namely, 'fix' biology, discharge patient) inevitably leads to a scenario where the patient is readmitted through relapse or resurgence, based on the same social and environmental conditions that pre-existed and contributed to the biological problem. In this scenario, the medic was treating the symptoms and not the cause. The medic is not healing; he or she is potentially maintaining the individual in a psychopathological state or problematic environment.

Within this context, the 'dogma' of medicine led to three perspectives on what encompasses medicine. The first, Engel termed 'reductionist' whereby human existence is entirely understood through physicochemical principles. The second was termed 'exclusionist', which was populated by medics who believed that anything that could not be explained by biological principles should be excluded from the category of disease. Such medics usually stated that individuals suffered from two categories of problems in life: one was the problems of living and the other was medical problems. The final perspective was psychiatry. It would appear that medicine was attempting to push psychiatry away from medicine and into another field. Engel (1977) argues that this led to a crisis of confidence in the field of psychiatry whereby two subgroups formed. One group adhered to the reductionist principle that all psychopathology was a problem with biology, usually the brain. The exclusionists responded to this attempted reconciliation by stating that this was the remit of a neurologist not a psychiatrist. The second group, which took Engel's perspective, rejected the biomedical model as a standalone theory for medicine and suggested that it should be replaced with a model that includes holistic information gained from the individual about their psychological and social wellbeing. To the reductionists they suggested that it is not possible to know whether a person is sick unless you ask them. In effect, the reductionist is not totally reliant on the biological tests. They must first know which tests and why. This could only be gained through talking to the patient, unless they wanted to advocate an expensive universal screening program for all illnesses. To the exclusionists the psychiatrists claimed arrogance – that it was impossible for them to decide what was worthy of being defined as a disease. It was not they who created the criteria for sickness; rather, it was society that decided who was ill and who needed 'help'. After 30 years of discussion, it would appear that the general consensus is that the biopsychosocial model has won the minds, if not the hearts, of the medical profession.

THE ROLE OF OTHER PROFESSIONALS

Fundamental to the biopsychosocial model was *not* that it should involve other professionals; rather, the model was created by medics, for medics to explore medical problems. It advocates that a holistic approach should be taken by the individual medic, and does not suggest that professionalisation of the three components of the model should be placed in independent streams. It is an integrated model and as such requires an individual to internalise the theory (Adler, 2009). Engel did not indicate that there were no distinctions between medical problems and problems with living. He simply defined medical problems as including components of psychology and sociology. This is the common misunderstanding of Engel's model. His only reference to non-medical professionals within his writings was to that of clinical psychologists:

> While the behavioral sciences have made some limited incursions into medical school teaching programs, it is mainly upon the psychiatrists, and to a lesser extent clinical psychologists, that the responsibility falls to develop approaches to the understanding of health and disease and patient care not readily accomplished within the more narrow framework and with the specialized techniques of traditional biomedicine. (Engel, 1977, pp. 133)

It is difficult to comprehend, based on the biopsychosocial model, why current health provision for chronic illness should include professionals from other disciplines outside of medicine. However, within every basic psychology textbook resides the answer. Current health provision policy has applied the work of a model designed to challenge the developing prejudices of medicine against one of its own sub-disciplines to the creation of a team of professionals working on specific aspects of a medical problem. Answering how this has developed is simple. The attitude of medical professionals does not correspond to their behaviour. Their behaviour is still aligned to the biomedical model (Alonso, 2004) and they have 'franchised' this element of the patients' care to other professional groups, while simultaneously remaining in control of all other forms of intervention for the purposes of health. The medic believes that both the social environment and the psychological composition of the individual are important, but their behaviour indicates that they do not perceive this to be their role or within their remit. For example, only 5% of the current undergraduate medical curriculum incorporates biopsychosocial principles (Adler, 2009) and some authors take this further to suggest that whole components of the model are not even considered at all (Schubert, 2010).

How this 'streaming' of professional involvement in gastroenterological cases has manifested is difficult to uncouple; however, it is unlikely that it is simply predicated on the beliefs, attitudes and practices of medical staff. Answers probably stem as much from the other professional groups declaring ownership of specific sectors within healthcare, through lobbying government agencies, coupled with medicine's desire to remain unified with molecular biology. It is a pragmatic alliance that abates the conflict between professional and personal attitudes. Adherents to the biopsychosocial model who reside outside of the medical profession must understand this arrangement. Stating that the service runs on this model is an implication that the patient is under the care of the medical team and that other professional groups are only engaged to consider specific components of the illness. Indeed, under the auspices of this model, other professionals are only involved because of current medical attitude. This approach to healthcare may also explain the disparate compositions of services around the world, as under the biopsychosocial model, medical teams have first refusal over what they feel they are able to implement without 'outside' professional involvement.

This concludes the historical context of the biopsychosocial model. There is a disparity between what Engel intended and what has been applied. Emergence of allied health professions that are specialised into a single aspect of health are arguably better placed to correct some dysfunctions than medics. The subsuming of this expertise into the healthcare system for specific problems should improve the outcome for the patients. Even within Engel's original paper, he acknowledges that the average medic is oblivious to behavioural technologies as they are predominantly published within psychology journals. The same argument could be made for nursing, dietetics, speech and language therapy and any other services allied to gastroenterology. However, an effective application of the model requires quality communication between the various professionals involved. Equally important is a strong case formulation, it would be counterproductive to effective implementation of biopsychosocial principles if three separate strands are created whereby each patient is screened, offered a formulation and an implementation strategy that conflicts or replicates the work of other involved groups. This would constitute a significant risk in the franchised environment where the 'bio', 'psycho' and 'social' elements of a patient's stay in hospital are dealt with by separate professional groups operating in isolation or sporadic consultation.

ACCEPTANCE OF THE MODEL: LIMITATIONS AND DISSENTION IN PRACTICE

Within the literature, there appears to be wide acceptance of the biopsychosocial model; especially within the allied health professionals. To say that the biopsychosocial model is completely accepted without dissenters or known limitations would be false. Dissent towards the biopsychosocial model resides in one of three categories, although it is acknowledged that the total dissent encompasses a very small minority of the total publications. The first of the three camps consists of the adherents of the biomedical model that still maintain that it is not the role of the medic to engage with the psychosocial components to his or her patients beyond simply exploring the context or impact of the biological dysfunction. The other two camps suggest that the biopsychosocial model does not stand up to scrutiny, either in a theoretical and/or practical context. These two camps suggest that the model is not novel and is too difficult to apply within many healthcare settings.

Theoretical dissent to the application of the biopsychosocial model claims that it does not really consider the psychosocial aspects. In effect, the model is 'BIOpsychosocial'. The inclusion of the other components allows the medic to continue to practise under the auspices of biomedicine and elevates conflict within medicine. Thus the true motivation for the adoption of the model is because it allows medicine to keep a hold of 'health' in the widest possible sense, to maintain their power and to subjugate other professionals with an interest in health (Armstrong, 1987).

> In each of these instances the role of psychosocial factors is clearly circumscribed. At no point do they challenge the dominance of the medical practitioner nor undermine or threaten the supremacy of the reductionist doctrine of the lesion contained in the biomedical model. Indeed, on the contrary, they strengthen biomedicine by ensuring that the patient – so often an awkward and unpredictable factor in the smooth operation of clinical work – is successfully 'managed'. The patient, would no longer be an impediment to diagnosis or treatment, no longer a malingerer or a recidivist when it came to compliance, but a helpful assistant to the clinician's application of a regime of biomedicine. (pp. 1214)

Armstrong's words are damning of the model. However, examination of the publications related to the biopsychosocial model reveals that Armstrong's position is not without substance. Most publications are letters or narrative reviews and nearly all call for a readjustment or revisiting of the principles of the biopsychosocial model. Coupled with the evidence that medical writers have not deviated from their biomedical position (Alonso, 2004), it would appear that the position held by medical professionals is mirrored in Armstrong's dissent.

Theoretical dissent is also evident towards the biopsychosocial model through the widely accepted claim that it provides circular causality in its arguments (Schubert, 2010) and therefore is too complex to apply. Moreover, the model cannot delineate between cause and effect and advocates a form of symbiosis or dualism that is difficult to uncouple or attribute to specific components in the presentation of an illness (Fava, 1996). One potential resolution that fits in with the historical context and attempts to implement the principles of the biopsychosocial model is the advice that has been offered by Freudenreich *et al.* (2010). Here the authors advocate that the medic consider the presentation of the patient under three topics called 'think neuroanatomically, think existentially and think dirty'. Under 'think neuroanatomically', it is advised that medics educate themselves to understand the neuroanatomical basis of behaviour. These authors suggest that 'thinking existentially' means that the medic should uncover the 'real' pain rather than the biological positioning of the pain – to find out the impact of their patient's problem rather than just its biological cause. Finally, 'thinking dirty' refers to not medicalising everything and to think deeper about the motives of the patient or those around them. These criteria would still indicate a very reductive application of the biopsychosocial model, as behaviour is not under the complete control of internally motivated events defined within neuroanatomy. Although this advice would fit well with a biomedical perspective, it would not be indicative of a group that readily accepts that some health problems manifest through environmental causes. It would be remiss to suggest that Freudenreich *et al.* (2010) were just advocating the biomedical components to the biopsychosocial model. They do accept that the 'psycho' component to the model has previously been subsumed as meaning 'psychiatric', which, in fact, goes against the principles of the model. Moreover, it would not be appropriate to overly criticise a practical clinical application of theoretical principles based on a model that has known weaknesses in this domain. Circular arguments and limited guidance on how to apply the model leaves practitioners that state they are adherents to the model not understanding its core concepts; such endorsements do not mean that there are any clear underlying principles on which adherents base their practice.

Limitations of the biomedical model have been referred to through the label of a physician- rather than a patient-centred approach. It is characterised by the medic's fears of emotional involvement and feelings of incompetence at dealing with a patient's emotional distress, among other things (Zimmermann and Tansella, 1996). Despite numerous calls, retraining and advocating an adoption of the biopsychosocial model, little has changed in relation to medics' attitudes, on average, in each decade since its inception (the seventies: e.g. Kahn *et al.*, 1979; the eighties: e.g. Putnam *et al.*, 1988; the nineties: e.g. Freedman, 1995; the two-thousands: e.g. Luthy *et al.*, 2007; the twenty-tens: e.g. Melchert, 2010). This is the biggest failure of the model. The repeated call to implement the model does not indicate therapeutic drift from its principles; instead, it would suggest reluctance among the medical profession to adopt the approach. Application of the biopsychosocial model in healthcare has been rationalised as simply understanding the factors that are determined to be predominantly psychological or social in nature rather than as an integrative approach (e.g. Luthy *et al.*, 2007). There are some distinct disadvantages to applying the theory in this manner. The model dictates that the individual comprises of factors that are influenced by each of the three domains. It does not suggest that some factors are only psychological or social. In effect, the model advocates that the illness is altered by each of the three factors interacting or more eloquently put by Lipowski (1974) as:

> It is generally agreed now that all diseases are multifactorial in origin ... Their relative weight may vary considerably from illness to illness, from individual to individual and from one episode to another of the same illness in the same person. (pp. 488)

This multifactorial origin does not lend to understanding which services are required for each individual. Moreover, it directly advocates that all factors should be measured. This has manifested in practice as an extended period of assessment where each professional group is required to assess the individual to determine whether they have a role within the individual's healthcare plan.

This slows down the access to treatment for many, as long waiting lists develop with the emphasis on getting the patient through the assessment process, rather than providing intervention. Although the model would advocate that biological dysfunction requires immediate attention in life-threatening situations, it does not offer direction for treating individuals with severe but stable conditions, as are frequently found within the gastroenterological setting. Indeed, this professional approach whereby there is a separation between the different elements of the model rather than an integrated approach has been shown to have a negative impact on children's recovery following admission to paediatric intensive care (Atkins *et al.*, 2012). In particular, it presents confusing messages to the parents, as the onus is on them to hold and integrate the various strands of their child's recovery. This would suggest that if the current iteration of the application of the biopsychosocial model persists, then it is important that professionals from differing backgrounds are able to effectively communicate a single, unified and agreed message to the families and patients or clients within their care. If the professionals cannot present such a message effectively, then it is likely to increase, rather than decrease, the anxiety within the family and lead to problems with the family's perceptions of professional competence, as the parents have to resolve which message is most valuable and what they consider to be the salient factors in their particular situation.

Despite the apparent difficulty to implement the biopsychosocial model among the wider medical profession, there is some compelling evidence for successful application in chronic conditions that require intensive multidisciplinary professional intervention and, in particular, in gastroenterological conditions. The remainder of this chapter will focus on the application of the biopsychosocial model to gastroenterology. In order to avoid overlap with other chapters within this book, this section will focus specifically on the application of the model, rather than a discussion on any specific topic.

BIOPSYCHOSOCIAL MODEL AND GASTROENTEROLOGICAL CONDITIONS

The biopsychosocial model and its application to gastroenterology has been championed by Professor Douglas Drossman (who wrote the Foreword for this book) over the last couple of decades (see Drossman, 1998; Drossman *et al.*, 1999; Levy *et al.*, 2006, for a detailed review). The variation between other areas of medicine and gastroenterological conditions is marked by the variation in the presentation of symptoms and the long-standing history of psychosocial factors impacting the digestive system. Whether the acceptance of the biopsychosocial model into gastroenterology is due to a difference in perspectives that the medical student who chooses this specialism adheres to or to the overwhelming evidence for the impact of psychosocial factors on the functioning of the stomach and intestines is left open to debate and further research.

Exploring the function of the gut from a biomedical perspective indicates overwhelming evidence for an interactional relationship between the gut and the brain, which together strive to control the regulation of appetite (see Harrold *et al.*, 2012, for a review). Appetite involves, in its most basic form, the regulation of available energy. Because of this fundamental necessity, every component of an organism's physiology has evolved towards the acquisition, accumulation, consumption and/or conservation of available energy. The biomedical model struggles to contend with the first component of appetite, as the acquisition of energy occurs through an interaction with the environment. Furthermore, energy is finite. Therefore, energy resources have to be shared among those individuals within the individual's family group. This places the role of eating behaviour (Dovey, 2010), and gastroenterology in particular (Drossman, 2010), firmly within the remit of the biopsychosocial model.

Drossman (1998) describes a series of adult referrals whereby large variation in symptoms and their impact are reported by patients presenting to his clinic. The general story indicates that individuals with serious conditions do not always report severe symptoms and those with minor afflictions sometimes suggest that their lives are unbearable. Furthermore, Drossman contends that it is only under exceptional circumstances that a disease is attributable to a specific medical illness. Evidence indicates that within gastroenterology only 10%–16% of patients are able to receive a definitive diagnosis for their symptoms (Kroenke and Mangelsdorff, 1989). For paediatric gastroenterology, little data is available; however, given the evidence, it would not be contentious to assume that the figure for attributing medical illness to symptoms is inflated. Moreover, the impact of the biopsychosocial model is even more pertinent, as the child is not often able to adequately verbalise their symptoms beyond 'my tummy hurts'. This constraint within the assessment processes means the clinician is reliant on the social components (i.e. the child's family) to provide more 'accurate' information on the child's biological and psychological symptoms. Therefore, for the paediatric gastroenterology team, the model would be more accurately termed the *'sociobiopsychological'* or *'sociopsychobiological'* model dependent on which professional is leading the assessment.

Reliance on parents to gain information brings with it additional limitations and variables. Numerous factors from parental anxiety, education level and motivations to familial composition and commitments all affect how the child's behaviour is perceived and thus what is reported to the physician and allied health professionals. Indeed, 'streamed' approaches to the biopsychosocial model may even exacerbate this reporting. Parents may assume what the professional wishes to hear based on their perceptions of what or who the professional is. For example, within a psychological assessment, the parents may focus only on their child's behaviour. This may manifest through implicit or explicit assumptions created by the therapist and/or the family. In contrast, the same family may report that their child is suffering from biological-related symptoms within the medical assessment. This can lead to difficulties in creating a combined formulation for the child and may also lead to confusion when professionals discuss a case after undertaking interviews in isolation.

What can the psychologist provide within the biopsychosocial model?

(*See* also Chapter 2.) From a purely psychological perspective, one factor that has received research attention within paediatric gastroenterology is that of the familial perceptions of 'sickness' and how this impacts on the child's behaviour and the parents reporting of their symptoms (Hyams, 1996). The behaviours that a family member adopts when 'feeling ill' differ markedly. It would appear that the family creates 'rules' around illness and being 'ill enough' (Whitehead *et al.*, 1994). Where some families suggest that any illness merits absence from school, others push the child to continue with their daily activities despite reporting symptoms. Interestingly, this appears to be mediated by the parents' own conditions, as parents with a previous history of functional gastrointestinal disorders are more likely to take their child out of school (Levy *et al.*, 2004). This approach does not appear to alter dependent on whether the child has a chronic or acute illness. In effect, it is rule-governed behaviour that a member of that family is expected to show when ill. This behavioural marker provides the psychologist under the biopsychosocial model with their first target.

The target of the psychologist when first confronted with a child suffering from a gastroenterological complaint is to explore what they habitually do, as a group, when ill. If a strategy of avoidance or escape is found whereby a family member is expected to withdraw, then it is important that the family is aware that illness-related decline is not entirely determined by biological complaints (Hyams, 1999). It should be stressed, and more so in chronic conditions, that the child should be encouraged to maintain his or her daily activities in order to maintain developmental trajectories to meet his or her milestones. Markers within this family therapeutic process would be to actively engage with their anxieties, the parent's or family's history of similar conditions, perception of disability, avoiding maladaptive coping strategies and to instil a programme of positive behaviour support for the child. The child, irrespective of his or her diagnosis, should be given the opportunity, as long as it is deemed age-appropriate and medically safe to do so, to engage in any and all activities. Inability to partake in specific activities should ideally be determined by specific evidence or the child's reluctance. It is important that the family and other professionals involved understand that by maintaining this view throughout it is less likely the child's development will be defined by his or her condition and allow the child to transition following recovery or cope with his or her condition better on a day-to-day basis. One obvious example of this is engaging with protocols that help the child connect with food and oral eating, even if the child is tube-dependent. Obvious caveats would be if there was a risk of aspiration or the child was not physically capable of oral eating. Another example would be that the child should continue his or her education even when reporting symptoms, with the educational programme adapting to the child's needs rather than removing the child altogether. This programme would ideally be a delivered on a generic basis; it is almost irrelevant which condition the child has within the spectrum of gastroenterological conditions, as these factors could potentially severely limit a child's development even if the child's complaint is only acute.

Following this primary objective, the psychologist, under the auspices of the biopsychosocial model, should work on a plan to help the child transition from his or her biomedical complaints once having recovered. The psychological components to the biopsychosocial model within paediatric gastroenterology should focus on preserving developmental milestones as much as possible.

For example, some children with specific gastrointestinal conditions may require being tube-fed. There is a high risk of tube-dependency in children when tube-feeding starts before 12 months of age (Senez *et al.*, 1996; Dello Strologo *et al.*, 1997). It is generally accepted within the biomedical approach that the placement of a gastrostomy tube is warranted if the condition is likely to be chronic. The general premise to this is biopsychosocial in nature, with the placement of the tube helping to limit aversive experience with food (Bazyk, 1990). However, adopting this approach is not without its consequences, unless carefully managed. Aversion to an experience or stimulus can extend from a fearful interaction brought about by consequential causality in the child's learning history that this will cause pain. This pain and oral eating learning history would lead to avoidant-related behaviours through food acting as a punisher to the child and may develop into a phobia. Equally, a child may have an aversion to a stimulus through having little or no experience with an object. Within the context of food and eating behaviour this phenomenon is understood under the term 'food neophobia' (Dovey *et al.*, 2008). Therefore, in this case, the psychologist within the gastroenterology team should focus on gaining a balance between no experience with oral eating and at the same time limiting the potential for aversive experiences (*see* also Chapter 13). Through the act of learning to self-feed, the child will transition through several stages that will naturally desensitise him or her to the tactile or 'messy' aspects of eating and to enjoy the variation in tastes and textures of different foods. The act of desensitisation can be inferred through several different sensory-related disorders that we often see in clinic. These are those that are sensory defensive (Dovey and Martin, 2012) or oral sensory defensive (Dodrill *et al.*, 2004; Dovey *et al.*, 2013). The psychologist, through instilling a behavioural programme embedded within the child's care package, ensures that the tube-feeding regimen remains as a maintenance rather than developing to become a dependency. The main goal of the psychologist would be to ensure that when the time comes for transition to oral eating the child is ready. Ignoring this essential development may lead to a child that exhibits a variety of problem behaviours in the presence of food or when instructed to eat orally. It may even lead to a child that has not sufficiently understood the act of eating and that this behaviour is simply something that others do, rather than what *they* do.

Case Example

'A' was a 4-year-old child with Smith–Magenis's syndrome that had led to severe developmental delay as well as a variety of gastroenterological complaints. At the time of referral the gastrological complaints had been rectified. The behaviours the child exhibited around food and when hungry were specific barriers to prohibit her from successfully transitioning to oral feeding. First, when hungry she would 'point to her stomach'. Staff and family believed that this was a sign that she felt hungry. She also engaged in a variety of other behaviours around food including bruxia following licking any food item, which lasted for several minutes, pretending that anyone who asked her to open her mouth did not exist, engaging in tantrums when presented with foods, and vomiting when encouraged to eat or drink. Closer examination of her behaviours indicated that she did not point to her stomach but to her percutaneous endoscopic gastrostomy tube. She was effectively saying that she wanted the tube, not that she was hungry. She had learnt that the placing of the tube removed the uncomfortable gastric feelings associated with being hungry. Functional analysis of her other behaviours indicated that bruxia was internally motivated (most likely to calm her down when anxious) and that the tantrums and vomiting were escape-motivated. What this case highlights is that a variety of problem behaviours had developed as a consequence of the placing of the tube and that these effectively stemmed from fear brought about by not understanding the necessity of eating behaviour.

This case example also highlights another factor that has been shown to affect transition from tube dependency – that of developmental delay (Bazyk, 1990). It would appear that the vast majority of children are expected to transition from tube dependency to oral eating under a structured programme within 58 days. Those who fail are characterised as having learning difficulties and complex medical problems. For these children, transition to oral eating has not been very successful within the wider literature. Failure to transition to oral feeding in children with gastroenterological complaints has been surprisingly difficult to both define and find within the literature. Within the biopsychsocial model, such behaviours would be any factor that can be directly or indirectly attributed to interfering with either eating or transitioning. By taking this broad perspective to identifying these problems or competing behaviours suggests that the practitioner could potentially be caught in a perpetual cycle of assessment, which may delay intervention.

Implementing a version of Freudenreich *et al.*'s (2010) principles, then advice for implementing the biopsychosocial model in practice would advocate vigilance over assessment. An understanding of the child and his or her family, as well as what is possible within the bounds of current practice pressures, should provide enough information to formulate what could potentially hold the child back in transitioning. Psychologists attached to a multidisciplinary team situated within gastroenterology and who are aligned to the biopsychosocial model should bear in mind the following key statements when practicing. These have been separated into three subsections based on their prospective recipients within the setting.

Other professionals

- The biopsychosocial model suggests that the three components should be internalised within all practitioners involved. Therefore, the psychologist should actively engage with other professionals to highlight and aid understanding of the 'psycho' and 'social' suffix.
- Psychologists should themselves be prepared to learn and fully understand all components of the 'bio' and 'social' components to gastroenterology. Individuals who suggest that these areas are outside of their expertise or that these subjects are not within their 'remit' are not adhering to the edicts of the biopsychosocial model. Instead, they are operating within a behavioural model.
- Psychology is not just practised by psychologists. The biopsychosocial model would suggest that behavioural technologies should be shared and implemented by all of the professionals in the team. It is impossible to know when a psychological-related matter might arise and all members of the team should be prepared for such occurrences and should have the confidence and knowledge to confront them at presentation. A model of referral based on a problem being 'outside of the expertise' of a professional that encounters it is not a model that adheres to the principles outlined in the current chapter.

The family

- Understanding the attitudes, perceptions and behaviours of what a particular family expects from a member who is ill, as well as their members' history of chronic conditions, is integral to ensuring that the child's development is not unduly interrupted or defined by his or her medical condition.
- Helping the family to internalise and learn about the child's condition as well as interpret the 'message' that is being given by the multi-professional team is important. This may be done as an antecedent to engaging with the family through ensuring the professionals have a single story and unified understanding of the child's condition, or it may be done directly with the family after they have been given information by professionals. It is important that the family does not place undue emphasis on any 'bio', 'psycho' or 'social' aspects of the child's condition. Under the biopsychosocial model the family must understand that it is integrated and all are equally important with some moderate variation at different stages of their child's recovery.
- Working with the wider family to understand and explicitly engage with their anxieties, perception of disability, and methods of coping with stress and distress is important. The main objective of this action is to ensure that everyone understands the action of a positive behaviour support model for the child so that implicit beliefs or prejudices do not overtly prohibit

aspects of the child's life that are not curtailed by his or her gastroenterological condition.

The child

- Within the biopsychosocial model, it is important that the condition of the child does not unduly affect his or her development. By creating and instilling a plan that allows the child to engage in mealtimes, toileting and so forth in particular and all activities those children without the condition habitually engage with. It is not enough to simply state this; explicit tasks should be created and adapted for each child.

- Ensure that the child becomes suitably desensitised to food- and toileting-related stimuli in his or her environment in an age-appropriate manner. The child should be actively encouraged to use as much of his or her biology within the bounds of his or her dysfunction.

- Assess, monitor and intervene as early as possible with problematic behaviours as they develop. These are likely to be functional in nature and related to specific events or learned experiences. Alternatively, it is important that a child does not learn the 'wrong' lessons from consequential learning while eating, defecating, and so forth.

SUMMARY

It is difficult to imagine a clinic engaging with children and young people with gastroenterological conditions that would not adhere to the biopsychosocial model. It is equally obvious that a child will transition through bio, psycho and social aspects in relation to which is impacting most on the child's recovery or achieving his or her maximal outcome. However, the most effective application of the biopsychosocial model would be ensuring that all three components are being assessed, with plans developed and implementation of interventions undertaken at the earliest and safest possible moment. To work towards this goal, it is essential that professionals are unified throughout the process. Operating separate clinics and/or interviewing patients or clients in isolation, according to the research base, will undermine the intention of the services to function as an integrated team. All professional groups should be involved at all times and the individual patient care package should control which professional is 'leading' at that particular time.

It would be at this point that theoretical purists would call for reapplication of the principles of the biopsychosocial model and an overhaul of the education of health professionals. History plus pragmatism would suggest that this is not going to be effective. In the absence of internal motivation to change, then an external control is necessary to ensure adoption of the principles outlined within this chapter. The role of the psychologist may be to ensure that the patient/client receives the entirety of the biopsychosocial model. Other professionals struggle to deal with the emotional distress surrounding illness and death and there is an ever-present danger of a 'reversion to professional type'.

This would be to hide within the auspices of the biomedical model and the focus on 'data-derived' deductive reasoning. This is motivated by escape behaviours in the professional who feels out of his or her depth. Such behaviours are understandable but they are not conducive to the best possible healing environment. If the clinic wishes to adhere to the biopsychosocial model, and the evidence-base would suggest they should, it is then imperative that the behaviour of all the individuals involved is aligned to the attitudes of the approach. The psychologist could have a specific focus on the divide between attitude and behaviour and draw attention to it when it becomes pertinent to do so – after all, this is one of the components of psychological therapies. However, this would transgress further upon Engel's intentions when he first formulated the biopsychosocial model. To truly comprehend the biopsychosocial model is to understand that it is applied to the professionals in the setting and not to the patients or clients. It is not for the patients or clients to be happy with the model, only for them to be happy that their wider needs are being met. A professional operating within the biopsychosocial model will find it difficult not to meet all the 'needs' of their patients or clients. In contrast, those operating within the biomedical model will constantly come across distressed children and families claiming that their children are not getting better and their 'needs' are not being met.

REFERENCES

Adler RH. Engel's biopsychosocial model is still relevant today. *J Psychosom Res.* 2009; **67**(6): 607–11.

Alonso Y. The biopsychosocial model in medical research: the evolution of the health concept over the last two decades. *Patient Educ Couns.* 2004; **53**(2): 239–44.

Armstrong A. Theoretical tentions in biopsychosocial medicine. *Soc Sci Med.* 1987; **25**(11): 1213–18.

Atkins E, Colville G, John M. A 'biopsychosocial' model for recovery: a grounded theory study of families' journeys after a paediatric intensive care admission. *Intensive Crit Care Nurs.* 2012; **28**(3): 133–40.

Bazyk S. Factors associated with the transition to oral feeding in infants fed by nasogastric tubes. *Am J Occup Ther.* 1990: **44**(12): 1070–8.

Corsini RJ, Wedding D, editors. *Current Psychotherapies.* 8th ed. Belmont, CA: Thomson Brooks/Cole; 2008.

Dello Strologo L, Principato F, Sinibaldi D, *et al.* Feeding dysfunction in infants with severe chronic renal failure after long-term nasogastric tube feeding. *Pediatr Nephrol.* 1997; **11**(1): 84–6.

Dodrill P, McMahon S, Ward E, *et al.* Long-term oral sensitivity and feeding skills of low-risk pre-term infants. *Early Hum Dev.* 2004; **76**(1): 23–37.

Dovey TM. *Eating Behaviour.* Maidenhead, UK: Open University Press; 2010.

Dovey TM, Aldridge VA, Martin CI. Measuring oral sensitivity in clinical practice: a quick and reliable behavioural method. *Dysphagia.* 2013; **28**(4): 501–10.

Dovey TM, Martin CI. A parent-led contingent reward desensitisation invention for children with a feeding problem resulting from sensory defensiveness. *Infant Child Adolesc Nutr.* 2012; **4**(6): 384–93.

Dovey TM, Staples PA, Gibson EL, *et al.* Food neophobia and picky/fussy eating: a review. *Appetite.* 2008: **50**(2–3): 181–93.

Drossman DA. Presidential address: gastrointestinal illness and the biopsychosocial model. *Psychosom Med.* 1998; **60**(3): 258–67.

Drossman DA. Biopsychosocial issues in gastrointestinal illness. In: Feldman M, Friedman LS, Brandt LJ, editors. *Sleisenger and Fordtran's Gastrointestinal and Liver Disease: pathophysiology, diagnosis, management.* Philadelphia, PA: Saunders; 2010. pp. 121–138.

Drossman DA, Creed FH, Olden KW, *et al.* Psychosocial aspects of the functional gastrointestinal disorders. *Gut.* 1999; **45**(Suppl. 2): 1125–30.

Engel GL. The need for a new medical model: a challenge for biomedicine. *Science.* 1977; **196**(4286): 129–36.

Engel GL. From biomedical to biopsychosocial: being scientific in the human domain. *Psychosomatics.* 1997; **38**(6): 521–8.

Fava GA. Beyond the biopsychosocial model: psychological characterization of medical illness. *J Psychosom Res.* 1996; **40**(2): 117–20.

Freedman AM. The biopsychosocial paradigm and the future of psychiatry. *Compr Psychiatry.* 1995; **36**(6): 397–406.

Freudenreich O, Kontos N, Querques J. The muddles of medicine: a practical, clinical addendum to the biopsychosocial model. *Psychosomatics.* 2010; **51**(5): 365–9.

Harrold JA, Dovey TM, Blundell JE, *et al.* CNS regulation of appetite. *Neuropharmacology.* 2012; **63**(1): 3–17.

Hyams JS. Crohn's disease in children. *Pediatr Clin North Am.* 1996; **43**: 255–77.

Hyams JS. Functional gastrointestinal disorders. *Curr Opin Pediatr.* 1999; **11**: 375–8.

Kahn GS, Cohen B, Jason H. The teaching of interpersonal skills in U.S. medical schools. *J Med Educ.* 1979; **54**(1): 29–35.

Kroenke K, Mangelsdorff AD. Common symptoms in ambulatory care: incidence, evaluation, therapy, and outcome. *Am J Med.* 1989: **86**(3): 262–6.

Levy RL, Olden KW, Naliboff BD, *et al.* Psychosocial aspects of the functional gastrointestinal disorder. *Gastroenterology.* 2006; **130**(5): 1447–58.

Levy RL, Whitehead WE, Walker LS, *et al.* Increased somatic complaints and health-care utilization in children: effects of parent IBS status and parent response to gastrointestinal symptoms. *Am J Gastroenterol.* 2004; **99**(12): 1–10.

Lipowski ZJ. Physical illness and psychopathology. *Int J Psychiatry Med.* 1974; **5**(4): 483–97.

Luthy C, Cedraschi C, Rutschmann OT, *et al.* Managing postacute hospital care: a case for biopsychosocial needs. *J Psychosom Res.* 2007; **62**(5): 513–19.

Melchert TP. The growing need for a unified biopsychosocial approach in mental health care. *Procedia Soc Behav Sci.* 2010; **5**: 356–61.

Putnam SM, Stiles WB, Jacob MC, *et al.* Teaching the medical interview: an intervention study. *J Gen Intern Med.* 1988; **3**(1): 38–47.

Schubert C. Biopsychosocial research revisited. *J Psychosom Res.* 2010; **68**(4): 389–90.

Senez C, Guys JM, Mancini J, *et al.* Weaning children from tube to oral feeding. *Childs Nerv Syst.* 1996; **12**(10): 590–4.

Whitehead WE, Cromwell MD, Heller BR, *et al.* Modeling and reinforcement of the sick role during childhood predicts adult illness behaviour. *Psychosom Med.* 1994; **56**(6): 541–50.

Zimmermann C, Tansella M. Psychosocial factors and physical illness in primary care: promoting the biopsychosocial model in medical practice. *J Psychosom Res.* 1996; **40**(4): 351–8.

PART II

Management and intervention

CHAPTER 8

Management of functional constipation in children

Caroline E Danda and Paul E Hyman

INTRODUCTION

Disorders of defecation are common in paediatric practice. One might expect that clinicians would understand and treat these benign problems with efficiency and excellence. However, understanding and treating disorders of defecation is confounded by the cultural views of clinicians and parents towards faeces. Many adults and children find discussions of bowel habits distasteful, shameful and embarrassing. Consequently, there are misunderstandings that have been perpetuated by poor communications. The purpose of this chapter is to define the disorders of defecation occurring during childhood and to describe how to manage infant dyschezia and functional constipation from a biopsychosocial perspective.

During the past decade an international group of experts met to define symptom-based criteria for the diagnosis of paediatric functional gastrointestinal disorders, including functional defecation disorders. In this context, functional meant that there were signs and symptoms without easily identified disease pathology. Functional symptoms occur within the expected range of the body's behaviour and without tissue damage, like a runner's leg cramp or shivering when you are cold.

Infant dyschezia was diagnosed in healthy infants less than 6 months of age who exhibit at least 10 minutes of straining and crying before successful passage of soft stool (Milla *et al.*, 2006). Functional constipation was diagnosed after at least 1 month of at least two of these features:

1. two or fewer stools per week
2. at least one episode per week of incontinence after the acquisition of toileting skills
3. excessive stool retention
4. painful or hard bowel movements

5. a large faecal mass in the rectum
6. history of large-diameter stools which may obstruct the toilet.

Non-retentive faecal incontinence was diagnosed in a child with a developmental age of at least 4 years with at least 2 months of all these features (Di Lorenzo *et al.*, 2006):
1. defecation into places inappropriate to the social context at least once per month
2. no evidence of an inflammatory, anatomic, metabolic or neoplastic process that explains the symptoms
3. no evidence of faecal retention.

In contrast to the functional gastrointestinal disorders, the term encopresis is a psychiatric term to describe deposition of stool into places inappropriate to the sociocultural context (APA, 1994). Faecal incontinence is a feature of about half the children with functional constipation and all of the children with non-retentive faecal incontinence.

STANDARD MEDICAL TREATMENT

Infant dyschezia

Successful defecation requires two acts: increasing intra-abdominal pressure by contracting the abdominal wall muscles, and relaxing the anal sphincter and pelvic floor muscles. It appears that defecation is an instinct that is present at birth and that this instinct fades over the first weeks and months of life, like the rooting reflex and the Moro reflex (crying in response to a sudden loss of support or perceived falling). When the instinct is gone, the infant must learn to coordinate the act of defecation. The infant's cry increases intra-abdominal pressure, but there is no defecation until the infant relaxes the pelvic floor.

Most infants learn to defecate without much fussing, but a few present to their clinician with symptoms of screaming for 10 minutes or more before passing soft stool a few times daily. These crying bouts alarm parents. The clinician completes a thorough physical examination with the parents watching and concludes that the infant is healthy. The clinician makes the diagnosis of infant dyschezia with symptom-based criteria. No testing is necessary or desirable. Clinicians who prescribe suppositories are making a mistake. With suppositories, the infant learns to defecate with a cue from outside the body, and problems with recognition of internal cues may linger. Infant dyschezia is a transient problem, lasting a few days or a few weeks. Parents should be reassured that the problem will resolve itself (Hyman *et al.*, 2009).

Functional constipation

There are only two reasons why infants, toddlers and children refuse to defecate: either it hurts to defecate or they are afraid to defecate because of past painful or scary events. There are three common triggers for functional constipation. First, when the breastfed child moves to formula or solid food, stools change from soft to hard pebbles that hurt when they stretch the anus. Second, during toilet training when the child learns to hold on to stool to maintain continence, the child may overshoot the goal and struggle to pass a large, hard stool at infrequent intervals. Third, when a child attends school there are social pressures to hold on to stools and avoid having a bowel movement in the school lavatory.

The majority of children with functional constipation have symptoms that begin before first grade. The fear of repeated painful defecation prevents the child from relaxing the pelvic floor when there is an urge to defecate. Instead, infants and toddlers contract their pelvic floors and make every effort to retain colon contents. When there is a patient with functional constipation or soiling beginning later in the first or early in the second decade, there is a possibility of psychological problems or sexual abuse triggering the syndrome.

Functional constipation is diagnosed using symptom-based criteria. Laboratory and X-ray studies are unnecessary in most cases. However, warning signs of disease such as failure to thrive, persistent abdominal distension, unexplained fevers, Down's syndrome, bilious vomiting or spinal dysraphism should prompt a thorough evaluation for disease. Hirschsprung's disease (a lack of nerve innervation of the large intestine resulting in inability to move faecal matter through) occurs every 5 to 6000 births. Functional constipation occurs in about 5% of children. Chances that the next child who presents with constipation has Hirschsprung's disease are slim.

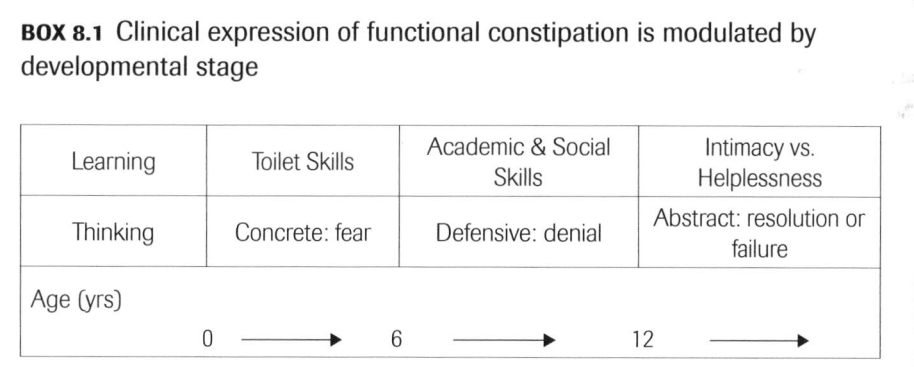

BOX 8.1 Clinical expression of functional constipation is modulated by developmental stage

Learning	Toilet Skills	Academic & Social Skills	Intimacy vs. Helplessness
Thinking	Concrete: fear	Defensive: denial	Abstract: resolution or failure

Age (yrs)

0 ⟶ 6 ⟶ 12 ⟶

When there is a large, hard stool in the rectum, the child becomes irritable and eats less than usual, perhaps to avoid the gastrocolonic response, the increase in colon contractions that accompanies a meal. High-amplitude propagating contractions begin in the ascending colon and propagate to the sigmoid, pushing the luminal contents in front of it and creating an urge to defecate. The normal response is to relax the pelvic floor to allow defecation, but in functional constipation children tighten their pelvic floor muscles because of fear, which creates painful high pressure in the colon. Toddlers demonstrate retentive posturing several times a day, stiffening and straightening their legs while standing with support from a parent, table or chair. Parents will often misinterpret retentive posturing as straining to defecate rather than working to avoid defecation. Older children who deny defecation problems learn to hide their retentive posturing. They may hide soiled underwear and drop dried stool around the house. They often feign nonchalance about bowel movements and avoid discussing the problem.

Everyone agrees that treatment for functional constipation includes education for the child and family, elimination of the rectal faecal mass, and maintenance of soft stools and regular bowel habits (NASPGHAN, 2006). However, there is wide-ranging opinion concerning the best way to achieve these objectives. Regardless of the methods, medical interventions are effective in 50%–60% of children. The response rate to enemas and oral laxatives are no better than to oral laxatives alone (Bongers *et al.*, 2009), suggesting that enemas are not necessary components to treatment. On the other hand, for school-aged children who have failed oral laxatives but are cooperative, a series of enemas may be effective (Collins, 2011).

Education consists of explaining the act and demystifying the legends of defecation. Toxins do not go from the colon back into the body, the colon never bursts, and holding your stools inside is uncomfortable but almost never dangerous. During the first 5 years of life the problem is all about fear. Toddlers and preschoolers have magical thinking and do not know what causes their pain, because they cannot see their anus. When a child is afraid, the pelvic floor cannot relax. If the child cannot relax the pelvic floor, there is no defecation. Constipated toddlers often run away to be alone to defecate. During 5–10 years of age, children may be ashamed of the problem and use denial to defend themselves. The child may report that he or she does not feel an urge to defecate, and does not feel stool leak onto his or her perineum, or smell the leaked stool. In reality, sensation is intact, and the child will feel high-amplitude propagating colon contractions, the 90-second event that triggers an urge to defecate (Firestone Baum *et al.*, 2013). Therefore, the child is employing denial as an escape-motivated behaviour to avoid confronting defecation.

Well-meaning but uninformed clinicians have a higher likelihood to accept the inaccurate child reports and frighten parents by telling them that the colon is stretched and the sensation nerves may have died. Most children will endorse a different reality when confronted. Faecal incontinence occurs because every child must pass gas 20 or 30 times a day. The sensitive anoderm lining the bottom of the digestive tract can tell the difference between the hard stool mass and gas, and the difference between the hard stool mass and liquid. The anoderm cannot discriminate between gas and liquid. Liquid stool leaks out when the child passes gas. The child is mortified.

There are several choices for evacuating the rectal faecal mass. Daily oral polyethelene glycol is often the most benign treatment. Regardless of the size of the faecal mass, daily polyethelene glycol will melt away any impaction over a few days or a few weeks. The advantage of this non-punitive, child-friendly choice is that it helps the child to learn control of the pelvic floor. Many clinicians and parents lack the patience for daily polyethelene glycol, and use repeated enemas until clear. However, repeated enemas may reinforce pain and unpleasantness associated with defecating and do not necessarily help children resume normal defecation. When consulted for a large faecal impaction from functional constipation, the paediatric gastroenterologist may elect to admit the child for an overnight 'clean-out'. Clean-out consists of placing a nasogastric feeding tube for continuous drip of a colon lavage solution at a rate expected to evacuate the stool overnight. Oral midazolam 0.5 mg/kg before placing the nasogastric tube and intravenous needle relaxes the child and provides amnesia for the procedures. If a child has more than one admission for clean-out, it suggests that there is a problem with adherence to the maintenance treatment plan and indicates the need for adjunctive treatment with a psychologist.

Maintenance treatment is daily oral polyethelene glycol titrated to stool consistency like chocolate soft serve ice cream, oatmeal, apple sauce or mustard. Maintenance treatment can continue for many months. In infants and toddlers, the goal is to assure painless defecation until several months after toilet-training is complete. In older children, maintenance treatment may last years. Relapses are common and faecal impaction returns.

Treatment is successful in 50%–60% of children referred to a gastroenterologist. Medical clinicians interviewing patients who have failed previous interventions must assess a number of confounding factors: (1) parent adherence to providing daily polyethelene glycol and an environment conducive to toilet learning, (2) child's motivation to change and (3) child's ability to change. Learning problems and developmental disabilities may prolong toilet learning or prolong functional constipation. Children with Down's syndrome or those on the autism spectrum may require more resources and effort to treat. A medical clinician may find it helpful to consult with a psychologist to evaluate and treat the cause for treatment failure.

COMPREHENSIVE BEHAVIOURAL METHODS

The majority of the cases of toileting refusal result from functional constipation and painful defecation, which interrupt the normal developmental process of toilet training. Children with toileting refusal are more likely to be resistant to medical treatment alone for functional constipation (Taubman and Buzby, 1997). Children with toileting refusal benefit from adjunct behavioural strategies and/or working with a psychologist who can provide more intensive assistance to help children overcome their fear and re-learn or master defecation for the first time. Toilet training is re-learnt as a gradual process that involves shaping and rewarding appropriate toileting behaviours and decreasing fear.

Multiple studies support the efficacy of combined medical and behavioural methods in helping children resume normal bowel habits and functioning (Brazzelli et al., 2011; Brooks et al., 2000; Cox et al., 1998). Comprehensive behavioural methods work in conjunction with appropriate medical treatment.

That is, parents and children first must understand the nature of condition and be assured of painless pooping. Parents of children who fail medical treatment may have a negative view of their child and feel that their child is defecating inappropriately on purpose (Young *et al.*, 1995). The medical clinician provides effective reassurance and dispels myths; particularly that working with a psychologist does not imply the child is emotionally disturbed. Rather, the psychologist helps the child engage in a corrective learning experience for toileting.

Components of comprehensive behavioural methods include skill building, positive reinforcement and bowel recording. Skill building occurs in conjunction with the education the medical clinician has already provided. Education may need to be repeated to the child in child-friendly language. To ensure understanding, the child can then describe what happens when he or she holds back his or her poo. Illustrations and diagrams are especially helpful. In addition, the child may benefit from instruction about basic defecation dynamics. Children with a history of functional constipation may inadvertently learn to tighten both their abdominal muscles and the muscles in their bottom to inhibit and avoid painful defecation (Loening-Baucke *et al.*, 1987). Clinicians educate children about defecation dynamics, or the need to simultaneously relax their bottom while contracting their tummy muscles.

First, clinicians instruct children to practise tightening and relaxing their bottom so the children can feel the difference. Children sit upright in a chair and practise this for a few minutes at a time, usually with a parent to model and make it a pleasant time. Once children learn to relax their bottom, they learn to contract their abdominal muscles. They place a hand on their tummies, take a deep breath in, hold it and push it down, while keeping the lower half of their body relaxed. Children initially practice this simulation daily. Depending on the comfort level of the child, the muscle relaxation and tightening practice starts in a chair, then moves to a toilet when clothed, and then finally unclothed on the toilet. Practising defecation dynamics can also be combined with regular toilet sits (as described later in this chapter), depending on the comfort level of the child with the sitting on the toilet.

Any barriers to toileting, such the recognising the sensation to defecate, the inability to open a door, undress, get on the toilet or communicate the need to go, must also be remedied. Children are educated that the feeling in their tummy, which they sometimes interpret as hurting, is their body's way of telling them it is time to let go of the poo in the potty – it's just a little squeeze. This information is best delivered using a combination of modelling and illustrations of the body. Parents can reinforce a simple word or phrase or gesture children can use to communicate the need to defecate, particularly if they need assistance in undressing or getting onto the toilet. If parents recognise a face a child makes or does, parents simply comment on it ('Oh, it looks like you need to go poop') in a matter-of-fact tone, rather than have the child admit they have to defecate. In order to promote proper defecation dynamics, a footstool is placed in front of the toilet. Having a firm place for a child's feet makes it easier to push. Parents should also consider modelling appropriate toileting behaviour, by announcing that their tummies are telling them it is time to let the poop go and, if comfortable, allow children to remain in the bathroom while the parent defecates so they can see that it is not a painful process. The entire defecation process can also be modelled using dolls.

Once the child has the appropriate instruction in defecation dynamics and barriers have been addressed, goals are set to help children overcome the fear and re-learn toileting behaviours. Goals are set using successive approximation. Target behaviours gradually move the child towards the normal use of the toilet. Hiding or requesting to defecate in a nappy is commonly associated with toileting refusal (Taubman, 1997; Taubman et al., 2003). In these cases, target behaviours might include having the child indicate the need to go, having the child go to the bathroom to defecate in the nappy, eventually moving closer to the toilet and even on the toilet prior to the nappy coming off. Additional goals might include simply approaching toilet, sitting on the toilet with clothing on, removal of clothing for toileting and proper body posture on the toilet. Time spent in the bathroom might be accompanied by reading, music or dolls, or it might be time spent with a parent. The goal is to increase positive associations with and mastery of with toileting behaviours.

When children no longer fear being in the bathroom or sitting on the toilet, regularly scheduled toilet sits are encouraged. To maximise the possibility of defecating during toilet sits, children are encouraged to sit on the toilet upon waking and after every meal to make use of the gastrocolonic reflex that occurs most often at these times. Exercise can also stimulate to gastrocolonic reflex. The maximum time for toilet sits is 5–10 minutes. Boys are encouraged to sit while urinating to increase opportunity to defecate. Sitting on the toilet should be enjoyable as already indicated. Any behaviour that brings a child closer to normal defecation and use of the toilet is rewarded and praised, at least informally, and sometimes more formally with tangible rewards.

Case Study 1

Three-year-old G was born to a 15-year-old woman. He was bottle-fed and enjoyed normal growth and development. However, his daily care was divided between maternal grandparents, the parents of the mother's current boyfriend and the mother. None of G's caretakers recalls when he began to have enormous stools at infrequent intervals. For several days before passing a bowel movement, G became irritable and his appetite decreased. Defecation took several hours, as the terrified toddler attempted to prevent defecation. He became tearful, diaphoretic and he trembled with anticipation of a painful passage of a hard, wide stool. After passing the stool, G returned to his routine of normal eating and play. Several times every day he would stiffen his lower extremities while holding on to a chair or a person. He would not speak, but had a faraway look in his eyes. These stiffening, staring episodes lasted about 2 minutes. G resumed his routine behaviours immediately following these episodes.

When G was 2½ years old, caretakers became alarmed when G's abdomen became protuberant when he was nearing another stool-retentive crisis. They took him to an emergency room where the staff took an X-ray, did a rectal examination, made a diagnosis of faecal impaction and treated G with multiple enemas. This episode so traumatised G that his caretakers were unable to seek further medical care. When G realised a doctor visit was imminent, he screamed with fear and became combative. The multiple household members taking care of G were divided about what to do. They recognised that G needed medical care, but G's behaviour made evaluations impossible. The caretakers tried a variety of over-the-counter treatments for constipation, but treatment was inconsistent.

G presented to Children's Hospital Gastroenterology Clinic when he was 3½. His screaming in the waiting room and hallways was unceasing. The gastrointestinal fellow obtained a history and made a symptom-based diagnosis of functional constipation. She prescribed daily polyethelene glycol. She did not do an X-ray, a rectal exam or even attempt to examine the child at the first visit. She arranged for a follow-up visit in 1 week at the hospital playground, a short distance from the clinic.

At the playground G was initially pensive and suspicious of the examiner. The examiner sat on the ground at eye level with G. Minutes passed as G played on the slides. His family members clustered around the examiner and engaged in an update on G's progress. Finally, G approached the examiner and agreed to allow an exam of his abdomen. Return visits were arranged for the playground every week. With each passing week, the caretakers became more adherent to the medication schedule, and G became less worried about visits to see the examiner. During the next visit G and his family walked from the playground to the waiting room. G allowed the examiner to palpate G's abdomen in the waiting room. During the next visit, G and his family walked to the clinic and with the examiner to a clinic room. At that point, G was still in nappies, but having one or two soft bowel movements daily without fear or retentive posturing. The examiner considered that toilet training might get started because G's fear of painful defecation was over.

When a child has problems with defecation, parents may become very anxious, and family life starts to revolve around toileting concerns to the exclusion of attending to other behaviours. In addition, the struggle over toileting can lead to power struggles and negativity related to other tasks as well. Children may experience feelings of low self-efficacy and competency. As such, it is imperative to provide positive reinforcement and attention to desirable behaviours, both related to the toileting and in general. In general, behaviour that receives attention leads to more of the same behaviour, whether the attention is 'positive' (e.g. praise) or 'negative' (e.g. yelling, lecturing) or whether the behaviour receiving the attention is a desired or an unwanted behaviour. Parents should focus on catching their child being good in a variety of settings, being as specific as possible in their praise (e.g. 'I like the way you put your clothes on yourself; You did a great job choosing your clothes or putting them on by yourself;

Thank you for using your words to ask for help.'). The emphasis on praise for toileting and non-toileting behaviours restores a positive atmosphere in the home and decreases the stress surrounding problems in toileting. As positive reinforcement increases, parents can use punishment or aversive consequences sparingly, if at all. A natural and logical consequence for soiling is to have the child to participate in cleaning up (e.g. put soiled clothing away, gets new clothing, bathe). Above all, a child should never be shamed or embarrassed for having toileting accidents or forced to admit an accident. Rather, a matter-of-fact manner and tone is used when addressing a toileting. The information about parent responding and encouraging successful toileting can be summarised in a handout and provided to the parents (*see* Handout 1 from 'Handouts from Chapter 8' in Part III).

The use of a token economy more formally reinforces and provides external motivation for behaviours that support toileting. Such a reward system is particularly important for children who have denied a problem and do not appear to have internal motivation to change their toileting behaviours. For other children, a reward system makes re-learning toileting more fun. A token economy awards the child a sticker or token for each agreed upon behaviour. The token economy focuses on target behaviours needed for successful toileting (e.g. communicating need to go, communicating soiled underwear so can be changed, participate in clean-up, toilet sits, practising bowel relaxation and tightening) as well as end point (e.g. clean underwear, poop in potty). Sometimes the stickers themselves can be reward enough, particularly for younger children, but often they are 'cashed in' to buy a specific reward. Popular token economies for young children include using a dot-to-dot, making a 'pizza' and adding a pepperoni for each behaviour completed, drawing flowers and adding a petal for each behaviour, and so forth. For the latter reward systems, a larger reward (e.g. stuffed animal, truck or train, special outing) can be earned once a dot-to-dot, slice of pizza or flower is complete. Younger children might also like using a grab bag with a variety of prizes. A child earns a draw from the bag every time a certain number of stickers are earned. Older children may prefer the use of a 'store' that has small rewards (e.g. stay up 10 minutes later, choose dessert, choose dinner, special playtime with parent), medium rewards (e.g. drink or treat at convenience store or at an outing, art or craft activity, book, download music, play date) and large rewards to buy (e.g. friend spend the night, movie, trip to the zoo). Using these types of reward system ensures that there are immediate and short- and long-term rewards to maximise the effectiveness and maintain a child's interest. In addition to the reward routine, recording stool frequency, consistency, volume and accidents can be invaluable in determining appropriate doses of polyethelene glycol, best times for toilet sits, treatment compliance and overall progress (*see* 'Handouts from Chapter 8' in Part III, 3.2g).

Evidence suggests that such behavioural methods can be delivered individually, in a group format and even via the web (Brazzelli *et al.*, 2011; Brooks *et al.*, 2000; Ritterband *et al.*, 2003). The delivery system and intensity of follow-up should be based on each individual child. For example, a child with a difficult or anxious temperament may need more support and a more gradual approach and positive reinforcement for appropriate toileting behaviours than children with other temperaments.

ADDITIONAL STRATEGIES

Biofeedback includes exercises related to the external sphincter muscles, training in discrimination of rectal sensations, and training in the synchronisation of internal and external sphincter responses. Treatment studies have found mixed results, with some evidence that biofeedback training can help children learn appropriate defecation dynamics more quickly (Brooks *et al.*, 2000). However, instruction and modelling of appropriate defecation dynamics can be equally effective (Cox *et al.*, 1998; Borowitz *et al.*, 2002). Given the more invasive nature and lack of availability of clinicians trained in anorectal biofeedback, recommendations for biofeedback should be limited to children with clear problems with defecation dynamics or discriminating sensations, such as those with developmental delays, or those who have failed combined medical and behavioural treatments.

Evidence does not support fibre supplementation or forced dietary changes in the treatment of constipation (NASPGHAN, 2006). In fact, if a child is already constipated and withholding, additional fibre may bulk up the stools further, leading to painful defecation rather than ameliorating it. Getting a child to eat adequate fibre may also result in additional power struggles and negativity, particularly with young children who are often picky eaters and want to assert their independence. At the same time, a well-balanced diet is strongly recommended, as is drinking adequate fluids, as part of a healthy diet rather than as necessary to relieve the encopresis.

ADDITIONAL CONSIDERATIONS

The majority of children with defecation disorders are not emotionally disturbed. Studies using rating scales to evaluate children's emotional and behavioural functioning found that although children with encopresis have more behaviour problems than control children, scores remain within the normative range (Young *et al.*, 1995; Loening-Baucke, 1987; Gabel *et al.*, 1986). Children with toileting refusal trended towards having more difficult temperaments (Blum *et al.*, 1997). Recent studies assessing self-esteem in children with encopresis and soiling have found no differences (Cox *et al.*, 2002; Joinson *et al.*, 2005). Emotional and behavioural issues may be secondary to the functional constipation rather than causing the constipation or problems in toileting. Certainly, being constipated can cause irritability, and struggles related to soiling over which the child may not have control can lead to poor self-esteem and perceived noncompliance.

At the same time, two studies found a higher incidence of mental health disorders in children with encopresis and soiling (Cox *et al.*, 2002; Johnston and

Wright, 1993), indicating that a subset of children with functional constipation and soiling (approximately 25%) may have clinically significant emotional or behavioural problems. The presence of co-existing behaviour problems is often associated with poorer treatment outcome (Levine and Bakow, 1976). In general, children should be able to follow approximately 70%–80% of instructions in a timely manner. If a child has problems complying with general commands, they are less likely to follow through with toileting-specific instructions and toileting may become yet another battle of control. In these instances, children and parents should be referred to a psychologist for parent training and behaviour management prior to embarking on addressing toilet-training.

Children with attention deficit hyperactivity disorder (ADHD) may not attend to body signals as readily as other children or 'wait until the last minute' to defecate or urinate, leading to more soiling accidents (Golubchik and Wiezman, 2009). Children who are impulsive and active may also prematurely leave the toilet after an initial defecation, leading to unintentional stool withholding. Children with ADHD or poor attention to body signals should be reinforced for attending to and recognising body signals for defecation as part of their target behaviours. In addition, the children are also given the expectation that if they do not leave an activity soon enough to toilet, then that activity will be restricted for a period of time. Some case studies suggest that treatment of ADHD with medication helped resolve toileting problems (Bilgic, 2011; Golubchik and Wiezman, 2009).

Case Study 2

T was an 11-year-old male presenting with a previous diagnosis of Asperger's disorder and past history of constipation, withholding and current soiling in underwear. The child had never been fully bowel trained and had a history of withholding bowel movements since the age of 1. Full medical work-up, including colonoscopy, indicated no medical explanation for symptoms of constipation and withholding. T had daily leaks from his bowel, with large accidents happening three to four times a day. Stools were very loose. The current regimen included three capfuls of Miralax and toilet sits every 30 minutes. T expressed motivation to avoid becoming constipated, to avoid pain associated with large bowel movements and to avoid returning to the hospital for an enema. Initial assessment supported a diagnosis of Asperger's syndrome and also indicated difficulties focusing, paying attention and staying on task and some difficulty with overall compliance. Despite some motivation to avoid having a large bowel movement or going to the hospital, he showed limited interest in actual toileting behaviours. T had difficulty cleaning up after himself after having a soiling accident. Although not clinically significant, the child exhibited non-compliance in other areas at home.

Mother and child participated in a five-session protocol, including the assessment. After the initial assessment, psychoeducation was provided about the physiology of defecation, withholding, and defecation dynamics, using illustrations. Information was gathered to develop a token economy. The nurse was also consulted regarding appropriate dosage of Miralax to achieve stools with slightly thicker consistency. We problem-solved with parents about how to assist T in cleaning up (e.g. parent would assist in removing pull-up to decrease amount of faecal matter smeared on body and pre-portioned wipes provided to decrease amount of toilet paper used). Target behaviours included toilet sits, bowel movement in toilet, clean underpants (every hour), wiping bottom on own, initiating clean-up, washing hands and doing muscle relaxation/tightening exercises. Two sessions focused on continued behavioural analysis, developing and adjusting reward system and behaviour plan, and helping the parent learn to monitor and shape small changes (e.g. longer periods for clean underwear, more independence in initiating toileting behaviours). Initially, the child had a meltdown because he had not earned one of the prizes he wanted; however, the next day, he began sitting on the toilet voluntarily and began trying to have a bowel movement in the toilet. He was clearly proud of his accomplishments and agreed to start wearing underwear on a limited basis. The behaviour plan was communicated to the school. Parent and child participated in one booster or relapse prevention session to strategise on how to further address any new problem behaviours that arose or that could happen in future.

LONG-TERM OUTCOMES AND FUTURE DIRECTIONS

Early intervention is much more effective in preventing chronic functional constipation. The longer a child practises maladaptive toilet behaviours, the longer rehabilitation takes. It behooves the experts to train the clinicians in primary care how to recognise and treat childhood functional constipation.

About 10% of children with functional constipation take the illness into adult life with them. Subjects in this longitudinal study had no psychiatric diagnoses. One possibility is that they became hopeless about the problem. Another possibility is that after a decade or more of dilated colon due to withholding behaviour, colon smooth muscle has been replaced by fibrous tissue and the colon no longer moves. In such cases, there should be referral to a centre that performs colon motility testing. For a small group of patients, total colectomy and ileoproctostomy may be a good option. Before surgery it is imperative to train the patient how to use the pelvic floor muscles and anal sphincter, so that retentive behaviours are not repeated. In this operation, the end of the small intestine is moved to the top of the rectum. The rectum serves as a storage area, as it did before surgery. Although diarrhoea may be a problem complicating the first weeks after surgery, adaptation to a normal bowel habit occurs in a few months.

It is little more than a decade since the publication of paediatric Rome criteria, including symptom-based diagnostic criteria for functional constipation. The Rome criteria stimulated new research but have had little impact on primary care physicians. There is an opportunity for education. So much suffering could be avoided by early appropriate interventions.

In addition, functional constipation is more common in obese children and more difficult to treat. Diet is not important for the treatment of functional constipation, but diet is important for preventing functional constipation. There is an opportunity for early intervention to prevent childhood obesity.

SUMMARY

In summary, the majority of children with functional constipation and encopresis are likely to be treated effectively with medical management of constipation combined with basic education and behavioural methods. A small subset may need more traditional psychological intervention combined with medical-behavioural treatment of soiling and toilet-training. Assessment should include evaluation of a child's emotional well-being and temperament, cognitive and developmental level, behavioural compliance and family functioning. Particularly for those children who were not successful with standard medical treatment, clinicians can evaluate emotional and behavioural functioning using a standardised rating scale such as the Child Behaviour Checklist or the Behaviour Assessment Scale for Children. Another broad-band option would be the Swanson, Nolan and Pelham–IV rating scale, which provides specific assessment of behavioural and attention issues and is available in the public domain. Many of the same combined medical and behavioural strategies can be used with children with developmental delays or other physical abnormalities. However, language may need to be modified to be developmentally appropriate and shaping toileting behaviours may involve more steps.

REFERENCES

American Psychiatric Association (APA). *Diagnostic and Statistical Manual of Mental Disorders.* Washington, DC: APA; 1994.

Bilgic A. The possible effect of methylphenidate on secondary encopresis in children with attention-deficit/hyperactivity disorder. *Prog Neuropsychopharmacol Biol Psychiatry.* 2011; 35(2): 647.

Blum NJ, Taubman B, Osborne ML. Behavioral characteristics of children with stool toileting refusal. *Pediatrics.* 1997; 99(1): 50–3.

Bongers MEJ, van der Berg MM, Reistma JB, *et al.* A randomized controlled trial of enemas in combination with oral laxative therapy in children with chronic constipation. *Clin Gastroenterol Hepatol.* 2009; 7(10): 1069–74.

Borowitz SM, Cox DJ, Sutphen JL, *et al.* Treatment of childhood encopresis: a randomized trial comparing three treatment protocols. *J Pediatr Gastroenterol Nutr.* 2002; 34(4): 378–84.

Brazzelli M, Griffiths PV, Cody JD, *et al.* Behavioural and cognitive interventions with or without other treatments for the management of faecal incontinence in children. *Cochrane Database Syst Rev.* 2011; (12): CD002240.

Brooks RC, Copen RM, Cox DJ, *et al.* Review of the treatment literature for encopresis, functional constipation, and stool-toileting refusal. *Ann Behav Med.* 2000; 22(3): 260–7.

Collins RW. *The Clean Kid Manual V: treatments for bowel and bladder control.* Spring Lake, MI: Soiling Solutions; 2011.

Constipation Guideline Committee of the North American Society for Pediatric Gastroenterology, Hepatology and Nutrition (NASPGHAN). Evaluation and treatment of constipation in infants and children: recommendations of the North American Society for Pediatric Gastroenterology, Hepatology and Nutrition. *J Pediatr Gastroenterol Nutr.* 2006; **43**(3): e1–13.

Cox DJ, Morris JB, Borowitz SM, *et al.* Psychological differences between children with and without chronic encopresis. *J Pediatr Psychol.* 2002; **27**(7): 585–91.

Cox DJ, Sutphen J, Borowitz S, *et al.* Contribution of behavior therapy and biofeedback to laxative therapy in the treatment of pediatric encopresis. *Ann Behav Med.* 1998; **20**(2): 70–6.

Di Lorenzo C, Rasquin A, Forbes D, *et al.* In: Drossman DA, editor. *The Functional Gastrointestinal Disorders.* 3rd ed. McLean, VA: Degnon; 2006. pp. 762–5.

Firestone Baum C, John A, Srinivasan K, *et al.* Colon manometry proves that perception of the urge to defecate is present in children with functional constipation who deny sensation. *J Pediatr Gastroenterol Nutr.* 2013; **56**(1): 19–22.

Gabel S, Hegedus AM, Wald A, *et al.* Prevalence of behavior problems and mental health utilization among encopretic children: implications for behavioral pediatrics. *J Dev Behav Pediatr.* 1986; **7**(5): 293–7.

Golubchik P, Wiezman A. Attention-deficit hyperactivity disorder, methylphenidate, and primary encopresis. *Psychosomatics.* 2009; **50**(2): 178.

Hyman PE, Cocjin J, Oller M. Infant dyschezia. *Clin Pediatr (Phila).* 2009; **48**(4): 438–9.

Johnston BD, Wright JA. Attentional dysfunction in children with encopresis. *J Dev Behav Pediatr.* 1993; **14**(6): 381–5.

Joinson C, Heron J, Buyler R, *et al.* Avon Longitudinal Study of Parents and Children Study Team. Psychological differences between children with and without soiling problems. *Pediatrics.* 2005; **117**(5): 1575–84.

Levine MD, Bakow H. Children with encopresis: a study of treatment outcome. *Pediatrics.* 1976; **58**(6): 845–52.

Loening-Baucke VA, Cruikshank B, Savage C. Defecation dynamics and behavior profiles in encopretic children. *Pediatrics.* 1987; **80**(5): 672–9.

Milla PJ, Hyman PE, Benninga MA, *et al.* Childhood functional gastrointestinal disorders: neonate/toddler. In: Drossman DA, editor. *The Functional Gastrointestinal Disorders.* 3rd ed. McLean, VA: Degnon; 2006. pp. 707–9.

Ritterband LM, Cox DJ, Walker LS, *et al.* An Internet intervention as adjunctive therapy for pediatric encopresis. *J Consult Clin Psychol.* 2003; **71**(5): 910–17.

Taubman B. Toilet training and toileting refusal for stool only: a prospective study. *Pediatrics.* 1997; **99**(1): 54–8.

Taubman B, Blum NJ, Nemeth N. Children who hide while defecating before they have completed toilet training: a prospective study. *Arch Pediatr Adolesc Med.* 2003: **157**(12): 1190–2.

Taubman B, Buzby M. Overflow encopresis and stool toileting refusal during toilet training: a prospective study on the effect of therapeutic efficacy. *J Pediatr.* 1997; **131**(5): 768–71.

Young MH, Brennen LC, Baker RD, *et al.* Functional encopresis: symptom reduction and behavioral improvement. *J Dev Behav Pediatr.* 1995; **16**(4): 226–32.

CHAPTER 9

Interdisciplinary intervention in adolescents with rumination syndrome

*Anthony Alioto, Carlo Di Lorenzo and
Michela I Parzanese*

INTRODUCTION

Rumination syndrome (RS) represents the involuntary regurgitation of recently ingested food from the stomach to the mouth, where it is either expelled or chewed again and re-swallowed (Olden, 2001). Within the last few decades, RS was mainly considered a condition found only in profoundly intellectually delayed infants or adults, with an almost equal prevalence in the two groups of 6%–10% (Fredericks *et al.*, 1998; Khan *et al.*, 2000; Thumshirn *et al.*, 1998). More recently, it has become clear that individuals who are otherwise healthy and not cognitively impaired can also be affected by this disorder (Green *et al.*, 2011). RS is considered a rare condition, mainly because of the paucity of published studies and the unawareness of this entity by many physicians. Individuals affected by RS often are misdiagnosed and typically undergo unnecessary extensive, invasive and costly testing (Chial *et al.*, 2003; Talley, 2011).

The diagnosis of RS is based on the recently revised Rome III Diagnostic Criteria for RS, which must include all the following listed symptoms, occurring at least once per week for a minimum of 2 months (Rasquin *et al.*, 2006; Talley 2011).

1. Repeated painless regurgitation and re-chewing or expulsion of food that
   a. begins soon after ingestion of a meal
   b. does not occur during sleep
   c. does not respond to standard treatment for gastro-oesophageal reflux.
2. No retching.
3. No evidence of an inflammatory, anatomic, metabolic or neoplastic process that explains the subject's symptoms.

These criteria must be fulfilled for the last 3 months, with symptom onset at least 6 months prior to diagnosis

Several authors have documented the onset of rumination as occurring around the time of a stressor such as a mucosal disease or viral infection. In addition, stressors such as emotional arousal or a psychological stressor (e.g. loss, abuse) may precede the onset of rumination symptoms and, consequentially, the more 'full blown' RS (Chial *et al.*, 2003; Reis, 1994). The current chapter serves as a review of the existent literature with regard to pathophysiology, assessment and treatment. Building up on this, we describe our interdisciplinary approach to assessment and treatment, and we provide a case example to highlight individual aspects of treatment.

REVIEW OF THE CURRENT LITERATURE
Pathophysiology and medical treatments

The act of rumination is driven by a rise in intra-abdominal and intragastric pressure associated with a relaxation of the lower oesophageal sphincter (LES) leading to the reflux of the gastric content into the oesophagus. Manometric studies demonstrate that when a patient ruminates, there is a simultaneous increase in intraluminal pressure at every level of the gastrointestinal tract that is consistent with an increase in intra-abdominal pressure due to an external event (i.e. the contraction of the abdominal muscles) (Gourcerol *et al.*, 2011). However, the precise mechanisms generating the reflux at the gastro-oesophageal junction during the rise in intra-gastric pressure remain unknown. Once the regurgitant reaches the oropharynx, most patients can make a conscious decision about whether to re-swallow or spit out (O'Brien *et al.*, 1995). Many patients engage in both activities, depending on the social situation and amount of regurgitant at the time of rumination.

Rumination has been conceptualised as a learnt adaptation of the belch reflex and it has been suggested that the gastro-oesophageal junction moves from the abdominal cavity into the thorax creating a 'pseudo-hernia'. Gourcerol *et al.* (2011) have proposed that this displacement of the gastro-oesophageal junction into the thorax, occurring before the rise in intra-oesophageal pressure, explains the mechanism of voluntary regurgitations occurring during rumination. An impaired gastric accommodation and a decreased threshold for triggering a transient LES relaxation also have been demonstrated in adult patients with RS (Thumshirn *et al.*, 1998). In contrast to what occurs in ruminant animals, the presence of an antiperistalsis in the human oesophagus has not been demonstrated.

Some forms of RS may be associated with a phenomenon called 'supragastric vomiting'. Fernandez *et al.* (2010) highlighted the parallel between rumination and this entity, which is characterised by instantaneous vomiting of any ingested solid food or liquid (but not saliva). Similar to the 'supragastric belching' reported in a previous study (Bredenoord *et al.*, 2003), radiographic contrast studies and manometry with impedance tests show that before swallowing a bolus of food, patients take a deep breath, trap the air in the oesophagus, and then regurgitate the material from the oesophagus (Bredenoord et al., 2004).

There is no single medical intervention that has proven efficacy in improving the rumination behaviour itself. Before a diagnosis of rumination is made, many patients are futilely treated with medications aimed at reducing gastric acid secretion or accelerating gastric emptying. Surgical interventions should be avoided in a condition that has a significant behavioural component. Recently, the gamma-aminobutyric acid (GABA)$_B$ agonist baclofen has been shown to reduce postprandial flow events (regurgitation or belching) in adult patients with rumination and supragastric belching (Blondeau et al., 2012). The mechanism of action of baclofen is not completely understood but it has been speculated that it may enhance LES function, reduce swallowing frequency, affect straining behaviour and affect primary vagal afferent nerves (Hornby, 2002; Page and Blackshaw, 1999).

Behavioural and psychological factors and treatments

In the existing literature, several behavioural and psychological factors have been identified as contributing to or maintaining RS, and interventions have focused on amelioration of these factors. First, many authors have conceptualised RS in terms of a learned 'habit,' and therefore have utilised strategies that have been empirically supported in the treatment of habit disorders (Chitkara et al., 2006; Dalton 3rd and Czyzewski, 2009; Green, et al, 2011; Wagaman et al., 1998). This 'habit' may be reinforced by the sense of relief that patients experience after food has been expelled (Fairburn and Cooper, 1984). Consequently, behavioural interventions similar to those utilised in the treatment of habit disorders have been proposed and utilised in the treatment of rumination. Several authors have discussed the importance of providing strategies for improving self-control over the behavioural manifestation of rumination. As rumination involves contraction of the abdominal wall, diaphragmatic breathing has been utilised to provide abdominal muscle relaxation (Chitkara et al., 2006). Other authors have employed progressive muscle relaxation in order to achieve general relaxation (Wagaman et al., 1998) or even as a competing response to the behaviour of abdominal wall contraction or rumination (Chial et al., 2003; Tack et al., 2011). The use of biofeedback has been described by several authors as a beneficial intervention in patients with RS (Chial et al., 2003; Olden, 2001; Soykan et al., 1997), often with minimal description of the specific biofeedback modality employed or the proposed mechanism by which the biofeedback allowed for improvement.

Second, psychological factors have been determined to play a role in the development and maintenance of RS. Many patients experience anxiety simply around the fact that their disorder associated with the vomiting has not been diagnosed, and treatments offered have not proven beneficial. Indeed, accurate diagnosis and reassurance have been found to provide considerable relief to families and patients (Banez and Gallagher, 2006; Khan et al., 2000). Education about RS may allow for a reduction in anxiety, as patients understand that no structural or intrinsic motility problems exist. Accurate description of the disorder also may allow patients to have a more active role in their own treatment.

A subset of patients with RS also has co-morbid emotional difficulties including depression, anxiety, histories of abuse and life stressors (Chial *et al.*, 2003; Soykan *et al.*, 1997). The relationship between emotional state, autonomic nervous system activation and the experience of pain has been widely recognised (Beidel *et al.*, 1991; Fernandez *et al.*, 2010). While these co-morbid conditions are unlikely to be the cause of RS, treatment from a biopsychosocial perspective dictates that co-morbid emotional challenges must be addressed as part of treatment (Guthrie and Thompson, 2002).

THE INTERDISCIPLINARY APPROACH TO ASSESSMENT AND TREATMENT

Building upon the current knowledge base and treatments that have demonstrated empirical support, professionals from several disciplines at our institution developed an inpatient programme for patients with severe RS who often required enteral or parenteral nutrition (see Green *et al.*, 2011).

The sections below provide a more in-depth presentation of the assessment and treatment approach in our inpatient programme.

Assessment
Medical

The diagnosis of RS is based on the previously listed Rome III diagnostic criteria. As with most other functional disorders, rumination is a diagnosis of exclusion, after efforts to identify metabolic, infectious, neoplastic and structural diseases have been exhausted (Hyman *et al.*, 2006). RS needs to be distinguished from gastro-oesophageal reflux, achalasia, gastroparesis and cyclical vomiting syndrome (Talley, 2011) (*see* Table 9.1).

The diagnosis of RS should be easily obtained when the clinical history reveals the timing of regurgitation to be during or immediately after the meal, and the regurgitation to be effortless, factors that should be considered pathognomonic for this condition. Often, the patients describe a preceding sensation of pressure or the need to belch, an increase in nausea, or the experience of some discomfort just before the regurgitation. The regurgitated material is easily recognised as food by the patients, and as having a normal taste. Some patients report other functional symptoms such as heartburn, diarrhoea or constipation and abdominal pain. Weight loss, another prominent feature of RS, can make distinguishing rumination from gastroparesis or eating disorders more challenging (Bredenoord *et al.*, 2003; Di Lorenzo and Youssef, 2010; Hyman *et al.*, 2006).

Radiographic contrast studies and an esophagogastroduodenoscopy usually are necessary to rule out organic diseases that can cause emesis, such as congenital anatomic defects or eosinophilic oesophagitis. A 24-hour oesophageal pH test may be used to identify the pattern of reflux (occurring soon after eating and not at night in patients with RS).

A test that often provides added diagnostic value is gastroduodenal manometry, an invasive test requiring significant technical and interpretive expertise. While manometry is not necessary in order to diagnose RS, it may be beneficial in 'clinching' the diagnosis when the patients, their family or the medical providers still need to be convinced that RS is the appropriate diagnosis (Di Lorenzo and Youssef, 2010). Recent data have shown that the combined use of high-resolution manometry and stationary oesophageal impedance also provide excellent diagnostic accuracy (Kessing *et al.*, 2011; Rommel et al, 2010). The manometric pattern associated with RS is characterised by a rise in intra-gastric pressure (spikes termed 'R waves') generated by a voluntary contraction of the abdominal wall musculature, preceded or coincident with retrograde intra-oesophageal passage of gastric contents that can be detected by impedance (Amarnath *et al.*, 1986).

TABLE 9.1 Differential diagnosis of the most common gastrointestinal conditions presenting in adolescents with recurrent vomiting

Gastrointestinal condition	Vomiting	Gastric emptying	Esophagitis	Prokinetics	Fundoplication
Rumination syndrome	Soon after meals, not at night	Normal or delayed	No	Rarely helpful	Not helpful
Gastro-oesophageal reflux	After meal and at night	Normal	Possible	Helpful	Helpful
Gastroparesis	Hours after eating	Delayed	No	Helpful	Not helpful
Cyclical vomiting	Intermittent	Normal between 'episodes'	May be severe during 'episodes'	Not helpful	Contraindicated
Achalasia	Hours after eating and when lying down	Normal	Mild, due to food stasis	Not helpful	Contraindicated

Clinical nutrition

Prior to the patient's admission, the patient completes a 3-day food journal. Along with this data, the registered dietitian (RD) on the team conducts an initial evaluation of current height, weight and body mass index as well as weight history. The RD calculates the patient's estimated nutritional needs (with regard to calories, protein and fluid), assesses the patient's current and previous intake (either by mouth, total parental nutrition or tube-feeds), and reviews nutrition-related laboratory values.

Psychological and behavioural

After the diagnosis of RS is presented to the family, the psychologist meets with the family and continues the discussion of RS, focusing on what the family has heard from past providers, what they have 'heard' from our medical team during the current visit, and clarifying any misunderstandings. Many families have had past experiences with providers who also have suggested that the symptoms are suggestive of a functional disorder and not suggestive of organic disease. Unfortunately, the family and patient frequently understand presentation of this information as the problem being purely 'psychological' and 'all in their head'. For the most part, these diagnostic suggestions are rejected, and the family presents as wary of the mental health component of the initial evaluation. Families then tend to minimise or even deny any concerns or past history of anxiety and/or depression, eating disorders, involvement with mental health or past abuse during the initial consultation.

RS is discussed in terms of the problem having started with a triggering event that may have caused damage to the functioning of the gastrointestinal tract, but that has since evolved into a learnt behavioural response that feels impossible to alter. It is explained clearly that by 'behavioural,' we are not implying that the patient is purposely engaging in the behaviour (i.e. malingering). Instead, it is a behaviour that the body has learnt and is then reinforced by the feeling of relief after food is expelled. This behaviour can be modified and 'unlearnt'.

The initial consultation also focuses on family dynamics and the reason for wanting to engage in treatment. Occasionally, the duration of rumination symptoms has resulted in significant family stress, with parents more interested than the adolescent in having the adolescent participate in treatment. It is emphasised that the decision to engage in treatment must be the adolescent's. Patient enthusiasm toward treatment should be considered a favourable prognostic sign. Family supportiveness or conflict is taken into consideration in treatment planning.

Several studies have documented the co-existence of functional and psychiatric challenges such as anxiety and depression as well as physical reactivity to stress. Therefore, several aspects of psychosocial functioning are assessed, including personality and psychological variables, somatic symptoms, abdominal pain, functional disability and a behavioural evaluation of the actual rumination and vomiting.

- *Psychological functioning.* To assess general psychological functioning and personality features, patients complete either the *Minnesota Multiphasic Personality Inventory – A (MMPI-A) or the MMPI-2*, depending on their age (Butcher and Williams, 1992). The *MMPI-A/MMPI-2* is a self-report inventory containing 478 (*MMPI-A*) or 567 (*MMPI-2*) descriptive statements on which patients indicate whether each statement is true or false for them. This widely used objective personality assessment provides the psychologist with information about the patient's approach to completion of the measure (i.e. validity), diagnostic and treatment considerations, and aspects of the patient's personality and psychological functioning they may not have wanted to share with the clinician initially.

- *Somatic symptomatology*. Patients complete the Children's Somatization Inventory – 24 (CSI-24), a measure that assesses the perceived severity of 24 non-specific somatic symptoms in the past 2 weeks (Walker *et al.*, 2009). Utilisation of this measure assists in determination of whether the patient's somatic concerns are purely gastrointestinal in nature, or if there are other more general somatic concerns present (e.g. headaches, other pains, fatigue).
- *Abdominal pain*. Patients complete the Abdominal Pain Index (API), a four-item self-report measure, consisting of four items used to assess the frequency, daily occurrence, general duration, and intensity of episodes of abdominal pain experienced in the past 2 weeks (Walker *et al.*, 1997).
- *Health-related quality of life*. Patients complete the PedsQL 4.0 Generic Core Scales (Varni *et al.*, 2003). The PedsQL is a 23-item measure that assesses perceptions of health-related quality of life, encompassing (1) physical functioning, (2) emotional functioning, (3) social functioning and (4) school functioning. The instructions ask how much of a problem each item has been for the past 1 month. Patient reports on this measure enable our team to understand how functional the patient has been with their ongoing rumination problems present. Each subdomain score ranges from 0 (very low quality of life) to 100 (very high quality of life).
- *Observation of eating and rumination*. Perhaps the most important portion of the psychological or behavioural evaluation is the observation of the patient's vomiting. Many patients have shared that nobody has ever actually watched their vomiting occur. Observation is done in a controlled manner. We first ask the patient how much food or liquid typically will result in rumination. While some patients explain that only a sip of water or a bite of food will result in vomiting, others state that vomiting does not occur until they stop eating a meal. In fact, the latter patients often have adopted the mealtime strategy of overeating during meals, anticipating that vomiting will occur, and hoping that at least some food will remain ingested after vomiting, thereby allowing weight to be maintained.

For patients who regurgitate immediately after one bite or one sip of water (i.e. the more 'classic' presentation of RS), their meals are characterised by several trials of one bite or sip at a time and observing the repercussions. Patients are asked to ingest the bite or sip and attend to their abdominal wall contraction upon rumination. This initial session allows patients to increase physical awareness while also allowing the team to observe the immediacy and force of the vomiting. With successive bites or sips of water, patients often are asked to attempt to re-swallow the emesis once it is regurgitated into their mouth to obtain an initial sense of the patient's control over the vomiting. Vomiting is acceptable during the initial evaluation.

For patients who are able to eat a significant portion of food and then ruminate, the observation is somewhat more involved. Before commencement of eating, patients are asked to describe the sensations that typically lead up to or occur immediately prior to vomiting. Patients typically describe an increase in nausea, pain, bloating or 'food coming up their throat'. Prior to eating, patients are asked to give a baseline rating (scale of 0–10) of each sensation they experience prior to vomiting. Utilising a chart with 5-minute increments, patients are asked to take in a predetermined amount of food or fluid (e.g. one ounce of water, one bite of a cracker) and then provide a rating of each sensation every 5 minutes. Rumination waves, belching, re-swallowing and vomiting are noted on the chart as well. These data allow the patient to better understand the relationship between physical sensations and the vomiting behaviour. Similar to the evaluation of the patient with more 'classic' RS, patients are asked to attempt to re-swallow the emesis after one episode of rumination. After vomiting occurs, sensations continue to be tracked for several minutes in order to determine if vomiting results in a reduction of the uncomfortable sensations. By assessing the role of these symptoms in the patient's rumination, the treatment team can focus on amelioration of these symptoms throughout the patient's rehabilitation.

Child life

The child life specialist (CCLS) assesses family and peer supports, interests, and any restrictions that patient may have on daily activity. The CCLS assesses the patient's and family's understanding of the diagnosis of rumination and the goals of the programme. Other factors evaluated include the social impact that the patient's rumination (and possibly enteral or parenteral feedings) have had on social interactions, the patient's expectations for the programme, and their approach to the programme on the initial day (e.g. apprehension, enthusiasm). Finally, the CCLS examines the patient's ability to express their thoughts and feelings in a developmentally appropriate manner.

Massage therapy

During their initial evaluation the massage therapist provides education about massage, the modes of massage therapy often used in treatment and the role of massage in treating rumination (e.g. to 'calm' the central nervous system, to promote increased body awareness and to focus on the abdominal space and help the patient 'open' this space). The initial evaluation also involves some initial massage to assess the patient's openness to massage, their anxiety, posture, palpation and response to touch.

Therapeutic recreation

The therapeutic recreation specialist (CTRS) meets with the patient in order to better understand the patient's typical daily schedule, leisure interests and social supports. The CTRS often asks for the patient's own narrative of his or her past and current medical difficulties. The CTRS assesses the patient's activity level prior to the onset of rumination.

BOX 9.1 Case Study – Brianna, a 16-year-old girl with chronic vomiting

At the time of evaluation, Brianna was referred to our centre for motility testing to better understand her challenges with recurrent vomiting. In addition to understanding the vomiting, she and her family were interested in determining if a gastric pacemaker would provide added benefit.

One year prior to motility testing, Brianna had hip surgery and soon after she had a viral infection that resulted in vomiting several times each day. After the viral infection had subsided, the vomiting continued and became even more frequent over the next few months. Vomiting would last for hours after eating and did not occur during sleep. She had been seen by various specialists, and initially was diagnosed with *Helicobacter pylori* infection and treated with medications that seemed to only exacerbate the vomiting. Because of her rapidly decreasing oral intake, nasojejunal (NJ) feeds were started. An outside gastrointestinal specialist had suggested gastroparesis as a likely diagnosis.

Brianna was an excellent student. Even though she had missed a significant amount of school, she was able to remain caught up and continued with excellent grades. She had been involved in outpatient psychological services for 4 months to assist with coping with her illness.

Medical

Brianna had received very extensive testing, which included multiple radiologic tests (upper gastrointestinal series with small bowel follow through, ultrasound of the abdomen, computed tomography of the abdomen and pelvis, nuclear medicine gastric emptying test, magnetic resonance imaging of the brain), three upper gastrointestinal endoscopies, two colonoscopies and multiple laboratory tests, with the only abnormality being a mild delay in gastric emptying (a common finding in patients with RS due to the constant regurgitation and re-swallowing of the test meal). She had been treated with multiple acid suppressing medications, prokinetic and anti-nausea drugs, and on admission she was receiving amitriptyline at bedtime and ondansetron on an as-needed basis for nausea.

Clinical nutrition

Upon admission, Brianna was determined to be at 95% of her desirable weight, with a body mass index at 19.2. She was receiving all her calories through an NJ feeding catheter. The RD estimated her daily energy and fluid needs to be approximately 2000 kcal/day and 2200 mL/day, respectively. Brianna was determined to have been a healthy eater pre-morbidly with no specific dietary restrictions in place. Her NJ feeds regimen was reviewed and recommendations were made to the team regarding daily management.

Psychological and behavioural

Brianna and her family were engaged in the consultations with the psychologist, and seemed to have a solid understanding of the biopsychosocial interpretation of Brianna's difficulties with rumination. They did not feel that further testing was required to determine any other possible organic diagnoses that would explain her vomiting.

On the CSI-24, Brianna's report yielded a raw score of 17, with only three of the 24 items endorsed as significant (using a cut-off point, dichotomising responses of 0, 1, and 2 and not significant, responses of 3 or 4 as significant). These three items were (1) nausea and upset stomach, (2) abdominal pain and (3) food making her sick. On the API-4, Brianna rated her abdominal pain over the prior 2 weeks and reported that the pain occurred every day, was constant throughout the day, and was rated to be a '4–5 out of 10' intensity. Brianna completed the PedsQL to document her impressions of her quality of life in several domains. With subdomain score ranges from 0 (very low quality of life) to 100 (very high quality of life), Brianna's overall report yielded a Psychosocial Health Summary Score of 72. Subscale scores were as follows: 44 (Physical Health), 70 (Emotional Functioning), 85 (Social Functioning) and 60 (School Functioning). Brianna's report on the MMPI-A yielded a valid protocol. Her report generated clinically significant elevations (i.e. t-score >65) on three of the clinical scales (1, 2 and 3), with the R scale yielding a t-score of 63. Her profile was suggestive of an adolescent who likely responded to stress by developing somatic symptomatology (e.g. headaches, chest pain, vague symptoms) and who may have little insight into her behaviour. Her profile also suggested that she may be non-assertive and may not openly express anger or negative feelings. Individuals who report similarly are able to interact with other people easily and not experience significant anxiety in social settings. Even so, interpersonal relationships may tend to be superficial.

During the initial mealtime observation, it was determined that an intake amount of even one Cheerio was enough to elicit rumination and vomiting. As Brianna focused on re-swallowing and keeping down the Cheerio, data collection included tracking the number of rumination waves over the initial mealtime (two 5-minute trials) to obtain a baseline. Over the course of the first 5 minutes, slight abdominal contractions were seen, but no regurgitation into the mouth was observed. Another Cheerio was ingested, rumination into the mouth occurred several times, but Brianna was able to avoid overt vomiting. She was asked to track waves that occurred over the next few hours, to increase her awareness of how the rumination contractions diminish over time (for this first session, waves terminated at around the 2-hour point).

Child life

Evaluation by the CCLS revealed that Brianna had many friends and family providing support during the hospitalisation. She had multiple diversionary items available to her, including her laptop computer and phone. No specific concerns were noted regarding coping with hospitalisation.

Massage therapy

The massage therapist focused the initial evaluation on massaging the lower extremities and determined that all of Brianna's muscle groups were tense upon palpation. Several massage strategies were introduced during the initial evaluation, including muscular kneading, circular friction, passive touch and deep tissue rocking. The therapist found Brianna to be content, able to rest quietly and open to receiving massage. Brianna verbalised relief at the end of the session.

Therapeutic recreation

The CTRS met with Brianna to obtain her narrative of her medical history, current challenges and functional limitations. Brianna shared that since commencement of her rumination and weight loss, she found herself unable to participate in age-appropriate activities because of loss of strength and stamina. She experienced continuous abdominal pain and nausea throughout the day. Brianna was only able to attend school for half a day because of these reductions in functionality. At times, she has needed to utilise a wheelchair.

Treatment
Medical

Although RS was considered benign in the past (Levine *et al.*, 1983) it is now clear that it can result in serious health risks including weight loss, dehydration, and electrolyte abnormalities (Fredericks *et al.*, 1998). Oftentimes, it is necessary for adolescents to receive enteral or parenteral nutrition to restore excessive caloric depletion prior to any intervention (Khan *et al.*, 2000).

TABLE 9.2 Common symptoms reported by patients with rumination syndrome and medications utilised

Symptom	Medication
Abdominal pain	Anticholinergics (hyoscyamine, dicyclomine)
Nausea	Ondansetron
Early satiety	Cyproheptadine
Postprandial discomfort	Amitriptyline, cyproheptadine, iberogast, intra-pyloric injection of botulin toxin
Excessive belching	Baclofen
Bloating or distension	Cycles of intraluminal antibiotics to treat and prevent possible bacterial overgrowth
Constipation	Stool softeners or stimulant laxatives as needed
Poor sleep	Amitriptyline, cyproheptadine, melatonin

As described earlier, there is no single medical intervention that has proven efficacy in improving the rumination behaviour itself. Even so, there is a role for drug treatment in many patients with this condition. The use of medications can be beneficial in improving symptoms that either co-exist with or precede the act of rumination. Table 9.2 summarises the medications that we often use as adjuvants to the behavioural intervention. The medical team also focuses on the management of the patient's fluids and tube-feeds, and works along with the team in determining the appropriate rate at which to reduce these as the patient makes progress with oral intake.

Clinical nutrition

During the admission, enteral feedings are monitored and recommendations made throughout the admission. The patient's oral caloric intake and fluid intake is recorded daily and information is provided to the medical team with regard to changes in enteral feedings. As the patient progresses in treatment, and foods for mealtimes are selected based on calories, the RD provides patient education regarding calorie counting and provides calorie counts for all foods on the hospital menu. Finally, the RD works with the patient and family regarding calorie and fluid goals for discharge, along with recommendations for eating that meet the patient's particular dietary needs (e.g. vegetarianism, specific food allergies).

Psychological and behavioural

Similar to the discussion and explanation of RS at the time of the initial assessment, these issues are discussed once again in detail. The topics are revisited not only to keep the important aspects of the disorder salient, but also to tie these concepts to the aspects of treatment introduced.

FEEDING INTERVENTION

Meals are completed in the patient's room, and patients may opt to eat in their beds or in a chair. At the time of the first treatment 'meal' (after the observation meal), it is explained that no emesis basins, cups, bottles or other items that have been used for emesis capture in the past are allowed to be present. This intervention is important, as it removes the visual 'cue' to vomit, and removes any 'safety net' that the patient may have felt was present when the urge to vomit presented itself.

Patients have three time periods per day set aside to focus on feeding treatment. Mealtimes are designed to be 2 hours in duration to allow for late-arriving meals and so that patients do not feel rushed during their feeding treatment. The initial use of small feeding trials seems to provide several benefits to patients. First, frequent, small eating or drinking trials allow for repeated re-exposure to a stressful stimulus (i.e. actual eating or drinking and/or anticipatory anxiety about eating or drinking). Second, smaller amounts of food and fluid are more manageable as patients focus on re-swallowing their food and not expelling the emesis. Finally, this measured approach provides patients with a sense of self-efficacy as they make progress and have successful experiences with keeping food down.

During the mealtime, patients are prescribed specific amounts or bites of the particular food item and/or specific quantities of fluid to consume during four

5-minute intervals. This is done to allow the patient to begin pacing themselves during meals, and to manage the abdominal wall contractions/rumination with gradually increasing amounts of food or fluid.

Patients complete a tracking sheet of their trials as they work on their meal, recording data such as the number of rumination 'waves' that occur during each 5-minute interval, a rating of specific sensations on a 0–10 scale (e.g. bloating), and whether or not the food remained 'down' by the end of the interval or if it was vomited 'out.' Typically, patients complete four or five 5-minute trials during a mealtime session.

For patients who have difficulty keeping very little down, starting with simple carbohydrate foods (e.g. crackers, cereals) and gradually working up to more 'complex' foods (e.g. pancakes, sandwiches) allows patients to perceive their own progress while starting with foods that are easier to digest. For patients who are able to eat larger amounts initially, most foods on the hospital menu are permitted, but the focus is on the amount of these foods. For all patients, food and fluid trials are integrated.

Teaching patients to re-swallow emesis that has gone into the mouth (but not expelled) is an important component of the intervention. After the rumination behaviour, expulsion of the food or fluid typically results in a reduction of the unpleasant symptoms that preceded the rumination (e.g. nausea, pain). After time, the expulsion of the food may develop a reinforcing quality (Lang *et al.*, 2011; Rapp and Vollmer, 2005). Re-swallowing of the ruminated food allows the patient to recognise that even with the food remaining in the stomach, the unpleasant symptoms diminish on their own. In addition, re-swallowing allows patients to experience a sense of 'control' over a behaviour that has, up until now, felt to be completely uncontrollable.

As patients work on the goal of keeping increasingly larger amounts of food and fluid down, strategies for self-management are taught and practised. Many authors have promoted the use of diaphragmatic breathing as an integral part of treatment for RS. At our centre, diaphragmatic, effortless breathing is taught as well. Even though some patients may 'feel' and report they are relaxed, their sense of relaxation may or may not correlate with autonomic nervous system 'relaxation.' Therefore, biofeedback is utilised to assist in mastery of diaphragmatic, effortless breathing as well as autonomic nervous system self-regulation, with modalities of feedback typically including heart rate variability and skin temperature.

While many patients find the use of effortless breathing beneficial, others find effortless breathing difficult to achieve but discover that different strategies allow for support during mealtimes. Adjunctive strategies have included engagement in video games, crafts, listening to music, reading children's books aloud, or even ambulating around the hospital unit during mealtimes.

PSYCHOLOGICAL SUPPORT

In addition to the behavioural aspects of the treatment, psychological issues are addressed as well. On a more general level, we address coping with hospitalisation, stressors in the patient's life (including internal stressors such as perfectionistic tendencies) and functional disability. On a more specific level, the MMPI-A or MMPI-2 is reviewed with the patient to provide a 'jumping off' point for discussion of self-reported difficulties such as anxiety, depression or somatisation in response to stress. Often, issues become more salient during the course of treatment as the patient and family become more comfortable with the team, and as the team observes the patient's response to the treatment (e.g. becoming overly distressed when mealtimes do not go 'perfectly').

Child life

Child life interventions during the hospitalisation typically focus on adjustment to the hospital setting and self-expression. The CCLS assists in providing predictability to the patient's admission by collaborating with the team and developing the daily schedule of therapies for the patient's entire inpatient admission. The CCLS also provides the patient with diversionary activities to utilise during mealtimes.

Massage therapy

The massage therapist typically focuses on strategies specific to the patient's needs (e.g. co-existing headaches) as well as the more general goals of assistance with relaxation, nausea, pain, and abdominal wall contractions. Common modes of therapy utilised include Swedish massage, acupressure, craniosacral therapy, healing touch, myofacial, trigger point, and aromatherapy. Self-care strategies are taught and practised.

Therapeutic recreation

During treatment, the CTRS focuses on gross motor skills, ambulation, and improving the patient's stamina. Breathing exercises and stretching are utilised to achieve many of these goals as well as to address the patient's specific challenges with the rumination behaviour.

BOX 9.2 Brianna's interdisciplinary treatment protocol

Medical

During her admission, Brianna continued to take the medications she found helpful prior to the hospitalisation (amitriptyline at bedtime, and ondansetron on an as-needed basis). We also added dicyclomine and polyethylene glycol 3350 on an as-needed basis for abdominal cramping and constipation, respectively. Intravenous fluids were started and NJ feedings were decreased to half the previous volume in order to increase hunger while keeping her hydrated. After 5 days of treatment the feedings were discontinued and the feeding tube was removed on the seventh day of the hospitalisation. On the day of admission her weight was 54.4 kg and on the day of discharge it was 54.9 kg.

Clinical nutrition

Throughout treatment, recommendations were made with regard to the gradual weaning from NJ feeds. As Brianna progressed, calorie counting was taught so that Brianna could begin making her own selections for meals. Other topics discussed with Brianna included food selections (especially around vegetarian meals), portion sizes, selection of foods at home, daily caloric goals and how to maintain her goals in the home and school settings.

Psychological and behavioural

Initial 'meals' consisted of four 5-minute trials of one Cheerio ingested at the start of each trial. As Brianna made progress keeping down this amount, trials increased in size (e.g. two Cheerios per trial) and variety, and fluids were added to each trial (e.g. two Cheerios and one ounce of water).

Within 4 days of treatment, Brianna was eating approximately 1000 kcal/day. With this progress, the focus during mealtimes transitioned to calorie-based selections (e.g. selection of any foods and drinks that would total approximately 300 calories for the lunch meal). For her final day in the programme, Brianna was requested to eat any foods she wanted, from either inside or outside of the hospital, as long as she was monitoring her caloric and fluid intake. Rumination contractions did continue, but she was able to manage these well with no emesis. Throughout treatment, abdominal contractions were noted to be less intense, less frequent and continuing for less time after termination of the meal.

During her mealtimes, Brianna utilised several biofeedback apparatuses and modalities. Aspects of respiration and skin temperature (a proxy measure of blood flow and cardiovascular response) were self-regulated utilising the ProComp Infiniti hardware and BioGraph Infiniti software from Thought Technology Ltd, Montreal, Canada. To further develop self-regulation training, Brianna utilised the Alive and Dual Drive software developed by Somatic Vision, Encinitas, California. Distraction strategies such as reading aloud and ambulation soon after eating were introduced. As treatment progressed, Brianna was asked to select the strategies that were most useful to her.

In addition to the focus on feeding therapies, the psychology postdoctoral fellow met regularly with Brianna in a more 'traditional' psychotherapy role. Utilising her MMPI-A profile as way of identifying possible areas for discussion, Brianna was able to discuss stressors in her life and her own recognition of how her body responds to these stressors.

Child life

The CCLS focused sessions on self-expression utilising both discussions as well as structured activities. Of note was the creation of a plaster of Paris 'cast mask' in which Brianna cut and pasted words on the inside of the mask that represented her challenges and struggles prior to admission on the inside, and words that represent her recent successes on the outside. Therapy was provided three times a week.

Massage therapy

The massage therapist met with Brianna two to three times a week. During the massage session, the massage therapist utilised a variety of methods to assist with pain, general relaxation and specific relaxation of the abdominal wall, including Swedish massage, craniosacral massage, acupressure, healing touch and aromatherapy.

Therapeutic recreation

The CTRS focused treatment on increasing Brianna's stamina as well as assisting her ability to walk (as Brianna seemed to have developed a foot-shuffling gait pattern during her period of illness). In addition to increasing stamina, the CTRS utilised stretching exercises on a Bosu ball and reinforced diaphragmatic breathing exercises. Therapy was provided three times per week.

Brianna was discharged 9 days after admission. At the time of discharge, she was able to keep down enough calories and fluid to maintain her weight and hydration. Some rumination waves did continue to occur, but Brianna felt that they were easily managed.

WHAT WE HAVE LEARNT

Over the years of working with diverse patients with severe RS, our group has had the opportunity to learn from our successes as well as our challenges. Several suggestions are offered based on these experiences.

1. Recognise that each patient with RS has a different presentation. The differences may be with regard to the specific types or amounts of food or fluid that trigger the rumination, the timing and intensity of rumination, symptoms that accompany the rumination, and the way in which rumination is managed by the patient.

2. Observation of the rumination is crucial. Given the aforementioned differences in the rumination behaviour and presentation, simply understanding that the patient has 'rumination syndrome' does not allow for development of a specific treatment plan that meets that patient's needs.

3. Education is an especially important component of treatment. Education involves not only presenting the diagnosis of rumination but also explaining it in terms of the biopsychosocial model, discussing past diagnoses and how they relate, and discussing other more organic 'rule outs' that already have been considered. The diagnosis of RS must be clear, and the patient and family must be on the 'same page' in order to engage and progress in treatment. In our experience, the patient's and/or family's continued search and consideration of organic causes for the vomiting is a poor prognostic indicator.

4. Patient and family acceptance of the diagnosis of RS is essential to the success of treatment. If there is still a doubt about other conditions being responsible for the symptoms, a diagnostic test such as gastroduodenal

manometry or oesophageal manometry with impedance are justified to convince beyond any doubt that the child indeed has RS.

5. Never underestimate the family's ability to obtain information about RS prior to and during your work with the family. The Internet has allowed families to have unfettered access to scholarly journals, postings about RS and even the ability to interact with other patients who have received the diagnosis of RS through blogs and chat rooms. While some information may prove to be relevant and useful, much information is incorrect, not appropriate to the case at hand (e.g. reading about rumination in young children with developmental disabilities), and may prove to be detrimental to the family's understanding of the diagnosis and treatment.

6. Addressing other somatic symptoms through targeted use of pharmaco-therapy is very important. Constipation, sleeping difficulties, headaches, dizziness and other functional symptoms are very common in adolescents with RS and may interfere with the success of treatment by distracting the care providers and the patients. Often the act of rumination occurs in response to abdominal discomfort (cramping, early satiety, nausea, bloat-ing). Alleviating such symptoms may increase the patient confidence in the treatment plan.

7. Be patient. All of our patients have progressed at different rates. While some patients demonstrate improvement on the first day of treatment, others may take several days before any signs of improvement are noted.

SUMMARY

We have outlined in this chapter the results of several years of diligent work with an enthusiastic group of medical providers committed to improving the care of patients with RS. RS in adolescents should be easy to diagnose and it is treatable. Unfortunately, we continue to encounter many patients with RS who have been misdiagnosed and have been ineffectively treated. Clearly, much work needs to be done to educate medical providers on the pathophysiology, clinical presentation and appropriate interventions in patients with this condi-tion. Rehabilitating a patient with RS to a full oral diet requires a tremendous investment of time and energy from a committed team of providers. Even so, in our careers we rarely have experienced as much personal gratification as we have in observing adolescents going from not being able to keep down one Cheerio to eating a full meal without vomiting in a matter of days.

REFERENCES

Amarnath RP, Abell TL, Malagelada JR. The rumination syndrome in adults: a characteristic manometric pattern. *Ann Intern Med.* 1986; **105**(4): 513–18.

Banez GA, Gallagher HM. Recurrent abdominal pain. *Behav Modif.* 2006; **30**(1): 50–71.

Beidel DC, Christ MG, Long PJ. Somatic complaints in anxious children. *J Abnorm Child Psychol.* 1991; **19**(6): 659–70.

Blondeau K, Boecxstaens V, Rommel N, *et al.* Baclofen improves symptoms and reduces postprandial flow events in patients with rumination and supragastric belching. *Clin Gastroenterol Hepatol.* 2012; **10**(4): 379–84.

Bredenoord AJ, Chial HJ, Camilleri M, *et al.* Gastric accommodation and emptying in evaluation of patients with upper gastrointestinal symptoms. *Clin Gastroenterol Hepatol.* 2003; **1**(4): 264–72.

Bredenoord AJ, Weusten BL, Sifrim D, *et al.* Aerophagia, gastric, and supragastric belching: a study using intraluminal electrical impedance monitoring. *Gut.* 2004; **53**(11): 1561–5.

Butcher JN, Williams CL. *MMPI-2/MMPI-A: essentials of interpretation.* Minneapolis: University of Minnesota Press; 1992.

Chial HJ, Camilleri M, Williams DE, *et al.* Rumination syndrome in children and adolescents: diagnosis, treatment, and prognosis. *Pediatrics.* 2003; **111**(1): 158–62.

Chitkara D, Van Tilburg M, Whitehead WE, *et al.* Teaching diaphragmatic breathing for rumination syndrome. *Am J Gastroenterol.* 2006; **101**(11): 2449–52.

Dalton WT 3rd, Czyzewski D. Behavioral treatment of habitual rumination: Case reports. *Dig Dis Sci.* 2009; **54**(8): 1804–7.

Di Lorenzo C, Youssef NN. Diagnosis and management of intestinal motility disorders. *Semin Pediatr Surg.* 2010; **19**(1): 50–8.

Fairburn CG, Cooper PJ. Rumination in bulimia nervosa. *BMJ.* 1984; **288**(6420): 826–7.

Fernandez S, Aspirot A, Kerzner B, *et al.* Do some adolescents with rumination syndrome have 'supragastric vomiting'? *J Pediatr Gastroenterol Nutr.* 2010; **50**(1): 103–5.

Fredericks DW, Carr JE, Williams WL. Overview of the treatment of rumination disorder for adults in a residential setting. *J Behav Ther Exp Psychiatry.* 1998; **29**(1): 31–40.

Gourcerol G, Dechelotte P, Ducrotte P, *et al.* Rumination syndrome: when the lower oesophageal sphincter rises. *Dig Liver Dis.* 2011; **43**(7): 571–4.

Green AD, Alioto A, Mousa H, *et al.* Severe pediatric rumination syndrome: Successful interdisciplinary inpatient management. *J Pediatr Gastroenterol Nutr.* 2011; **52**(4): 414–18.

Guthrie E, Thompson D. Abdominal pain and functional gastrointestinal disorders. *BMJ.* 2002; **325**(7366): 701–3.

Hornby PJ, Abrahams TP, Partosoedarso ER. Central mechanisms of lower esophageal sphincter control. *Gastroenterol Clin North Am.* 2002; **31**(4): 11–20.

Hyman PE, Milla PJ, Benninga MA, *et al.* Childhood functional gastrointestinal disorders: neonate/toddler. *Gastroenterology.* 2006; **130**(5): 1519–26.

Kessing BF, Govaert F, Masclee AA, *et al.* Impedance measurements and high-resolution manometry help to better define rumination episodes. *Scand J Gastroenterol.* 2011; **46**(11): 1310–15.

Khan S, Hyman PE, Cocjin J, *et al.* Rumination syndrome in adolescents. *J Pediatr.* 2000; **136**(4): 528–31.

Lang R, Mulloy A, Giesbers S, *et al.* Behavioral interventions for rumination and operant vomiting in individuals with intellectual disabilities: a systematic review. *Res Dev Disabil.* 2011; **32**(6): 2193–205.

Levine DF, Wingate DL, Pfeffer JM, *et al.* Habitual rumination: a benign disorder. *BMJ.* 1983; **287**(6387): 255–6.

O'Brien MD, Bruce BK, Camilleri M. The rumination syndrome: clinical features rather than manometric diagnosis. *Gastroenterology.* 1995; **108**(4): 1024–9.

Olden K. Rumination. *Curr Treat Options Gastroenterol.* 2001; **4**(4): 351–8.

Page AJ, Blackshaw LA. GABA(B) receptors inhibit mechanosensitivity of primary afferent endings. *J Neurosci.* 1999; **19**(19): 8597–602.

Rapp JT, Vollmer TR. Stereotypy I: a review of behavioral assessment and treatment. *Res Dev Disabil.* 2005; **26**(6): 527–47.

Rasquin A, Di Lorenzo C, Forbes D, *et al.* Childhood functional gastrointestinal disorders: child/adolescent. *Gastroenterology.* 2006; **130**(5): 1527–37.

Reis S. Rumination in two developmentally normal children: case report and review of the literature. *J Fam Pract.* 1994; **38**(5): 521–3.

Rommel N, Tack J, Arts J, *et al*. Rumination or belching-regurgitation? Differential diagnosis using oesophageal impedance-manometry. *Neurogastroenterol Motil.* 2010; **22**(4): e97–104.

Soykan I, Chen J, Kendall BJ, *et al*. The rumination syndrome: clinical and manometric profile, therapy, and long-term outcome. *Dig Dis Sci.* 1997; **42**(9): 1866–72.

Tack J, Blondeau K, Boecxstaens V, *et al*. Review article: the pathophysiology, differential diagnosis, and management of rumination syndrome. *Aliment Pharmacol Ther.* 2011; **33**(7): 782–8.

Talley NJ. Rumination syndrome. *Gastroenterol Hepatol (N Y).* 2011; **7**(2): 117–18.

Thumshirn M, Camilleri M, Hanson RB, *et al*. Gastric mechanosensory and lower esophageal sphincter function in rumination syndrome. *Am J Physiol.* 1998; **275**(2 Pt. 1): G314–21.

Varni JW, Burwinkle TM, Seid M, *et al*. The PedsQL 4.0 as a pediatric population health measure: feasibility, reliability, and validity. *Ambul Pediatr.* 2003; **3**(6): 329–41.

Wagaman J, Williams D, Camilleri M. Behavioral intervention for the treatment of rumination. *J Pediatr Gastroenterol.* 1998; **27**(5): 596–8.

Walker LS, Beck JE, Garber J, *et al*. Children's somatization inventory: Psychometric properties of the revised form (CSI-24). *J Pediatr Psychol.* 2009; **34**(4): 430–40.

Walker LS, Smith CA, Garber J, *et al*. Development and validation of the Pain Response Inventory for children. *Psychol Assess.* 1997; **9**: 392–405.

CHAPTER 10

Autism spectrum disorders and gastrointestinal problems: current state of the research and implications for practice

*Keith E Williams, Douglas G Field
and Chandran P Alexander*

INTRODUCTION

Numerous studies have examined the presence of gastrointestinal problems in samples of children with autism spectrum disorders (ASDs). While some have speculated that these gastrointestinal problems are the result of features associated with ASD (e.g. limited diet, low muscle tone), others have speculated that the gastrointestinal problems and the underlying disease responsible for the gastrointestinal problems are causally related to, or even responsible for, the behavioural symptoms definitive of an ASD. This chapter will review the research involving gastrointestinal problems and ASDs, evaluate theories concerning how they are related, and discuss implications for practice.

THE RELATION BETWEEN DIET AND AUTISM

Examining grain consumption during the Second World War, F Curtis Dohan noted that the prevalence of schizophrenia was negatively correlated with the consumption of grains (Dohan, 1966) and further observed that some societies, whose diets were free of wheat, barley and rye, experienced fewer and less severe cases of schizophrenia (Dohan *et al.*, 1984). He speculated that coeliac disease, an immune-mediated enteropathy triggered by the ingestion of foods containing gluten, could be causally linked to schizophrenia (Dohan, 1966). He further theorised that genetic abnormalities permitted exorphins or the opioid peptides from some food proteins, especially gluten and casein, a milk protein, to move from the gut to the brain and cause symptoms of schizophrenia (Dohan, 1988). This theory was expanded to autism when Mary Goodwin and her colleagues noted a boy with coeliac disease was among a group of 65 children with autism whose communication skills were being studied (Goodwin and Goodwin, 1969). In a follow-up study, Goodwin and her colleagues studied 15 children with autism and found that seven of these children exhibited gastrointestinal symptoms including diarrhoea, abnormal stools, constipation, milk intolerance and, in one child, a diagnosis of coeliac disease (Goodwin et al., 1971). A connection between autism and opioid peptides derived from gluten and casein was also proposed after laboratory animals exhibited 'autistic behaviours' after being injected with small amounts of opioid peptides (Panksepp, 1979).

The Opioid Excess Theory has been refined and it has been hypothesised that the opioid peptides derived from gluten and casein are able to enter the bloodstream through the lumen of the intestine due to two biological deficits, inadequate production of enzymes to digest gluten and casein and increased gut permeability (Shattock et al., 1990). The presence of increased urinary peptides has been used to demonstrate the inadequate production of digestive enzymes in children with ASDs. While some studies have shown support for the Opioid Excess Theory by either demonstrating children with ASDs have higher urinary peptide levels than children without special needs (Cade et al., 2000) or showing decreases in urinary peptide levels after dietary restriction of gluten and casein (Reichelt et al., 1990), other studies have found no evidence of exogenous or endogenous peptides in the urine of children with ASDs (Cass et al., 2008; Le Couteur et al., 1988). The other biological deficit hypothesised by the Opioid Excess Theory, increased gut permeability, has been measured by permeability testing with a few studies showing increased permeability in children with ASDs (D'Eufemia et al., 1996; de Magistris et al., 2010). Again, evidence for the presence of this biological deficit is mixed, with several studies finding no difference in intestinal permeability between children with and without ASDs (Kemperman et al., 2008; Robertson et al., 2008).

The notion that the peptides resulting from the incomplete digestion of gluten and casein have adverse effects on brain maturation, causing social deficits in children with autism (Reichelt et al., 1991, 1997) has resulted in a dietary intervention, the gluten-free, casein-free diet, to correct this problem. A recent systematic review of the literature involving gluten-free and casein-free (GFCF) diets in the treatment of ASDs was conducted and the authors concluded that the lack of empirical evidence and the adverse consequences associated with the use of the diet did not justify its use unless the child experiences acute behavioural changes seemingly associated with the diet, or medical testing confirms the presence of an allergy or intolerance to gluten or casein (Mulloy et al., 2010, 2011). In their review, Mulloy and colleagues critically examined 19 studies in which GFCF diets were used with children with ASDs, including the research design and methodology used by each study. Multiple weaknesses including the lack of a research design, problems with sampling, a failure to measure the accuracy of intervention implementation, and a lack of inter-observer reliability for the measures of behaviour, were commonly found in the methodology of most of these studies. Of note, the three studies evaluated to be the most methodologically sound all produced negative results. The conclusion reached by this review was similar to the findings of a Cochrane review, which also found empirical evidence for the GFCF diet to be lacking (Milward *et al.*, 2009). A study published subsequent to the review of Mulloy and colleagues compared children with ASDs randomly assigned to either a GFCF diet condition or a healthy low-sugar diet condition (Johnson *et al.*, 2011). This study, conducted over a 3-month period, found no significant differences on measures of behaviour, language or the core features of autism between the two groups.

Despite the lack of empirical evidence, the GFCF diet is widely used, with up to 27% of children with ASDs adhering to the diet (Levy and Hyman, 2005). In a recent online survey, the parents of 387 children with ASDs were interviewed about their use of the GFCF diet (Pennesi and Klein, 2012). Seventy-six per cent of this sample reported having used the GFCF diet, with over 50% of the parents using the diet for longer than one year. There are, no doubt, many reasons for the diet's widespread usage, among them the belief that the GFCF diet is a risk-free intervention. For children who eat a wide range of food and are flexible about making dietary changes, it may be the case that the diet offers little risk. However, for many children with ASDs, food selectivity is a significant problem and increasing dietary variety is difficult (Schreck *et al.*, 2004; Williams *et al.*, 2010), which often means implementation of the GFCF diet results in further limiting the child's diet. Adverse health effects of the diet were shown in one study that found boys with ASDs on a casein-free diet showed reduced bone cortical thickness (Hediger *et al.*, 2008).

For parents who report improvement in their children's behaviour with the GFCF diet, it is important to consider possible reasons for these reports. A study involving the use of the GFCF diet in 13 children with ASDs failed to find improvements in language and behaviour using objective measures (Elder *et al.*, 2006), yet 7 of 13 families reported improvements in language and behaviour, suggesting the potential for parental placebo effects (Elder, 2008). In the Pennesi and Klein (2012) study, the parents whose children had either gastrointestinal problems or food allergies reported more improvement in behaviours indicative of autism, physiological symptoms, and social behaviours than parents of children without medical issues. It could be the case that the GFCF diet, which would preclude the consumption of many processed foods high in fat and low in fibre, while allowing fruits and vegetables, could produce improvement of conditions such as such as chronic constipation which in turn could decrease irritability, discomfort, or even pain, leading to subsequent improvements in various behaviours.

While the GFCF diet cannot be considered as an evidence-based intervention to be used with the entire population of children with ASD, practitioners will no doubt be asked about the diet by parents and other caregivers, who in some cases, will already be using the diet with their children. Parents who are using the diet or planning to use the diet should at the very least be encouraged to have their child monitored regularly by a healthcare professional and asked to consider whether further limitations of their child's diet could compromise their child's nutritional status (Elder, 2008). Families should also be made aware that the GFCF diet typically requires more time and effort for food preparation as well as foods that may be more expensive and less readily available (Elder, 2008).

Case Study 1: Bryan

Bryan, a 3-year-old male diagnosed with ASD, was referred to a feeding programme for refusal to eat textured foods and a limited diet. His mother reported he had never transitioned successfully to foods with texture and consumed only pureed foods. He drank large amounts of milk, mostly from a bottle. Developmentally, Bryan had not yet acquired any language and his mother reported frequent tantrums and irritability. Co-morbid medical problems included chronic diarrhoea and constant rashes. Bryan's mother further reported Bryan had not had a formed bowel movement in several years. Further investigation of the diarrhoea revealed a severe milk protein allergy. As a result, all milk protein was eliminated from Bryan's diet.

A behavioural intervention was used to teach Bryan to eat a wide variety of table foods and drink from an open cup, eliminating the need for both baby food and bottle drinking.

At a follow-up appointment 3 months after the initial visit, Bryan's mother reported a regular stooling pattern, no rashes, fewer tantrums and advances in development including improvements in speech and learning to ride a tricycle.

For all children with identifiable food allergies or intolerances, elimination of the offending foods is typically recommended. There is no evidence that children with ASDs suffer more from food allergies than other children, yet there is also no evidence they suffer less, and food allergies, especially milk protein, are common in the paediatric population. While all of the changes reported by Bryan's mother could be attributed to a change in diet, and some of these changes, particularly the elimination of the diarrhoea and rashes, can be more easily linked to the diet change, there are several possible factors involved in these changes. Certainly the decrease in tantrums and general improvement in his behaviour could be attributed to a reduction in gastrointestinal discomfort. However, these changes, as well as the improvement in language, could have been either the result of development or the therapy services being provided across the same period of time the dietary changes were being made. While some parents attribute improvements in their children's language, behaviour, or other areas of development to changes in diet, because the children are receiving other services that could impact their learning and behaviour, often during a period of in their lives when development proceeds rapidly, it is hard to determine what, if any, improvements are the result of dietary changes.

THE MMR VACCINE, GASTROINTESTINAL PROBLEMS AND AUTISM SPECTRUM DISORDERS

Although the possibility of a relationship between the gut and autism had been mentioned in the literature, there was not a significant focus on the relationship between gastrointestinal dysfunction and autism until after a news conference at which Andrew Wakefield speculated the measles, mumps and rubella (MMR) vaccine was responsible for autism. In an article published by Wakefield and his colleagues (1998) in the *Lancet*, 8 of 12 children who reportedly exhibited signs of autism within days of their MMR vaccines were also described as having lymphoid nodular hyperplasia on endoscopy; based upon this finding, it was speculated that the MMR vaccine caused inflammation that allowed certain proteins to escape the gastrointestinal system, reach the brain and adversely affect development (Wakefield *et al.*, 1998). In several subsequent publications, Wakefield and his colleagues suggested that the gastrointestinal inflammation found in children with regressive autism represents a new variant of inflammatory bowel disease and this variant was named 'autistic enterocolitis' (Wakefield *et al.*, 1998, 2005).

The hypothesis that the MMR vaccine is related to autism has been extensively evaluated from a range of perspectives. One approach has been the use of ecological studies that have studied the relationship between the MMR vaccine and autism. Examining vaccination data over a decade, a study from the United Kingdom found that at the rate of autism increase, the rate of MMR vaccination remained stable (Kaye *et al.*, 2001). One Canadian study examining a sample of 27 749 children even found that as autism rates increased, MMR vaccination rates decreased (Fombonne *et al.*, 2006). Thirteen ecological studies have failed to find a relationship between the MMR vaccine and autism (Gerber and Offit, 2009). Although Wakefield and his colleagues claimed to have found evidence of the measles virus in the children they studied (Kawashima *et al.*, 2000; Uhlmann *et al.*, 2002; Wakefield, 2002), other studies have not supported this finding. Three studies did not find evidence of measles virus in the blood of children with ASDs (Afzal *et al.*, 2006; D'Souza *et al.*, 2006; Baird *et al.*, 2008) and an additional study that compared the bowel biopsies of 25 children with autism and gastrointestinal problems with 13 children with gastrointestinal problems alone found only one child from each group exhibited the measles virus in their bowel samples (Hornig *et al.*, 2008). In addition to finding far fewer cases of measles virus in bowel samples than the studies by Wakefield and colleagues, this study also failed to find the appropriate temporal relations between the MMR vaccine, the onset of the gastrointestinal problems and the onset of autism. If the MMR vaccine is causally related to the development of autism, then the MMR vaccine should precede the onset of gastrointestinal problems, which should in turn precede the onset of autism. Hornig and colleagues

(2008) found this pattern in only 5 of the 25 children with autism. In addition to multiple lines of evidence contradicting Wakefield's hypothesised relations between the MMR vaccine, gastrointestinal problems and autism, the determination of the British General Medical Council's Fitness to Practise Panel that Dr Wakefield's name should be erased from the Medical Register based upon numerous findings of dishonesty and fraud (GMC, 2010) as well as subsequent evidence of fraud (Godlee *et al.*, 2011) brings serious doubt to the veracity of any claims made by Wakefield and his colleagues. The editors of the *Lancet* subsequently retracted the original research paper.

Secretin as a treatment for autism

At the same time as Wakefield's theory of an MMR-autism connection was bringing attention to a possible relationship between autism and the gastrointestinal system, another study suggested a connection between the gut and autism. A case series described the outcome of three children with ASDs and chronic diarrhoea who were administered a single infusion of secretin as part of a diagnostic endoscopy (Horvath *et al.*, 1998). In addition to resolution of their gastrointestinal symptoms, the parents of these three children reported improvements in their children's social skills and communication. Based upon these reported changes in the children's behaviours, Horvath and his colleagues suggested a link between the gastrointestinal and neurological systems in children with autism. After a television news story reporting the success of secretin in the treatment of autism, perhaps thousands of children with autism were treated with secretin (Sandler and Bodfish, 2000). Despite this initial positive result of the Horvath study, subsequent research failed to find any significant positive effects from secretin. A systematic review described seven randomised controlled trials and one prospective case series that all failed to demonstrate any significant effects from secretin (Krishnaswami *et al.*, 2011). These studies revealed that participants receiving secretin demonstrated no greater improvements in measures of language, cognition or autistic symptoms when compared with placebo. These results are consistent with a Cochrane review of intravenous secretin for ASDs that included 13 randomised studies and revealed no evidence for the efficacy of secretin in persons with ASDs (Williams *et al.*, 2005).

EXAMINATION OF GASTROINTESTINAL ISSUES AND AUTISM SPECTRUM DISORDERS

In an early study of gastrointestinal problems among children with autism, 36 children referred to a gastrointestinal service found gastro-oesophageal reflux in 69% of children, chronic gastritis in 42%, and chronic duodenitis in 67% (Horvath *et al.*, 1999). While this study revealed the majority of children with autism had gastrointestinal disease, this should not be surprising given the children were referred to a gastroenterology service due to gastrointestinal complaints. Other studies that have examined the incidence of gastrointestinal diseases in children with and without autism have not found that children with autism have higher rates of gastrointestinal problems. One of these studies examined the medical histories of 96 children with autism and 449 age- and gender-matched children without autism and found no significant differences between the two groups for coeliac disease, chronic gastroenteritis, regional enteritis, malabsorption, ulcerative colitis, food intolerance or frequent gastrointestinal symptoms (Black *et al.*, 2002). Another study examined the presence of gastrointestinal disease in 118 individuals diagnosed with infantile autism and 312 controls without autism over a 30-year span and found persons with autism were no more likely to have a defined gastrointestinal disease, including inflammatory diseases such as coeliac disease, than persons without autism (Mouridsen *et al.*, 2009).

While children with autism appear to be no more likely to be diagnosed with a gastrointestinal *disease* than children without autism, research indicates differences in the frequency of gastrointestinal *problems or symptoms*. In an epidemiologic sample of 15 500 preschoolers, 96 children with ASD were identified, with 19% of these children with ASD having gastrointestinal problems, compared with 9% for the remainder of the sample (Fombonne and Chakrabarti, 2001). In this study, constipation was the most common gastrointestinal problem among children with autism, a finding replicated in another study that examined the incidence of gastrointestinal disease in 121 children with autism and 242 age- and gender-matched children without autism (Ibrahim *et al.*, 2009). While Ibrahim and his colleagues did find a significantly higher incidence of constipation and feeding issues, there were no differences in the incidences of diarrhoea, abdominal bloating or discomfort or gastro-oesophageal reflux. Ibrahim and his colleagues also suggested that the increased incidence of constipation could be due more to a behavioural aetiology than a gastrointestinal disease, and other research seems to support this hypothesis. Children with ASDs have been found to eat fewer fruits and vegetables (Schreck *et al.*, 2004) and exhibit more stool withholding (Badalyan and Schwartz, 2011) than children without autism, and both of these behaviours could increase the probability of constipation.

Although the studies just reviewed generally found children with ASDs to have a higher frequency of gastrointestinal symptoms, especially constipation, than children without special needs, this finding is less evident when comparing children with ASDs and children with other special needs. One study included three age- and gender-matched groups: 50 children with autism, 50 children with developmental disabilities other than autism and 50 children without disabilities. The parents of these children were asked to compete a gastrointestinal symptom and feeding questionnaire (Valicenti-McDermott *et al.*, 2006). The results showed significantly more of the children with autism exhibited frequent vomiting, abnormal stools, a history of bulky stools, chronic constipation, use of laxatives and faecal encopresis than the children without disabilities, but when compared with children with developmental disabilities the between group differences were fewer, with more of the children with autism reported to have abnormal stools, a history of bulky stools and faecal encopresis. The children with autism were also found to have significantly more problems with food selectivity than children from either of the other two groups. The authors suggested these feeding issues could have contributed to the bowel problems prevalent among the children with autism, as their selective diets may have resulted in insufficient intake of fluid or fibre (Valicenti-McDermott *et al.*, 2006). Similar findings were obtained by another study in which parents of 51 children with autism, 35 children with other developmental disabilities and 112 children without disabilities were asked about their children's bowel symptoms and found children with autism were reported to have significantly more constipation, diarrhoea, abdominal distension and flatulence than children without disabilities, but none of these differences were found between the children with autism and the children with other special needs (Smith *et al.*, 2009).

Gastrointestinal disorders such as gastro-oesophageal reflux, various forms of dysmotility, and constipation are common in children with developmental disabilities, especially those with more significant neurological impairment such as cerebral palsy or spina bifida (Sullivan, 2008). The same forms of neurological impairment that make gastrointestinal problems more common in children with special needs than children with typical development are also found among children with ASDs. A summary of studies examining the relations between ASDs and gastrointestinal problems is found at the end of this chapter.

Case Study 2: John

John, a 17-year-old male diagnosed with autism, was admitted to the inpatient unit of a children's hospital for abdominal pain. He was diagnosed with severe constipation and anaemia. John's parents reported they were unaware of his stooling pattern but did report he did occasionally have extremely large stools. The nutritionist's evaluation revealed John's diet consisted exclusively of specific brands of potato chips, crackers and other snack foods. He drank chocolate milk and soft drinks, but no juice or water. John refused to take any medications.

A nasogastric tube was required to give the medication required for a bowel cleanout. A behavioural intervention was developed with two goals: increasing liquid intake and establishing oral intake of stool softeners. Reinforcement in the form of access to the Internet was provided, contingent upon consumption of a specific amount of watered-down soda. Stool softener was systematically faded into the drink until John was drinking the required daily dosage.

While constipation can result from numerous factors, in this case it was attributed to inadequate intake of fibre and fluids, and possibly stool withholding. While selective or picky eating is commonly described among toddlers and preschoolers in the general paediatric population, this problem appears to be common for children with ASDs of all ages, with multiple studies describing selective eating in not only younger children but also among school-aged children and adolescents (for review, Williams *et al.*, 2010).

BEHAVIOURAL SEQUELAE OF GASTROINTESTINAL SYMPTOMS

As behavioural problems are prevalent in children with autism, one study examined both the prevalence of gastrointestinal symptoms as well as their impact in a well-characterised sample of children of ASDs (Nikolov *et al.*, 2009). The results showed 23% of the children were positive for gastrointestinal symptoms and that these children had higher scores on measures of irritability, social withdrawal and anxiety. A second study examined behavioural characteristics that have been suggested to be expressions of gastrointestinal problems in a sample of children with ASDs of which 35 children had co-morbid gastrointestinal problems and 452 children did not (Maenner *et al.*, 2012). Five of these behavioural characteristics – sleep disturbance, abnormal eating habits, oppositional behaviours, tantrums and delayed motor milestones – were found significantly more often among children with gastrointestinal problems. Although these two studies showed that the children with autism who exhibited gastrointestinal symptoms had more behavioural problems than those without symptoms, this finding is not unique to children with autism. Children of typical development with gastrointestinal symptoms exhibit more symptoms suggestive of anxiety and depression (Mussel *et al.*, 2008) and typically developing children with constipation displayed both higher rates of internalising and externalising behaviours than children without symptoms (Van Dijk *et al.*, 2010). Again, gastrointestinal symptoms do not appear to play a role in ASD that is specific to this disorder.

SUMMARY

At the current time, the empirical evidence does not support the presence of a gastrointestinal disorder specific to autism, for example, an autistic entercolitis. Additionally, there is no support for interventions such as the GFCF diet or use of secretin, which are based on the notion that autism has a gastrointestinal aetiology. The one finding that was supported by multiple studies was an increased prevalence of constipation among children with ASDs. There are several factors that could account for this finding. As previously mentioned, the diets of children with ASD are often limited, with foods high in fibre such as fruits and vegetables, being eaten less often. For children presenting to a clinic for feeding disorders, the children with ASDs were more likely to present with food selectivity than another other type of feeding problem (Field *et al.*, 2003). In addition to diet limitations, another behavioural aetiology, increased stool withholding, has also been found in children with ASD. As a neurodevelopmental disorder, ASD is the result of some form of nervous system dysfunction. For children who have nervous system dysfunction, hypotonia, problems with motor control and other forms of nervous system dysregulation are common and these children are more likely to have gastrointestinal problems such as constipation. Finally, constipation is also a know side effect of many classes of medications such as anticonvulsants, antispasmodics and antihistamines. Given the co-morbid medical issues found among children with autism such as epilepsy, cerebral palsy, nocturnal enuresis and sleep problems, the use of these medications are more common among children with ASDs (Kielinen *et al.*, 2004; Myers and Johnson, 2007).

Although the majority of studies have not found a clear connection between ASDs and a specific gastrointestinal disorder, this is not indication that gastrointestinal problems do not present a significant issue for many children with ASDs. Several behavioural problems, including tantrums and oppositional behaviours, were reported more often among the children with ASDs who presented with gastrointestinal problems than those without (Maenner *et al.*, 2012). In any child, gastrointestinal disorders such as functional abdominal pain or irritable bowel syndrome, or even gastrointestinal problems such as constipation, can worsen behaviour or disrupt sleep. For children with ASDs who cannot express pain or discomfort verbally, tantrums or other maladaptive behaviours, possibly even including aggression or self-injury, may be used in at least two ways: to communicate pain or to attenuate pain or discomfort. While some maladaptive behaviours may be triggered by the pain or discomfort secondary to a gastrointestinal problem and only occur when the gastrointestinal problem is present, this is not the only way in which behavioural issues are related to gastrointestinal problems. Behaviours do not occur in a vacuum, behaviours affect the environment in which they occur and are, in turn, controlled by various aspects of the environment. For example, caregivers, including parents, may react in a number of ways to their child's behaviour, including maladaptive behaviour. In some cases, caregivers will give their child attention contingent upon their child exhibiting a particular behaviour. For example, if the child cries, the parent may pick him up and comfort him. If this behaviour occurs over time and regardless of conditions, the child will learn that if he cries he is picked up by the parent, regardless of the aetiology of the crying. In other cases, parents may react to a particular behaviour by allowing the child to avoid less preferred activities or escape from demands; if the child whines or exhibits discomfort, the parent may allow the child to stay home from school. Alternatively, a parent may respond to a specific child behaviour by providing the child with a tangible object; a parent may give soda and crackers rather than the family meal if the child is holding his stomach. Thus, behaviours that were initially exhibited by children as a direct result of a gastrointestinal problem may become maintained over time by social variables. As gastrointestinal problems can both initiate and amplify maladaptive behaviours it will be important to identify and treat gastrointestinal issues sooner rather than later.

This said, not every child with an ASD will have gastrointestinal problems and there is no reason to conduct medical testing for possible gastrointestinal problems in children who are not exhibiting signs or symptoms. In a recent consensus report on the evaluation and treatment of gastrointestinal problems in individuals with ASDs, it was suggested that caregivers and others working with children with ASDs be taught the signs and symptoms of gastrointestinal problems so early effective treatment can be provided (Buie *et al.*, 2010). While recognising gastrointestinal problems in children who may have limited means of communication is necessary, it is further suggested that it is important to consider predisposing factors for gastrointestinal problems such as limited diet, poor fluid intake, and side effects of medications. Although not all behavioural problems found among children with ASD are causally related to gastrointestinal problems, the possibility of such a relationship should at least be considered when developing hypotheses about the factors that initiate and maintain these behaviour problems.

Some interventions for ASD were derived from a hypothesis that autism is related to gastrointestinal functioning. Although the use of some of these interventions, such as secretin, has dramatically declined, others such as the GFCF diet are still widely used by parents. As clinicians, it will be important to be able to discuss the use of these interventions. While children diagnosed with food allergies are typically prescribed a diet free of offending foods, many of the children who received the GFCF diet have not been identified with food allergies. For any child on this type of elimination diet, it is important that the parents ensure their child is receiving the micronutrients usually obtained from foods eliminated from the child's diet. While a GFCF diet may be healthy as it largely excludes processed foods that are high in calories and low in fibre and nutrients, it is only healthy if these processed foods are replaced by a variety of foods including fruits, vegetables and proteins. The research suggests that given the prevalence of food selectivity among children with ASDs, it may be difficult to make the changes necessary for implementation of restrictive diets in children with ASDs.

REFERENCES

Afzal MA, Ozoemena LC, O'Hare KA, *et al.* Absence of detectable measles virus genome sequence in blood of autistic children who have had their MMR vaccination during the routine childhood immunization schedule of UK. *Med Virol.* 2006; **78**: 623–30.

Badalyan V, Schwartz RH. Mealtime feeding behaviors and gastrointestinal dysfunction in children with classic autism compared to normal sibling controls. *Open J Pediatr.* 2011; **2**: 150–60.

Baird G, Charman T, Pickles A, *et al.* Regression, developmental trajectory and associated problems in disorders in the autism spectrum: the SNAP study. *J Autism Dev Disord.* 2008; **38**(10): 1827–36.

Black C, Kaye JA, Jick H. Relation of childhood gastrointestinal disorders to autism: nested case-control study using data from the UK General Practice Research Database. *BMJ.* 2002; **325**(7361): 419–21.

Buie T, Campbell DB, Fuchs G. *et al.* Evaluation, diagnosis, and treatment of gastrointestinal disorders in individuals with ASDs: a consensus report. *Pediatrics.* 2010; **125**(Suppl. 1): S1–18.

Cade R, Privette M, Fregly M, *et al.* Autism and schizophrenia: intestinal disorders. *Nutr Neurosci.* 2000; **2**: 57–72.

Cass H, Gringras P, March J, *et al.* Absence of urinary opioid peptides in children with autism. *Arch Dis Child.* 2008; **93**(9): 745–50.

De Magistris L, Familiari V, Pascotto A, *et al.* Alterations of the intestinal barrier in patients with autism spectrum disorders and in their first-degree relatives. *J Pediatr Gastroenterol Nutr.* 2010; **51**(4): 418–24.

D'Eufemia P, Celli M, Finocchiaro R, *et al.* Abnormal intestinal permeability in children with autism. *Acta Paediactr.* 1996; **85**(9): 1076–9.

D'Souza Y, Fombonne E, Ward BJ. No evidence of persisting measles virus in peripheral blood mononuclear cells from children with autism spectrum disorder. *Pediatrics.* 2006; **118**(4): 1664–75.

Dohan FC. Cereals and schizophrenia data and hypothesis. *Acta Psychiatr Scand.* 1966; **42**(2): 125–52.

Dohan FC. Genetic hypothesis of idiopathic schizophrenia: its exorphin connection. *Schizophr Bull.* 1988; **14**(4): 489–94.

Dohan FC, Harper EH, Clark MH, *et al.* Is schizophrenia rare if grain is rare? *Biol Psychiatry.* 1984; **19**(3): 385–99.

Elder JH. The gluten-free, casein-free diet in autism: an overview with clinical implications. *Nutr Clin Pract.* 2008; **23**(6): 583–88.

Elder JH, Shankar M, Shuster J, *et al.* The gluten-free, casein-free diet in autism: results of a preliminary double blind clinical trial. *J Autism Dev Disord.* 2006; **36**(3): 413–20.

Field D, Garland M, Williams K. Correlates of specific childhood feeding problems. *J Pediatr Child Health.* 2003; **39**(4): 299–304.

Fombonne E, Chakrabarti S. No evidence for a new variant of measles-mumps-rubella-induced autism. *Pediatrics.* 2001; **108**(4): e58.

Fombonne E, Zakarian R, Bennett A, *et al.* Pervasive developmental disorders in Montreal, Quebec, Canada: prevalence and links with immunizations. *Pediatrics.* 2006; **118**(1): e139–50.

Gerber J, Offit PA. Vaccines and autism: a tale of shifting hypotheses. *Clin Infect Dis.* 2009; **48**(4): 456–61.

General Medical Council (GMC). *Transcripts of hearings of fitness to practice panel (misconduct) in the case of Wakefield, Walker-Smith, and Murch.* 16 July 2007 to 24 May 2010. London: GMC; 2010.

Godlee F, Smith J, Marcovitch H. Wakefield's article linking MMR vaccine and autism was fraudulent. *BMJ.* 2011; **342**: c7452.

Goodwin MS, Cowen MA, Goodwin TC. Malabsorption and cerebral dysfunction: a multivariate and comparative study of autistic children. *J Autism Child Schizophr.* 1971; **1**(1): 48–62.

Goodwin MS, Goodwin TC. In a dark mirror. *Ment Hyg.* 1969; **53**(4): 550–63.

Hediger ML, England LJ, Molloy CA, *et al.* Reduced bone cortical thickness in boys with autism or autism spectrum disorder. *J Autism Dev Disord.* 2008; **38**(5): 848–56.

Hornig M, Briese T, Buie T, *et al.* Lack of association between measles virus vaccine and autism with enteropathy: a case-control study. *PLoS One.* 2008; **3**(9): e3140.

Horvath K, Papadimitriou JC, Rabsztyn A, *et al.* Gastrointestinal abnormalities in children with autistic disorder. *J Pediatr.* 1999; **135**(5): 559–63.

Horvath K, Stefanatos G, Sokolski KN, *et al.* Improved social and language skills after secretin administration in patients with autism spectrum disorders. *J Asso Acad Minor Phys.* 1998; **9**(1): 9–15.

Ibrahim SH, Voigt RG, Katusic SK, *et al.* Incidence of gastrointestinal symptoms in children with autism: a population-based study. *Pediatrics.* 2009; **124**(2): 680–6.

Johnson CR, Handen BL, Zimmer M, *et al.* Effects of gluten free/casein free diet in young children with autism: a pilot study. *J Dev Phys Disabil.* 2011; **23**: 213–25.

Kawashima H, Mori T, Kashiwagi Y, *et al.* Detection and sequencing of measles virus from peripheral mononuclear cells from patients with inflammatory bowel disease and autism. *Dig Dis Sci.* 2000; **45**(4): 723–9.

Kaye JA, Melero-Montes M, Jick H. Mumps, measles, and rubella vaccine and the incidence of autism recorded by general practitioners. *BMJ.* 2001; **322**(7284): 460–3.

Kemperman RFJ, Muskiet FD, Boutier I, *et al.* Brief report: normal intestinal permeability at elevated platelet serotonin levels in a subgroup of children with pervasive developmental disorders in Curacao (the Netherlands Antilles). *J Autism Dev Disord.* 2008; **38**(2): 401–6.

Kielinen M, Rantala H, Timonen E, *et al.* Associated medical disorders and disabilities in children with autistic disorder: a population-based study. *Autism.* 2004; **8**(1): 49–60.

Krishnaswami S, McPheeters ML, Veenstra-Vanderweele J. A systematic review of secretin for children with autism spectrum disorders. *Pediatrics.* 2011; **127**(5): e1322–5.

Le Couteur A, Trygstad O, Evered C, *et al.* Infantile autism and urinary excretion of peptides and protein-associated peptide complexes. *J Autism Dev Disord.* 1988; **18**(2): 181–90.

Levy SE, Hyman SL. Novel treatments for autistic spectrum disorders. *Dev Disabil Res Rev.* 2005; **11**(2): 131–42.

Maenner MJ, Arneson CL, Levy SE, *et al.* Brief report: association between behavioral features and gastrointestinal problems among children with autism spectrum disorder. *J Autism Dev Disord.* 2012; **42**(7): 1520–5.

Milward C, Ferrier M, Calver SJ, *et al.* Gluten- and casein-free diets for autistic spectrum disorder. *Cochrane Database Syst Rev.* 2009; (2): CD003498.

Molloy CA, Manning-Courtney P. Prevalence of chronic gastrointestinal symptoms in children with autism and autistic spectrum disorders. *Autism.* 2003; **7**(2): 165–71.

Mouridsen SE, Rich B, Isager T. A longitudinal study of gastrointestinal diseases in individuals diagnosed with infantile autism as children. *Child Care Health Dev.* 2009; **36**(3): 437–43.

Mulloy A, Lang R, O'Reilly M, *et al.* Gluten-free and casein-free diets in the treatment of autism spectrum disorders: a systematic review. *Res Autism Spectr Disord.* 2010; **4**(3): 328–39.

Mulloy A, Lang R, O'Reilly M, *et al.* Addendum to 'gluten-free and casein-free diets in treatment of autism spectrum disorders: a systematic review'. *Res Autism Spectr Disord.* 2011; **5**(1): 86–8.

Mussel M, Kroenke K, Spitzer RL, *et al.* Gastrointestinal symptoms in primary care: prevalence and association with depression and anxiety. *J Psychosomat Res.* 2008; **64**(6): 605–12.

Myers S, Johnson CS; American Academy of Pediatrics Council on Children with Disabilities. Management of children with autism spectrum disorders. *Pediatrics.* 2007; **120**(5): 1162–82.

Nikolov RN, Bearss KE, Lettinga J, *et al.* Gastrointestinal symptoms in a sample of children with pervasive developmental disorders. *J Autism Dev Disord.* 2009; **39**(3): 405–13.

Panksepp J. A neurochemical theory of autism. *Trends Neurosci.* 1979; **2**: 174–7.

Pennesi CM, Klein LC. Effectiveness of the gluten-free, casein-free diet for children diagnosed with autism spectrum disorder: based on parental report. *Nutr Neurosci.* 2012; **15**(2): 85–91.

Reichelt KL, Ekrem J, Scott H. Gluten, milk proteins, and autism: dietary intervention effects on behavior and peptide secretion. *J App Nutr.* 1990; **42**: 1–11.

Reichelt KL, Knivsberg AM, Lind G, *et al.* Probable etiology and possible treatment of children autism. *Brain Dysfunct.* 1991; **4**: 308–19.

Reichelt WH, Knivsberg A, Nødland M, *et al.* Urinary peptide levels and patterns in autistic children, from seven countries, and the effect of dietary intervention after four years. *Dev Brain Dysfunct.* 1997; **10**: 44–55.

Robertson MA, Sigalet DL, Holst JJ, *et al.* Intestinal permeability and glucagon-like peptide-2 in children with autism: a controlled pilot study. *J Autism Dev Disord.* 2008; **38**(6): 1066–71.

Sandler AD, Bodfish JW. Placebo effects in autism: lessons from secretin. *J Dev Behav Pediatr.* 2000; **21**(5): 347–50.

Schreck KA, Williams K, Smith AF. A comparison of eating behaviors between children with and without autism. *J Autism Dev Disord.* 2004; 34(4): 433–8.

Shattock P, Kennedy A, Rowell F, *et al.* Role of neuropeptides in autism and their relationships with classic neurotransmitters. *Brain Dysfunct.* 1990; 3(5–6): 328–45.

Smith RA, Farnworth H, Wright B, *et al.* Are there more bowel symptoms in children with autism compared to normal children and children with other developmental and neurological disorders? *Autism.* 2009; 13(4): 343–55.

Sullivan PB. Gastrointestinal disorders in children with neurodevelopmental disabilities. *Dev Disabil Res.* 2008; 14(2): 128–36.

Taylor B, Miller E, Lingam R, *et al.* Measles, mumps, and rubella vaccination and bowel problems or developmental regression in children with autism: population study. *BMJ.* 2002; 324(7334): 393–6.

Uhlmann V, Martin CM, Sheils O, *et al.* Potential viral pathogenic mechanism for new variant inflammatory bowel disease. *Mol Pathol.* 2002; 55(2): 84–90.

Valicenti-McDermott M, McVicar K, Rapin I, *et al.* Frequency of gastrointestinal symptoms in children with autistic spectrum disorders and association with family history of autoimmune disease. *J Dev Behav Pediatr.* 2006; 27(2 Suppl.): S128–36.

Valicenti-McDermott MD, McVicar K, Cohen HJ, *et al.* Gastrointestinal symptoms in children with an autism spectrum disorder and language regression. *Pediatr Neurol.* 2008; 39(6): 392–8. doi: 10.1016/j.pediatrneurol.2008.07.019.

Van Dijk M, Benninga MA, Grootenhuis MA, *et al.* Prevalence and associated clinical characteristics of behavior problems in constipated children. *Pediatrics.* 2010; 125(2): e309–17.

Wakefield AJ. The gut-brain axis in childhood developmental disorders. *J Pediatr Gastroenterol Nutr.* 2002; 34(Suppl. 1): S14–17.

Wakefield AJ, Ashwood P, Limb K, *et al.* The significance of ileo-colonic lymphoid nodular hyperplasia in children with autistic spectrum disorder. *Eur J Gastroenterol Hepatol.* 2005; 17(8): 827–36.

Wakefield AJ, Murch SH, Anthony A, *et al.* Retracted: Ileal-lymphoid-nodular hyperplasia, non-specific colitis, and pervasive developmental disorder in children. *Lancet.* 1998; 351(9103): 637–41.

Wang LW, Tancredi DJ, Thomas DW. The prevalence of gastrointestinal problems in children across the United States with autism spectrum disorders from families with multiple affected members. *J Dev Behav Pediatr.* 2011; 32(5): 351–60. doi: 10.1097/DBP.0b013e31821bd06a.

Williams KE, Field DG, Seiverling L. Food refusal in children: a review of the literature. *Res Dev Disabil.* 2010; 31(3): 625–33.

Williams KJ, Wray JJ, Wheeler DM. Intravenous secretin for autism spectrum disorder. *Cochrane Database Syst Rev.* 2005; (3): CD003495.

Xue Ming, Brimacombe M, Chaaban J, *et al.* Autism spectrum disorders: concurrent clinical disorders. *J Child Neurol.* 2008; 23(1): 6–13. Epub 2007 Dec 3.

APPENDIX 1 Studies examining gastrointestinal (GI) problems among children with autism spectrum disorders (ASDs)

Study	Sample	Age (range)	Any GI symptom (%)	Constipation (%)	Diarrhoea (%)	GERD (%)	Comments
Fombonne and Chakrabarti (2001)	ASD = 96	41 mos (21–78 mos)	19	9.4	3.1	–	No relation between GI problems and developmental regression
Black, Kaye & Jick (2002)	ASD = 96 Non-ASD = 449	50 mos 49 mos	9 9	–	–	–	Examined only GI disorders, no differences in disorders between groups
Taylor, Miller, Lingam, et al. (2002)	ASD = 473		17	9	4	–	No evidence MMR vaccine associated with bowel problems
Molloy and Manning-Courtney (2003)	ASD = 137	55.6 mos (24–96 mos)	24.1	8.8	12.4	6.6	No association between GI problems and developmental regression
Ibrahim, Voigt, Katusic, et al. (2009)	ASD = 121 Non-ASD = 242	16.0 yrs (2.7–21.0 yrs) 17.4 yrs (3.8–21.0 yrs)	77.2 72.2	33.9 17.6	50.3 41.1	25.3 16.9	Measured cumulative incidence of GI problems to age 21; Constipation only problem found significantly more often in ASD
Xue Ming, Brimacombe, Chaaban, et al. (2008)	ASD = 160	(2–18 yrs)	59	16	23	11	No association between GI problems and developmental regression; Food intolerance associated with GI problems
Valicenti-McDermott, McVicar, Cohen, et al. (2008)	ASD lang. regress. ASD no lang. regress.	7.9 ± 5 10 ± 4.5	85 62	34 43	–	8 12	Children with language regression had more GI problems than children without language regression

Study	Sample	Age (range)	Any GI symptom (%)	Constipation (%)	Diarrhoea (%)	GERD (%)	Comments
Mouridsen, Rich & Isager (2009)	ASD = 118 Non-ASD = 336	5.4 yrs 2–15 yrs	30.5 30.7	– 	– 	– 	No differences between ASD and non-ASD in GI disease in longitudinal study
Nikolov, Bearss, Lettinga, *et al.* (2009)	ASD = 172	8.3 yrs (5–17 yrs)	22.7	8	3	2	ASD +GI problems showed more severity on measures of irritability, anxiety and social withdraw
Smith, Franworth, Wright, *et al.* (2009)	ASD = 51 Special school = 35 Regular school = 112	9.7 yrs 10.0 yrs 12.58 yrs	35 24 4	25 40 4	27 16 5	– 	ASD had more bowel problems than children in regular school, but not more than children enrolled in a special school More food selectivity in ASD than other groups
Badalyan and Schwartz (2011)	ASD = 211 Non-ASD = 160	7.9 yrs 7.7 yrs		29 0.6	11 0.2	14 0.7	Children with ASD significantly more likely to have constipation ASD more likely to have feeding problems
Maenner *et al.* (2011)	ASD = 487	8 yrs	7.2	– 	– 	– 	Children with GI problems had more sleep, eating and behaviour problems
Wang, Tancredi, & Thomas (2011)	ASD = 589 Siblings = 163	8.3 yrs (1–18 yrs) 8.9 yrs (1–18 yrs)	42 12	20 4	19 2	5 5	Children with ASD had more GI problems than unaffected siblings Autism severity related to more GI problems

GERD, gastro-oesophageal reflux disease; mos, months; yrs, years.

CHAPTER 11

Psychological well-being of children and young people with coeliac disease

Ruth A Howard and Gary Urquhart-Law

INTRODUCTION

Coeliac disease (CD) is not a food allergy. It is not a food intolerance. Instead, CD is a life-long autoimmune condition of the small intestine, triggered by the ingestion of the protein gluten found in wheat, barley and rye. The only treatment for CD is the elimination of gluten-containing food from the diet – a life-long gluten-free diet (GFD). Such strict dietary self-management is essential for the alleviation of medical symptoms, normal physical development, prevention of longer-term health complications, and for improved quality of life and well-being. For many, the GFD can be managed well and CD can be incorporated within day-to-day life (Kinos *et al.*, 2011) but, for a considerable number, a lifelong GFD can be difficult to accept and follow; it can present a considerable challenge and burden for children, adolescents and families.

This chapter first details the symptoms of CD in children and young people, the process for diagnosis and the requirements for a GFD. Second, the literature on the psychosocial impact and consequences of CD, and its treatment, on children, young people and families is presented. Third, recommendations are made for the assessment of dietary self-management, quality of life and psychological well-being, before, finally, presenting a case of CD, together with the assessment, formulation and intervention.

COELIAC DISEASE: DIAGNOSIS AND TREATMENT IN CHILDREN AND YOUNG PEOPLE

Symptoms

Tissue transglutaminase (tTG) is a naturally occurring enzyme present in us all, but people with CD develop anti-tTG antibodies that react to the ingestion of gluten and trigger an immune attack against the small intestine. The attack results in inflammation, damage and abnormality to the proximal mucosa of the small intestine. This results in stunted or even absent finger-like projections called villi – villous atrophy.

The structural damage to the small intestine, resolved on gluten withdrawal and recurring if gluten is reintroduced to the diet, restricts an individual's ability to absorb nutrients from food and leads to the wide spectrum of symptoms associated with CD. Traditionally, symptoms have been mainly recognised as gastrointestinal (GI); however, non-gastrointestinal (non-GI) symptoms can be reported. In 2012, the European Society for Paediatric Gastroenterology, Hepatology and Nutrition (Husby *et al.*, 2012) published its revised guidelines on the diagnosis of CD in children and young people, and the British Society of Paediatric Gastroenterology, Hepatology and Nutrition (BSPGHAN, 2006) have also produced guidelines for the diagnosis and management of CD in children. Table 11.1 highlights the main presenting symptoms of CD.

TABLE 11.1 Gastrointestinal and non-gastrointestinal symptoms of coeliac disease

'Classic' gastrointestinal symptoms	*'Atypical' non-gastrointestinal symptoms*
Chronic or intermittent diarrhoea	Failure to thrive
Bloating	Weight loss
Nausea	Stunted growth
Vomiting	Pubertal delay
Chronic abdominal pain and distension	Amenorrhoea or menstrual irregularities
Cramping	Iron-deficiency anaemia
Chronic constipation	Dental enamel defects
Poor weight gain or weight loss	Chronic fatigue
Wind and flatulence	Recurrent mouth ulcers
Irritability and lethargy	Skin rash (dermatitis herpetiformis–like rash)
	Unexplained fracture
	Bone density abnormalities
	Joint pain
	Abnormal liver function

Symptoms will differ between individuals in terms of type, severity and age (NICE, 2009; Polanco, 2008; Tanpowpong *et al.*, 2012), and many are similar to those presenting in other GI conditions, such as irritable bowel syndrome and inflammatory bowel disease. For younger children, 'classic' GI symptoms are commonly associated with CD and include weight loss, growth failure, vomiting, lethargy, abdominal bloating, abdominal pain and bowel movement changes. Short stature and anaemia are often more common than malabsorption symptoms in children (Fasano, 2005). Presentations for older children and adolescents can include few or no GI symptoms; such an 'atypical', non-GI, presentation testifies to the 'multi-system' nature of CD and can include headaches, mouth ulcers, menstrual irregularities and joint pain. A third phenotype is 'silent' CD (Rostrom *et al.*, 2006), in which individuals are completely asymptomatic but will evidence villous atrophy upon biopsy. The atypical and asymptomatic manifestations are becoming more commonly described in older children and adolescents.

The wide range of symptoms associated with CD makes it a challenge to diagnose. CD has been called an 'iceberg' phenomenon, testifying to the fact that only a minority of affected individuals are diagnosed (Bingley *et al.*, 2004; West *et al.*, 2007). The complexities of accurate diagnosis mean that children and young people can be investigated for other GI disorders and may be diagnosed with irritable bowel syndrome before CD is considered (Rashid *et al.*, 2005). Equally, those presenting with non-GI symptoms may be investigated for a wide range of conditions before CD is considered, assessed and diagnosed. The difficulty in diagnosing CD can lead not only to poor physical health but also to poor psychological well-being and quality of life.

In addition to the presence of various GI and non-GI symptoms, children and young people may also be at risk of CD if they have a first-degree relative with CD – the strong genetic component to the condition means that family members are encouraged to be tested after the diagnosis of a first-degree relative (Husby *et al.*, 2012; NICE, 2009). In addition, increased risk for CD is associated with the following diagnoses:

- type 1 diabetes mellitus
- Down's syndrome
- autoimmune thyroid disease
- Turner's syndrome
- Williams' syndrome
- selective immunoglobulin A deficiency
- autoimmune liver disease
- first-degree relatives with CD.

Diagnosis

Recent guidance on the awareness, recognition and diagnosis of CD was published by NICE (2009). The guideline states that if CD is suspected, a blood test should be carried out to look for coeliac antibodies, and the two most effective tests for this are:

1. tTG antibody
2. endomysial antibody.

An elevated level of these antibodies indicates the *likely* presence of CD; however, in order to confirm the diagnosis, a biopsy of the small intestine is taken via an endoscope in order to confirm damage to the villi, the so-called flat mucosal atrophy. The endoscopy procedure is carried out under sedation by a paediatric gastroenterologist and, if the diagnosis is positive, the child or young person will continue under the care of the specialist team. NICE (2009) stress the importance of continuing on a gluten-containing diet during the diagnostic process in order to maximise the likelihood of an accurate result.

Affecting around 1% of children and young people (Bingley *et al.*, 2004; Green and Cellier, 2007), and females more than males (ratio 2:1), there is no cure for CD. The only treatment for CD is strict self-management of a GFD.

Gluten-free diet

The GFD is the only treatment for CD and lifelong, strict, adherence is necessary to avoid longer-term health complications (e.g. osteoporosis, lymphoma, infertility). If followed correctly, the GFD will assist the damaged villi in the small intestine to regrow, to absorb nutrients and to restore gut health. For the majority of children and young people who commence on a GFD, symptoms of CD will reduce within a few weeks and after several months the lining of the gut will begin to regenerate, although the speed and eventual degree of histological improvement is unpredictable. The response to eating gluten by mistake can vary from person to person, but the usual symptoms of headache, tiredness, stomach pains and diarrhoea can last from a few hours to a few days (Coeliac UK, 2012).

The GFD requires the removal of all gluten-containing foods from the diet. This includes any foods containing wheat, barley and rye. Some children and young people will also need to remove oats from their diet, although for the majority of adults with CD, uncontaminated oats are safe to include in the diet – this should be discussed with the child or young person's healthcare team. The GFD is restrictive, especially in those cultures where foods are based largely on cereal products. For effective dietary self-management, gluten-containing bread, pasta, cake, biscuits and crackers need to be removed from the diet. In addition, many processed foods will also need to be removed from the diet, as they contain small amounts of gluten-containing products that enhance flavour and palatability. In terms of alcohol, which might be an issue for older adolescents, beer, lagers, stouts and ales contain gluten and should be avoided (spirit drinks are gluten-free). Despite this, many foods are naturally gluten-free and include:

- fresh meat and fish
- fruit and vegetables
- rice
- potatoes
- eggs
- cheese
- many yogurts
- beans and pulses.

For those children and young people with a medical diagnosis of CD, many gluten-free substitutes of everyday foods can be obtained on prescription (e.g. specially manufactured breads, crackers, pastas) or bought from supermarkets. The last decade has seen a rise in the availability and palatability of gluten-free alternatives for purchase. The removal of gluten-containing foods from the diet is a huge lifestyle change for children and young people and for families affected by CD. Most manage the change in behaviour, diet and life-style without undue difficulty, but for others the transition to a GFD, and its maintenance, can be associated with psychosocial difficulties, reduced well-being and a poor quality of life.

PSYCHOLOGICAL CONSEQUENCES OF LIVING AND MANAGING COELIAC DISEASE

Psychological well-being

Having CD and eating a GFD can affect a child's or young person's psycho-logical well-being. Psychological distress in the form of a range of emotional symptoms (including anxiety and depression) and behavioural difficulties has been reported, as have neurological and psychological disorders, includ-ing headaches, attention deficit hyperactivity disorder (Niederhofer and Pittschieler, 2006), tic and learning disorders. The pre-diagnosis and pre-GFD treatment phases are possible times of increased risk when psychological difficulties can present, and where a higher lifetime prevalence of major depres-sive disorder (31% vs. 7%) and disruptive behaviour disorders (28% vs. 3%) have been identified relative to non-CD matched controls (Pynnönen et al., 2004). Concerns with regard to shape, weight, body image and eating behav-iours have also been found in young women with CD (Karwautz et al., 2008). Interestingly, there is some indication that treatment with a GFD can improve depressive symptoms, behaviour and functioning (Pynnönen et al., 2005), including symptoms of attention deficit hyperactivity disorder (Niederhofer, 2011; Niederhofer and Pittschieler, 2006).

Older children and younger adolescents with CD on a strict GFD report significantly increased levels of depression (Children's Depression Inventory; Kovacs, 1982) and anxiety (Multidimensional Anxiety Scale for Children; March, 1997) in comparison with healthy age-matched controls (Mazzone et al., 2001). In addition, girls reported more internalising symptoms on the Child Behaviour Checklist (Achenbach, 1991), with boys reporting more externalising symptoms (Mazzone et al., 2011). These findings indicate that psychological difficulties are not necessarily resolved or lessened with the GFD (indeed, the GFD can exacerbate pre-existing difficulties or precipitate them), and they sug-gest that males and females differ in the manner in which they respond to CD and the challenges of treatment. The marked shift in dietary habits and degree of lifestyle change required for a strict GFD are proposed as one mechanism to explain the ongoing heightened anxiety, after diagnosis, in children and young people with CD.

In terms of parents of children and young people with CD, the litera-ture is inadequate. To date, only a handful of studies (e.g. Anson et al., 1990; Cederborg, et al., 2011; Jackson et al., 1985) have explored the thoughts and feelings of parents and the results show that, irrespective of the degree to which children and young people manage their diets, the majority report the dietary restrictions to be a burden, report difficulty in detecting gluten in food labels, and comment on social restrictions, such as the avoidance of travelling and eating out. Parents can also report heightened anxiety with regard to the possible long-term adverse effects of poorly managed CD. Thus, the impact of CD and the GFD on parental well-being requires assessment in clinic. Particular attention is required to examine the inter-relationships between parental functioning, child well-being, and self-management.

Overall, psychological well-being in young people with CD is complex and the results are mixed. However, managing a long-term condition is known to be commonly associated with psychological difficulties in children and young people (Hysing *et al.*, 2009) and should be assessed. For the healthcare professional, CD needs to be considered within the psychosocial developmental stage of the child or young person and viewed as an additional challenge that young people are required to cope with.

Quality of life

The findings that some children and young people can find the disease difficult to accept and the treatment a challenge to follow, together with stigma experiences (Olsson *et al.*, 2009), feelings of being different, feelings of isolation, embarrassment, anger and envy (Cinquetti *et al.*, 1999; Rashid *et al.*, 2005), has led researchers to explore the links between CD, the GFD and aspects of quality of life. A total of eight published studies have explored quality of life using questionnaires in children and young people with CD, and the results are equivocal. Methodological differences hinder definitive conclusions.

Some studies report a reduced quality of life in symptomatic young children (aged 2–4 years) at diagnosis, but with significant improvements in quality of life after 12 months on a GFD (Van Koppen *et al.*, 2009). Other studies report no difference in generic quality of life in comparison with healthy controls (Di Lorenzo *et al.*, 2012; Kolsteren *et al.*, 2001; Rashid *et al.*, 2005), and this is particularly so for those who report good dietary self-management (Pico *et al.*, 2012; Wagner *et al.*, 2008). The remaining studies report a reduced quality of life for children and young people with CD in comparison with healthy peers, but a better quality of life in comparison with other chronic paediatric illness groups (Van Doorn *et al.*, 2008). Byström *et al.* (2012) reported better health-related quality of life in those diagnosed before 5 years of age than those diagnosed later. The different types of information obtained from generic, disease-generic and disease-specific quality-of-life instruments, and the nature of comparisons that are made, explains the differences in outcomes reported (Loonen *et al.*, 2001).

Rosén *et al.* (2011) in their Swedish study concluded that clear health benefits of the GFD had to be weighed against social sacrifices necessary to manage the diet and that these factors were likely to affect the quality of life of children, young people and families. Other studies have demonstrated the importance of dietary self-management in enhancing quality of life, demonstrating an association between poorer dietary self-management and poorer quality of life. Wagner *et al.* (2008) found that poor dietary self-management was associated with lower general quality of life, more physical health problems, a greater sense of burden associated with CD, more family problems and more problems in leisure time for children and young people. They concluded that good dietary self-management is essential for good quality of life.

While most studies assess and report on the quality of life of children and young people with CD either alone or in comparison with non-CD peers (healthy matched peers or with children and young people with other chronic illnesses), only one study has been published that set out with the aim of improving quality of life (Bongiovanni et al., 2010). American children and young people with CD at a gluten-free camp for 7 days show significant improvements in self-reported 'well-being' (i.e. reduced frequency of GI symptoms), 'self-perception' (e.g. feeling less different or embarrassed), and 'emotional outlook' (e.g. less anger and frustration as a result of CD). The camp was specifically designed to reduce concern and preoccupation with foods and the social stigma of CD (Bongiovanni et al., 2010).

Quality of life within the family has been the subject of recent research (e.g. Di Lorenzo et al., 2012; Roma et al., 2010) and several domains of life have been shown to be affected by CD. Specifically, leisure activities, social functioning (such as relationships with friends), and the management of daily life with regard to gluten-free food are areas where difficulties can present. It has also been shown that good parental quality of life is associated with better quality of life in young people with CD (Anson et al., 1990; Knez et al., 2011b), thus illustrating the importance of support for the family when assessing and supporting children and young people with CD.

Overall, it would seem that the majority of children and young people, once diagnosed and following a GFD, report an improvement in quality of life to a level comparable to healthy controls. This is most likely because of children, young people and families having an explanation for their symptoms, commencing the GFD and experiencing an improvement in symptoms. However, for some children and young people, predominantly those receiving a diagnosis later on in childhood or during adolescence (and who may have been asymptomatic), the introduction of a GFD after many years on a diet full of gluten can precipitate a reduction in quality of life (Byström et al., 2012). Thus, the age of the child or young person, age at diagnosis, pre-diagnosis symptom profile, and degree of reported burden in following the GFD are factors important for assessing quality of life. Recommendations from children and young people themselves in terms of what would improve their quality of life, include better labelling of gluten-containing ingredients, more gluten-free foods in supermarkets, gluten-free choices on restaurant menus, earlier diagnosis, and better dietary advice and support (Rashid et al., 2005).

ASSESING SELF-MANAGEMENT, WELL-BEING AND QUALITY OF LIFE

CD and its treatment affects the individual child or young person as well as the family system. In considering what to assess and how, health professionals, working from a psychosocial perspective, must integrate models derived from, and developed for, children and young people with chronic health conditions as well as conceptual frameworks of health behaviour (Hagger, 2010) and paediatric self-management (Modi *et al.*, 2012). A multi-modal, multi-method, systemic approach is necessary in order to conceptualise the impact of CD upon the individual, the interplay between the different elements of the family system, and the relationships between the individual and family systems to the other domains of a child's or young person's functioning (i.e. healthcare and community systems, including peer relationships and school). All of this necessitates, on the part of the health professional, a good understanding of CD, the complex behaviour of self-management, the cognitive, emotional and social processes that influence self-management, and child and adolescent development.

Self-management of the gluten-free diet

Methodological variations, inconsistent definitions of self-management, methods of measurement used (e.g. self-report, proxy-report, biological markers) and differences in sampling have presented barriers to the accurate assessment of self-management in children and young people with CD. Across studies, figures show that between 45% and 95% report strict self-management to the GFD (i.e. not aware of taking gluten), with others eating gluten either occasionally or almost always (Errichiello *et al.*, 2010; Hopman *et al.*, 2006). The literature has identified a multitude of factors that have been associated with better and poorer dietary self-management in children and young people with CD (see Table 11.2).

The 'socially convenient' setting of home is where young people tend to find it easier to stick to the GFD (Olsson *et al.*, 2008). The home is a setting where CD is more visible and known to those around the young person and where the GFD menu has been negotiated and is, most probably, palatable. However, beyond the home setting, and more frequently a challenge for adolescents, are those social situations and scenarios where the invisibility of CD can be threatened, such as when eating out, visiting friends and travelling. It is in these 'socially situated dilemmas' (Olsson *et al.*, 2009) that children and young people can fear the reaction from others, when transgressions from the GFD occur, and where young people can restrict their integration into social and school environments (Errichiello *et al.*, 2010; Wagner *et al.*, 2008). In addition, for those who are motivated to keep to a strict GFD, there can be the additional worry that food labelled as 'gluten-free' has been contaminated by gluten-containing products, a not infrequent occurrence (Jadrešin *et al.*, 2008).

In a recent review of the literature on self-management of the GFD in children and young people with CD by our research group (Theodosi, 2009), no standardised questionnaires were identified. Instead, non-standardised questionnaires or daily diaries/food records, used either alone or in conjunction with biopsy and blood tests, were used to assess the degree of self-management to the GFD. Studies have not used the same methods, therefore limiting comparability. In addition, the time frames or recall periods used to assess gluten ingestion and to categorise the degree of self-management to the GFD varied between studies (e.g. gluten eaten 'once a month', 'once a week', 'several times per week', 'occasionally', 'small amounts').

TABLE 11.2 Factors associated with better and poorer self-management of the gluten-free diet (GFD)

Better GFD management	Poorer GFD management
Female	Male
Younger children (<13 years; probably because of parental influence over diet)	Older children (>13 years)
Earlier age at diagnosis (i.e. reduced length of time on a gluten-containing diet)	Later age at diagnosis
Presence of typical, unpleasant symptoms pre-diagnosis (symptom-detected individuals)	Asymptomatic pre-diagnosis (screening-detected individuals)
Number and type of symptoms after eating gluten	No symptoms or minor symptom severity after eating gluten
Attendance at check-ups	Non-attendance or reduced attendance at check-ups
Availability and palatability of gluten-free meals in school, restaurants and supermarkets	Poor availability and palpability of gluten-free meals outside of the home
Good coeliac disease-related knowledge in children, young people and parents	Poor coeliac disease-related knowledge in children, young people and parents
High self-efficacy for GFD in child, young person and parent or carer	Low self-efficacy for GFD in child, young person and parent or carer
Clear food labelling	Unclear or missing information on food labelling
Financial support for GFD available	Reduced or no financial support for GFD
Social support that includes others with coeliac disease	Isolation from others with coeliac disease
Involved and supportive parents or carers	Less involved parents or carers and those more worried about health generally
Satisfaction with one's healthcare team	Unhappiness with those professionals involved in one's healthcare

In terms of ongoing CD research at the University of Birmingham, to explore factors associated with self-management to the GFD, quality of life and well-being, a short four-item questionnaire has been developed by our research group to assess self-reported gluten intake in young people across home and out-of-home settings (Figure 11.1). Based on a sample of 112 young people with biopsy-confirmed CD, the internal reliability for the questionnaire is 0.90, a strong positive correlation has been found between dietary self-efficacy and dietary self-management ($r = 0.71$), and a moderate strength correlation with health-related quality of life. Thus, young people who reported more confidence in their ability to follow their GFD reported better self-management and improved quality of life.

In the last 2 weeks …	Never	Once or twice	A few times	Daily	All the time
How often have you knowingly eaten foods containing gluten while at home?					
How often have you knowingly eaten foods containing gluten when away from home?					
How well do you stick to your gluten-free diet when you are at home?					
How well do you stick to your gluten-free diet when you are away from home?					

FIGURE 11.1 Birmingham Coeliac Disease Self-Management Questionnaire (CD-SMQ)

The questionnaire shown in Figure 11.1 can serve as a useful guide to help assess the degree of self-management and identify potential problem areas that require further exploration and assessment (i.e. home vs. out-of-home settings and specific situations associated with transgressions in the GFD). In addition, a parent- or proxy-completed version can also be used to assess the degree of match or mismatch between the child or young person and his or her parent(s) or carer(s).

In addition to the GFD, a thorough assessment should include exploration of those factors known to be associated with self-management in paediatric health conditions, across both child or young person and family systems, including:

- CD-related knowledge[11]
- common-sense understanding (illness representations[11]) of CD (e.g. Leventhal et al., 1980)
- treatment representations[11] (i.e. the burden of the GFD, beliefs in the necessity of the GFD, and concerns about sticking to the GFD)
- confidence (self-efficacy[11]) in being able to stick to the GFD in the face of specific barriers and across different settings (Bandura, 1997)
- coping with CD (e.g. the CODI (coping with a disease) questionnaire; Petersen et al., 2004)
- degree and type of parental involvement and responsibility for GFD

---

11 CD-specific questionnaires, developed by the University of Birmingham coeliac disease research group as part of ongoing research, are available upon request from the authors.

- well-being and quality of life (e.g. the CDDUX questionnaire, the PedsQL (Pediatric Quality of Life Inventory), the KIDSCREEN-27 questionnaire).

Ultimately, an adequate understanding of dietary self-management in CD requires an appreciation of the intrapersonal and interpersonal dimensions of the task (Howard *et al.*, 2012).

Quality of life

To assess the experiences of children and young people with CD, specifically what they think and feel about their CD and its treatment, the 12-item disease-specific health-related quality-of-life measure CDDUX was developed (Van Doorn *et al.*, 2008). Building on the DUX-25, the generic health-related quality-of-life measure for children with chronic illness (Koopman *et al.*, 1998), the CDDUX elicits information about those aspects of life that are influenced by CD for children and young people aged 8–18 years. The CDDUX makes use of 5-point Likert 'smiley answer' categories as its response format. Its shortness, together with good reliability and validity statistics, makes it feasible for use either in routine clinical settings or as part of a more comprehensive assessment. Table 11.3 provides details on the CDDUX.

TABLE 11.3 CDDUX subscales and properties

CDDUX subscales	M (SD)[a] Child [Parent]	Alpha[a] Child [Parent]
Communication		
Three items ('Talking about coeliac disease with others my age, I find …'; 'Talking about coeliac disease I find …'; 'When I have to explain to others what coeliac disease is, I feel …')	59 (21) [53 (20)]	0.71 [0.85]
Having coeliac disease		
Three items ('When at school I am given food containing gluten, I find it …'; 'When someone offers me food that I can't have, I feel …'; 'When I think of food containing gluten, I feel …')	36 (21) [30 (18)]	0.77 [0.77]
Diet		
Six items (including 'Not being able to eat anything I want, I find …'; 'Having to follow a lifelong diet, I find …'; 'Not being able to eat all the things other people eat, I find …')	36 (16) [33 (18)]	0.88 [0.87]
Total	44 (15)	0.88
12 items	[39 (15)]	[0.88]

Note: [a]data taken from Van Doorn *et al.* (2008) and based on 512 children with coeliac disease and their parents in the Netherlands. Scores can range from 1 to 100; 1–20 is considered very bad; 21–40 is bad; 41–60 is neutral; 61–80 is good; and 81–100 is very good. M, mean; SD, standard deviation.

Research by Van Doorn *et al.* (2008) has shown that children and young people with CD have a 'bad to neutral experience' of their quality of life when using the CDDUX, which contrasts with a good perception of quality of life when a generic instrument is used. As the CDDUX assesses the consequences of CD on several aspects of daily life, and as children might evaluate these aspects of life negatively, this does not mean that their generic quality of life will be so. More recently, and in an independent sample, higher quality-of-life scores on the CDDUX have been reported in children and young people with better GFD self-management, and a moderate correlation was found between a generic health-related quality-of-life questionnaire – PedsQL (Generic Core Scales; Varni *et al.*, 2001) – and CDDUX scores (Pico *et al.*, 2012). Thus, the combination of disease-specific and generic quality-of-life instruments can be used; together they will provide a more comprehensive picture and help clinicians and researchers to evaluate the impact of CD, respond to the needs identified and monitor the effectiveness of clinical interventions.

In terms of other instruments that have been used to assess quality of life, health-related quality of life, subjective well-being, satisfaction with different areas of physical and psychosocial well-being, and more general emotional and behavioural functioning, the following list outlines a sample of measures used in children and young people with CD.

- *The Inventory of Life Quality in Children and Adolescents* (Mattejat and Remschmidt, 2006) – a nine-item self-rating scale, used in many European countries, to assess functioning across nine different areas in children and adolescents with chronic physical health conditions. The nine areas are (1) school, (2) family, (3) social peer contacts, (4) interests and leisure activities, (5) physical health, (6) psychological health, (7) overall quality of life, (8) disease-associated burden and (9) therapy-associated burden. Wagner *et al.* (2008) found that young people with poorer self-management of the GFD reported poorer physical, psychological and social quality of life than those with better self-management. More frequent transgressions in the GFD were associated with poorer quality of life. In contrast, those young people with strict self-management to the GFD reported good quality of life across all areas, equal to healthy controls.
- *KIDSCREEN-27* (Ravens-Sieberer *et al.*, 2007) – a 27-item measure assessing five health-related quality-of-life dimensions: (1) physical well-being, (2) psychological well-being, (3) autonomy and parent relations, (4) social support and peers and (5) school environment. Published alpha coefficients are reported as 0.61–0.74 for the various dimensions. The University of Birmingham CD research group has found that those young people with greater quality of life are those reporting significantly greater self-efficacy for the GFD ($r = 0.42$), more understanding of the GFD ($r = 0.34$), stronger beliefs in the ability of the GFD to control symptoms ($r = 0.24$) and better self-management ($r = 0.40$).
- *Strengths and Difficulties Questionnaire* (Goodman, 2001) is a well-validated and widely used measure of psychological well-being of children and adolescents. In addition to total score, it assesses functioning across five areas: (1) emotional problems, (2) conduct problems, (3) hyperactivity-inattention,

(4) peer problems and (5) a pro-social scale. Our research group has found the same pattern and strength of correlations between total Strengths and Difficulties Questionnaire scores and the variables associated with quality of life as measured by the KIDSCREEN-27.

A rigorous clinical interview of the child, young person and family will be required to tease apart those areas of functioning that might be more problematic for managing CD. Questioning should include how the child or young person is functioning in school (particularly in terms of his or her social relationships and interactions with peers, and management of the GFD during break and lunch times) and in his or her social relationships with peers outside of school. Self-imposed restrictions in both of these domains, in an attempt to hide CD, have been reported in the literature. The management of CD at home, while usually better, should be detailed and the nature and degree of parental involvement explored. Given the high levels of parental anxiety that can be present in CD, the way the family fosters a child's or young person's development in relation to dietary self-management is crucial for their developing self-efficacy and self-esteem, but it can be a source of disagreement and stress.

Altogether, a combined narrow- and broad-band approach to the assessment of quality of life and well-being is required in children and young people with CD so as to identify those individuals who have psychosocial needs, quality-of-life issues and/or psychological adjustment problems (Jozefiak *et al.*, 2010), which might go undetected in the absence of specific questioning. Clearly, the list of assessment instruments outlined here is not exhaustive and healthcare professionals can use the wide variety of questionnaires that would normally be used in the assessment of psychological well-being (e.g. Children's Depression Inventory, Child Behaviour Checklist). However, clinicians should be mindful of the overlap between GI and non-GI symptoms (which might be indicative of CD or poorly managed CD) and those somatic symptoms that can be indicative of psychological adjustment problems (e.g. tiredness, lethargy, stomach pains). Without careful consideration and questioning of the child or young person and family, there may be a risk of either over- or under-interpreting scores.

PSYCHOSOCIAL INTERVENTIONS
Young people with long-term health conditions are at greater risk of poor psychological well-being than their 'healthy' counterparts and therefore the psychosocial management of these people is vital if good outcomes are to be achieved. Physicians are encouraged to pay attention to the signs of poor self-management and poor psychological well-being, and to consider interventions that include the management of family dynamics, educational interventions and interventions that increase the young person's autonomy (Geist *et al.*, 2003). Geist *et al.*'s (2003) review, published 9 years ago, calls for further research into the efficacy of specific psychosocial interventions for young

people with long-terms conditions and yet to date no research has considered such interventions for young people with CD.

Given the lack of research specifically on interventions for young people with CD, it is necessary to draw from other areas of research. Studies considering the psychosocial consequences of CD occasionally make recommendations regarding psychosocial interventions, including the implementation of cognitive and self-management therapies (Argio *et al.*, 2012; Smith and Goodfellow, 2011), educational programmes (Ring Jacobsson *et al.*, 2012) and dietitian-led psychological support (Barratt *et al.*, 2011). For example, Argio *et al.* (2012) looked at psychiatric co-morbidities in 177 American women with CD who responded to a web-based survey. A significant proportion of the women met the criteria for depression (37%) and disordered eating (22%) and reported poorer quality of life and increased symptoms of CD, despite demonstrating good dietary self-management. This study provided further support for the growing evidence base that psychosocial interventions, in particular cognitive and self-management interventions, should be employed to enhance well-being among this group of individuals.

Acknowledging that GI disorders affect the family as a whole, parental support, in addition to that provided for the young person is recommended (Knez *et al.*, 2011a, 2011b). Knez and colleagues published two papers in 2011, both recommending psychosocial interventions for families where a young person has a GI disorder. They examined both parental quality of life and attachment styles and recommended support particularly for parents demonstrating insecure attachments. These papers highlight the need for psychological assessment within the arena of GI disease. Other research has made recommendations regarding the nature of support. Di Lorenzo *et al.* (2012) showed quality of life was impaired on dimensions of social life and leisure activities and recommended a multi-modal approach comprising a combination of CD-specific information coupled with strategies for managing social discomfort and increasing socialisation and leisure activities.

Hommel *et al.* (2010) concluded that psychosocial factors in patients and family members should be considered in GI clinics. They recommended a thorough psychosocial assessment and the use of *'adjunctive behavioural intervention'*, including problem-solving skills training, social skills intervention and the use of biofeedback. Consultation with a professional psychologist or referral to mental health services was also suggested.

In terms of research into interventions with adults with CD, Addolorato and colleagues, through providing adequate support (included counselling, stress management and problem-solving, particularly in relation to feelings of inadequacy and difference), showed that those receiving psychological intervention experienced a reduction in depression after 6 months (Addolorato *et al.*, 2004). Jacobsen *et al.* (2012) provided an intervention that covered three areas of support – an educational programme, problem-based learning, and information giving – with the aim of increasing dietary self-management and well-being. They found that psychological well-being increased, and that, similarly to the

Addolorato study, this was sustained at 6-month follow-up.

There remains a paucity of research considering the efficacy of psychosocial interventions with people with CD, and none has been published that specifically considers intervention for young people and their families. Therefore, in current clinical practice it is necessary to draw from other areas of applied research into interventions in long-term conditions in general, and specifically GI conditions. Interventions with a multi-modal focus are emerging as potential key support mechanisms for young people and families managing a GFD. However, further research is necessary in this area in order to understand more fully the efficacy of specific interventions and the mechanisms essential for a positive outcome.

The following case study illustrates a multi-modal intervention aimed at tackling a number of psychosocial difficulties within a family.

CASE STUDY 1
Genogram

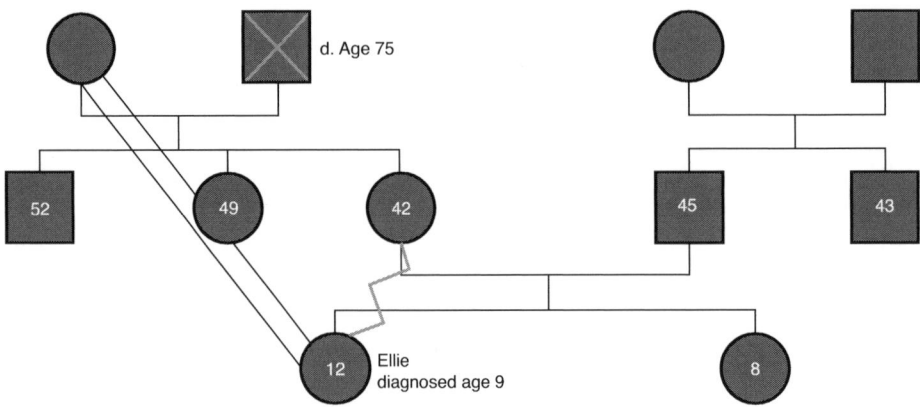

History of presenting problem
Ellie was diagnosed with CD at the age of 9. She had been experiencing mild symptoms of nausea, abdominal pain and fatigue for several years prior to the diagnosis and had always been considered a 'faddy eater'. After some initial anxieties, Ellie and her family coped well with the diagnosis (Ellie was in Year 5 at primary school) and GFD and, after only a few weeks, there was a noticeable improvement in her symptoms. No one else in the family was known to have CD. Ellie had a supportive group of friends in primary school and her mother worked closely with teaching and canteen staff to ensure that Ellie's new eating regimen was managed well in school.

At the time of referral Ellie was 12 and had recently completed her first year at secondary school. The school was some distance from home and only a handful of children from her primary school attended. Over the previous few months there had been a deterioration in Ellie's physical and emotional well-being. She had been complaining of nausea, particularly in the mornings, and was reluctant to go to school, missing the occasional day. Ellie and her mother had always worked together to manage Ellie's CD, with little input from her father. However, Ellie and her mother were exhibiting increased signs of anxiety and conflict around mealtimes. In addition to this, Ellie's mother had been finding it difficult to adjust to her daughter's increasing independence after starting secondary school.

Assessment

On assessment, Ellie and her mother presented as anxious and ill at ease with each other. Ellie, although reluctant to admit it at first, commented that she was worried about her CD as she became more aware of the long-term consequences of poor dietary self-management. However, she nevertheless felt she was managing her diet well and believed that the nausea was not entirely a result of possible gluten ingestion. Ellie later disclosed that there had been several transgressions from the GFD at school as she found it very difficult to tell her new school friends about her condition, and they had occasionally teased her about her eating habits. This was causing further anxiety during school time, as she felt different to her peers, leading her to turn down a number of social invitations from friends over the past year.

Ellie's mother reported no longer feeling in control of Ellie's diet and was anxious that her daughter might not be managing her diet well at school. Ellie was reluctant for her mother to become involved with school or to discuss Ellie's CD with teachers or canteen staff; this further exacerbated her mother's feelings of a lack of control. Because of increasing conflict with her mother, Ellie had sought support from her maternal grandmother, who had eventually suggested that further help for the family might be useful.

Psychological assessments indicated that for both Ellie and her mother there were increased levels of emotional problems (particularly anxiety and low mood) on the Strengths and Difficulties Questionnaire and the DASS-21 questionnaire (Lovibond and Lovibond, 1995), respectively. In addition, the Illness Perception Questionnaire-Revised (Moss-Morris et al., 2002) showed that both had a poor sense in their own personal control over CD, with Ellie reporting little belief in the power of treatment to help control symptoms of CD. Ellie scored high on perceived consequences of CD, indicating that she believed CD to interfere with many aspects of life. Ellie's self-efficacy for sticking to the GFD was low, particularly in out-of-home social situations; her mother completed a proxy-self-efficacy measure, which indicated that she also believed Ellie to have little confidence in sticking to the GFD and this worried her considerably.

Formulation

The *predisposing* factors in this case are Ellie's age at diagnosis and the relatively mild symptoms she reported pre-diagnosis. Thus, she came to CD and the GFD having spent a large portion of her childhood eating gluten-containing foods, without any severe physical consequences. In addition, and from the developmental history provided by mum, it appeared that there was a high degree of long-standing maternal overprotectiveness with regard to Ellie and her sister and high state maternal anxiety. The transition to secondary school seemed to be the *precipitating* factor for Ellie's deterioration in health, well-being and transgressions in the GFD.

The dissonance between wanting to 'fit in' and make new friends, and the skills and confidence necessary to manage the GFD, meant that Ellie chose to hide her CD from peers and teachers and occasionally consume gluten-containing foods. She believed that her headaches, tiredness and nausea were 'not too bad' and 'not too risky'. Ellie believed that in sticking to the GFD at home, this would compensate for any gluten-ingestion at school. These cognitive processes were serving to *perpetuate* the current transgressions in the GFD and, coupled with low confidence to talk to friends about her GFD, a growing awareness of longer-term health consequences, conflict with her mother in terms of dietary self-management, and increasing adolescent autonomy, were serving to maintain her anxiety and low mood, feelings of nausea and isolation in school.

Ellie's distancing from her mother, together with a high degree of maternal overprotectiveness, and the relative absence of her father as a source of parental support, were contributing to the maintenance of her mother's anxiety and stress. The *protective* factors in Ellie's case were the motivation of Ellie and mother to seek and accept help for the current situation. Ellie's mother very much wanted to begin a constructive dialogue with Ellie and school about how to move forward with her diet, and wanted to support Ellie to engage in social activities outside of the home. Previous to the current presentation, there is a positive history of good dietary self-management and parent–child problem-solving.

Intervention

A multi-modal intervention was used to manage the difficulties being experienced by Ellie and her mother, the aims of which were to:

- increase Ellie's sense of treatment and personal control
- reduce mother and child anxiety
- address and reduce family conflict
- increase self-efficacy for the diet, in particular when away from home.

Ellie and her mother were encouraged to share their feelings about their current situation, which Ellie was able to do through expressing her feelings of fear for longer-term health, but expressing her confusion as to what it could mean, and the sense of burden she had in sticking to the GFD. She also shared her beliefs about what 'bad' things she thought would happen if she disclosed her condition to her new friends at school or if her mother told the staff about her CD. In turn, Ellie's mother was able to share her feelings of anxiety about Ellie moving on to secondary school as well as her specific anxieties about her diet; this led to a shared and more considered understanding of the presenting difficulties between Ellie and her mother. Consequently, Ellie and her mother were able to agree on a number of behavioural experiments, set as 'home tasks', to start to address their feelings of conflict and anxiety. A session was also arranged for the family as a whole to discuss the difficulties and Ellie's father and sister attended this.

The following steps were achieved during the intervention.

- Ellie and her mother met with the Head of Year at school to discuss how to manage Ellie's CD. A plan was made for Ellie to receive ongoing support from the Head of Year, and for the two of them to discuss her dietary requirements with the canteen manager.
- After exploring and challenging her beliefs about what would happen if she spoke to friends, and rehearsing this through role-play, Ellie agreed to disclose her diagnosis with her closest friend at school. This led to her friend enabling her to discuss her condition with other pupils at school.
- Ellie and her mother organised a tea party with a group of Ellie's friends; Ellie took responsibility for deciding on the menu (in negotiation with mum) and they cooked the meal together.
- Ellie and her mother agreed to attend the local CD support group on a regular basis in order to increase their understanding and management of the condition and bolster their support networks.
- At the family session, conflict at mealtimes was discussed. Ellie's father agreed to take on certain aspects of managing Ellie's GFD within the home, and he and Ellie's younger sister agreed to attend occasional support group meetings to increase their understanding of CD.
- Ellie and her mother agreed strategies for regularly checking out Ellie's feelings regarding CD and the GFD, and also agreed that Ellie could continue to seek support from her grandmother.
- After tackling her dietary self-management at school, Ellie started to consider ways in which she could address her anxiety about eating away from home. She agreed to go to tea with a close friend, and sought support and information from members of the support group regarding eating in restaurants and away from home.

A programme of psychoeducation supported these aspects of the intervention. This included details of the symptoms of anxiety, and also the use of an education DVD for young people with CD produced by the University of Birmingham. The family was encouraged to attend an additional appointment with the paediatric gastroenterologist and dietitian to alleviate any anxieties about Ellie's physical well-being and to check her levels of coeliac antibodies.

Outcome

Six months on, anxiety levels had reduced for both Ellie and her mother and both reported less conflict within the family with regard to eating. Both felt better supported by family members and were finding positive benefits from attending the support group. Ellie's nausea had decreased and was evident only occasionally. However, Ellie's mother continued to experience some worries about Ellie's integration into secondary school. For Ellie, she had organised a number of social activities with friends over the previous few weeks, and she had been pleased about the response from pupils at school in relation to her CD; she was becoming more confident in herself and accepting of CD as part of her identity. She continued to have some low-level anxieties about lunchtimes at school, but these were improving. With help from members of the support group she had been for a meal at a local restaurant, and despite anxieties for her and her mother about managing the diet, this experience had been positive. Finally, the information provided by the DVD had given the family strategies for managing a planned holiday in the coming months.

Repeated measures of anxiety, self-efficacy and illness perceptions evidenced improvements, although Ellie's mother's levels of anxiety were elevated, but this was an area she was continuing to work on.

SUMMARY

This chapter has considered the psychosocial consequences for young people and their families of living with CD. It began by explaining the details of the diagnosis and management of the condition before exploring the psychosocial consequences of managing a GFD, covering issues of psychological well-being and quality of life. The assessment of psychological well-being and quality of life in CD were reviewed, before considering psychosocial interventions.

The area of psychological well-being, quality of life and CD is a developing one, and more attention needs to be paid to considering the efficacy of psychosocial interventions with young people and their families and integrating this into clinical practice. Knowledge can be drawn from interventions in other areas of paediatric psychology, and particularly in relation to the management of long-term conditions and other GI conditions, and it is recommended that clinical services consider the integration of psychological support into GI clinical and dietary care. However, further research as to the appropriate and effective nature of these interventions is needed.

Psychological support and intervention have been shown to play an important role across paediatric services, and CD should be no exception. With integrated psychological support, young people with CD and their families can achieve good dietary self-management and consequently good emotional and physical well-being.

REFERENCES

Achenbach T. *Manual for the CBCL/4-18 and Profile*. Burlington, VA: University of Vermont, Department of Psychiatry; 1991.

Addolorato G, De Lorenzi G, Abenavoli L, *et al.* Psychological support counselling improves gluten-free diet compliance in coeliac patients with affective disorders. *Aliment Pharmacol Ther.* 2004; **20**(7): 777–82.

Anson O, Weizman Z, Zeevi N. Celiac disease: parental knowledge and attitudes of dietary compliance. *Pediatrics.* 1990; **85**(1): 98–103.

Argio, D, Anskis AM, Smyth JM. Psychiatric comorbidities in women with celiac disease. *Chronic Illn.* 2012; **8**(1): 45–55.

Bandura A. *Self-efficacy: the exercise of control.* New York, NY: WH Freeman; 1997.

Barratt SM, Leeds JS, Sanders DS. Quality of life in coeliac disease is determined by perceived degree of difficulty adhering to a gluten-free diet, not the level of dietary adherence ultimately achieved. *J Gastrointestin Liver Dis.* 2011; **20**(3): 241–5.

Bingley P, Williams A, Norcross A, et al. Undiagnosed coeliac disease at age seven: population based prospective birth cohort study. *BMJ.* 2004; **328**(7435): 322–3.

Bongiovanni T, Clark A, Garnett E, et al. Impact of a gluten-free camp on quality of life of children and adolescents with celiac disease. *Pediatrics.* 2010; **125**(3): e525–9.

British Society of Paediatric Gastroenterology Hepatology and Nutrition (BSPGHAN). *Guidance for the Diagnosis and Management of Coeliac Disease in Children.* BSPGHAN; 2006. Available at: http://bspghan.org.uk/documents/Static/Coeliac%20Guidelines%202013.pdf (accessed 8 August 2012).

Byström I-M, Hollén E, Fälth-Magnusson K, et al. Health-related quality of life in children and adolescents with celiac disease: from the perspectives of children and parents. *Gastroenterol Res Pract.* 2012; **2012**: Article ID 986475.

Cederborg A-C, Hultman E, Magnusson K. Living with children who have coeliac disease: a parental perspective. *Child Care Health Dev.* 2011; **38**(4): 484–9.

Cinquetti M, Trabucchi C, Menegazzi N, et al. Psychological problems connected to dietary restrictions in the adolescent with coeliac disease. *Pediatr Med Chir.* 1999; **21**(6): 279–83.

Coeliac UK. *Coeliac Disease FAQs.* Buckinghamshire: Coeliac UK; 2012. Available at: www.coeliac.org.uk/coeliac-disease/coeliac-disease-faqs (accessed 8 August 2012).

Di Lorenzo C, Xikota J, Wayhs M, et al. Evaluation of the quality of life of children with celiac disease and their parents: a case-control study. *Qual Life Res.* 2012; **21**(1): 77–85.

Errichiello S, Esposito O, Mase R, et al. Celiac disease: predictors of compliance with a gluten-free diet in adolescents and young adults. *J Pediatr Gastroenterol Nutr.* 2010; **50**(1): 54–60.

Fasano A. Clinical presentation of celiac disease in the pediatric population. *Gastoenterology.* 2005; **128**(4 Suppl. 1): S68–73.

Geist R, Grdisa V, Otley A. Psychosocial issues in the child with chronic conditions. *Best Pract Res Clin Gastroenterol.* 2003; **17**(2): 141–52.

Goodman R. Psychometric properties of the Strengths and Difficulties Questionnaire. *J Am Acad Child Adolesc Psychiatry.* 2001; **40**(11): 1337–45.

Green PH, Cellier C. Celiac disease. *N Engl J Med.* 2007; **357**(17): 1731–43.

Hagger M. Health psychology review: advancing theory and research in health psychology and behavioural medicine. *Health Psychol Rev.* 2010; **4**(1): 1–5.

Hommel KA, McGraw KL, Ammerman RT, et al. Psychosocial functioning in children and adolescents with gastrointestinal complaints and disorders. *J Clin Psychol Med Settings.* 2010; **17**(2): 159–66.

Hopman E, le Cessie S, Von Blomberg B, et al. Nutritional management of the gluten-free diet in young people with celiac disease in the Netherlands. *J Pediatr Gastroenterol Nutr.* 2006; **43**(1): 102–8.

Howard RA, Urquhart-Law G, Petty JL. Coeliac disease: psychosocial factors in adults and children. In: Lloyd C, Heller T, editors. *Long-term Conditions: challenges in health and social care.* London: Sage; 2012. pp. 108–23.

Husby S, Koletzko S, Korponay-Szabo I, et al. European Society for Gastroenterology, Hepatology and Nutrition guidelines for the diagnosis of coeliac disease. *J Pediatr Gastroenterol Nutr.* 2012; **54**(1): 136–60.

Hysing M, Elgen I, Gillberg C, et al. Emotional and behavioural problems in subgroups of children with chronic illness: results from a large-scale population study. *Child Care Health Dev.* 2009; **35**(4): 527–33.

Jackson P, Glasgow J, Thom R. Parents' understanding of coeliac disease and diet. *Arch Dis Child.* 1985; **60**(7): 672–4.

Jacobsen PB, Wells KJ, Meade CD, *et al*. Effects of a brief multimedia psychoeducational intervention on the attitudes and interest of patients with cancer regarding clinical trial participation: a multicenter randomized controlled trial. *J Clin Oncol*. 2012; **30**(20): 2516–21.

Jadrešin O, Mišak Z, Kolaček S, *et al*. Compliance with gluten-free diet in children with coeliac disease. *J Pediatr Gastroenterol Nutr*. 2008; **47**(3): 344–8.

Jozefiak T, Larsson B, Wichstrøm L, *et al*. Quality of life as reported by children and parents: a comparison between students and child psychiatric outpatients. *Health Qual Life Outcomes*. 2010; **8**: 136.

Karwautz A, Wagner G, Berger G, *et al*. Eating pathology in adolescents with celiac disease. *Psychosomatics*. 2008; **49**(5): 399–406.

Kinos S, Kurppa K, Ukkola A, *et al*. Self-perceived burden of coeliac disease in children and their families: a nationwide prospective study. *J Pediatr Gastroenterol Nutr*. 2011; **52**: E131.

Knez R, Francisković T, Samarin RM, *et al*. Attachment style in parents of children with chronic gastrointestinal disease. *Coll Antropol*. 2011a; **35**(2): 125–30.

Knez R, Francisković T, Samarin R, *et al*. Parental quality of life in the framework of paediatric chronic gastrointestinal disease. *Coll Antropol*. 2011b; **35**(2): 275–80.

Kolsteren M, Koopman H, Schalekamp G, *et al*. Health-related quality of life in children with celiac disease. *J Pediatr*. 2001; **138**(4): 593–5.

Koopman H, Theunissen N, Vogels T, *et al*. The DUX-25: a short form questionnaire for measuring health-related quality of life of children with chronic illness. *Qual Health Res*. 1998; **7**: 619.

Kovacs M. *The Children's Depression Inventory: a self-rated depression scale of school-aged youngsters*. Pittsburgh, PA: University of Pittsburgh School of Medicine; 1982.

Leventhal H, Meyer D, Nerenz D. The common-sense representations of illness and danger. In: Rachman S, editor. *Medical Psychology*. Vol. 2. New York, NY: Pergamon; 1980. pp. 7–30.

Loonen H, Derkx B, Otley A. Measuring health-related quality of life of pediatric patients. *J Pediatr Gastroenterol Nutr*. 2001; **32**(5): 523–6.

Lovibond S, Lovibond P. *Manual for the Depression Anxiety and Stress Scales*. Sydney: Psychology Foundation; 1995.

March J. *Multidimensional Anxiety Scale for Children*. Tonawanda, NY: Multi-Health System; 1997.

Mattejat F, Remschmidt H. *Das Inventar zur Erfassung der Lebensqualität bei Kindern und Jugendlichen (ILK)* [*The Inventory of Life Quality in Children and Adolescents (ILC)*]. Bern: Verlag Hans Huber; 2006.

Mazzone L, Reale L, Spina M, *et al*. Compliant gluten-free children with celiac disease: an evaluation of psychological distress. *BMC Pediatr*. 2011; **11**: 46.

Modi A, Pai A, Hommel K, *et al*. Pediatric self-management: a framework for research, practice and policy. *Pediatrics*. 2012; **129**(2): e473–85.

Moss-Morris R, Weinman J, Petrie K, *et al*. The revised illness perception questionnaire (IPQ-R). *Psychol Health*. 2002; **17**(1): 1–16.

National Institute for Health and Care Excellence (NICE). *Coeliac Disease: recognition and assessment of coeliac disease; clinical guideline CG86*. London: NICE; 2009. http://guidance.nice.org.uk/CG86

Niederhofer H. Association of attention-deficit/hyperactivity disorder and celiac disease: a brief report. *Primary Care Companion for CNS Disorders*. 2011; **13**(3): PCC.10br01104.

Niederhofer H, Pittschieler K. Attention deficit hyperactivity-like disorder and celiac disease. *J Attention Disord*. 2006; **10**(2): 200–4.

Olsson C, Hornell A, Ivarsson A, *et al*. The everyday life of adolescent coeliacs: issues of importance for compliance with the gluten-free diet. *J Hum Nutr Diet*. 2008; **21**(4): 359–67.

Olsson C, Lyon P, Hornell A, *et al*. Food that makes you different: the stigma experienced by adolescents with celiac disease. *Qual Health Res*. 2009; **19**(7): 976–84.

Petersen C, Schmidt S, Bullinger M; the DISABKIDS Group. Brief report: development and pilot testing of a coping questionnaire for children and adolescents with chronic health conditions. *J Pediatr Psychol.* 2004; **29**(8): 635–40.

Pico M, Spirito M, Poizen M. Quality of life in children and adolescents with celiac disease: Argentinian version of the specific questionnaire CDDUX [Spanish]. *Acta Gastroenterol Latinoam.* 2012; **41**(1): 12–19.

Polanco I. Celiac disease. *J Pediatr Gastroenterol Nutr.* 2008; **47**: S3–6.

Pynnönen P, Isometsä E, Aronen E, *et al.* Mental disorders in adolescents with celiac disease. *Psychosomatics.* 2004; **45**(4): 325–35.

Pynnönen P, Isometsä E, Verkasalo M, *et al.* Gluten-free diet may alleviate depressive and behavioural symptoms in adolescents with coeliac disease: a prospective follow-up case-series study. *BMC Psychiatry.* 2005; **5**: 14.

Rashid M, Cranney A, Zarkadas M, *et al.* Celiac disease: evaluation of the diagnosis and dietary compliance in Canadian children. *Pediatrics.* 2005; **116**(6): e754–9.

Ravens-Sieberer U, Auquier P, Erhart M, *et al.* The KIDSCREEN-27 quality of life measure for children and adolescents: psychometric results from a cross-cultural survey in 13 European countries. *Qual Life Res.* 2007; **16**(8): 1347–56.

Ring Jacobsson L, Friedrichsen M, Goransson A, *et al.* Does a coeliac school increase psychological well-being in women suffering from coeliac disease, living on a gluten-free diet? *J Clin Nurs.* 2012; **21**(5–6): 766–75.

Roma E, Roubani A, Kolia *et al.* Dietary compliance and life style of children with celiac disease. *J Hum Nutr Diet.* 2010; **23**(2): 176–82.

Rosén A, Emmelin M, Carlsson A, *et al.* Mass screening for celiac disease from the perspective of newly diagnosed adolescents and their parents: a mixed-methods study. *BMC Public Health.* 2011; **11**: 822.

Rostrom A, Murray J, Kagnoff M. American Gastoenterological Association (AGA) Institute Technical Review on the diagnosis and management of celiac disease. *Gastroenterology.* 2006; **131**(6): 1981–2002.

Smith MM, Goodfellow L. The relationship between quality of life and coping strategies of adults with celiac disease adhering to a gluten-free diet. *Gastroenterol Nurs.* 2011; **34**(6): 460–8.

Tanpowpong P, Ingham T, Lampshire P, *et al.* New Zealand Asthma and Allergy Cohort Study Group. Coeliac disease and gluten avoidance in New Zealand children. *Arch Dis Child.* 2012; **97**(1): 12–16.

Theodosi E. Children, young people and coeliac disease [unpublished doctoral dissertation]. Birmingham: University of Birmingham; 2009.

Van Doorn R, Winkler L, Zwinderman K, *et al.* CDDUX: a disease-specific health-related quality-of-life questionnaire for children with celiac disease. *J Pediatr Gastroenterol Nutr.* 2008; **47**(2): 147–52.

Van Koppen E, Schweizer J, Csizmadia C, *et al.* Long-term health and quality of life consequences of mass screening for childhood celiac disease: a 10-year follow-up study. *Pediatrics.* 2009; **123**(4): e582–8.

Varni J, Seid M, Kurtin P. PedsQL 4.0: reliability and validity of the Pediatric Quality of Life Inventory version 4.0 generic core scales in healthy and patient populations. *Med Care.* 2001; **39**(8): 800–12.

Wagner G, Berger G, Sinnreich U, *et al.* Quality of life in adolescents with treated coeliac disease: influence of compliance and age at diagnosis. *J Pediatr Gastroenterol Nutr.* 2008; **47**(5): 555–61.

West J, Logan R, Hill P, *et al.* The iceberg of celiac disease: what is below the waterline? *Clin Gastroenterol Hepatol.* 2007; **5**(1): 59–62.

CHAPTER 12

Disable to enable: morbidity and quality-of-life challenges in adolescents with Crohn's disease

Gill Townson and Ella Mozdiak

INTRODUCTION

This chapter examines quality-of-life issues in adolescents with Crohn's disease. It outlines the demographics, clinical course and treatment of young patients with Crohn's disease. In order to appreciate how adolescents live with Crohn's disease and the many challenges these children, their families and carers face, it is important to understand what Crohn's disease is, how it may present and how it is diagnosed, as well as the various treatment options for this as yet incurable disease. Attention is paid here to the patient's perspective, including concerns over access to rapid diagnosis and specialist care, the healthcare professionals' perspectives – including education targeted at primary care and more time with specialist teams. Finally, how clinicians may incorporate understanding of Crohn's disease in the multidisciplinary care of adolescents with Crohn's disease encompassing the latest work on quality of life, as well as the use of patient focus groups, is also discussed. Although clinicians recognise that quality of life is impaired in chronic disease like Crohn's disease, many underestimate the degree of disability it causes.

A cross-European group has reported on the experiences of patients with Crohn's disease in 27 European countries (Van Assche *et al.*, 2010). It concluded that patients and healthcare professionals had to work together to highlight the need for high-quality care (incorporating the consequences of disability on long-term outcome of patients with Crohn's disease) to government bodies and policymakers (Wilson *et al.*, 1994). A discussion of a new measure, 'the disability index', was also included.

INCIDENCE, AETIOLOGY AND PROGNOSIS
Definition and aetiology

Described in 1932 by Burrill B Crohn, a New York physician, Crohn's disease is a chronic inflammatory condition that can affect any part of the gastrointestinal tract from the mouth to the anus, but which most commonly affects the terminal ileum and caecum. It is currently incurable and is characterised by discontinuous transmural granulomatous inflammation (Crohn, 1932). This results in ulceration of the bowel wall. The exact aetiology of Crohn's disease has not been established, but it is thought to be an interaction between genetic and environmental factors causing an exaggerated immune response in the gastrointestinal tract (Bouma and Strober, 2003). Many decades after it was first described, it is still unclear whether the disease develops as an appropriate response to an as yet unrecognised pathogen or whether it is the response that is inappropriate (Bamias *et al.*, 2005).

A large amount of work into the environmental triggers that may determine the development of Crohn's disease is being undertaken. Scientists are particularly interested in genetic markers associated with risk of developing the disease; however, no genes have been identified with enough association to justify routine use of genetic tests (Bouma and Strober, 2003). What is known is there is an increased prevalence if a family member is affected, and it has a strong association with smoking. Patients have higher overall mortality rates than average (Lichtenstein *et al.*, 2006).

Epidemiology and prognosis

Crohn's disease affects around 87,000 people in the United Kingdom (Bamias *et al.*, 2005). Twenty-five per cent present in adolescence and the median age of diagnosis is 29.5 years, with an equal sex ratio (IBD Standards Group, 2009). In Europe, there is a higher prevalence in northern than in southern European countries, but there has been an increase noted in southern countries in recent years (Bouma and Strober, 2003). It has a low incidence in Asia, Japan and South America (Bamias *et al.*, 2005). Smoking increases the risk of developing the disease by three to four times (Hanauer, 2006).

Crohn's disease follows an unpredictable relapsing and remitting course, with at least half of patients undergoing surgery at some stage (IBD Standards Group, 2009). It can be stricturing or fistulating, with perianal disease affecting up to a quarter of patients (Bamias *et al.*, 2005). There is an increased risk of colonic cancer, and bowel surveillance is recommended after 10 years of diagnosis in patients with colonic Crohn's (Stone *et al.*, 2003). Clinical course is dependent on the site affected, whether the disease is stricturing or fistulating and whether the perianal region is affected. There is a large variation in severity of the disease and response to treatment in each individual, but it is well recognised that when diagnosed in childhood, the disease has a more severe course (Henderson *et al.*, 2011).

PRESENTATION AND MANAGEMENT

Presentation

Diagnosis may be delayed because of the heterogeneous nature of presentation. Children and adolescents may present with intestinal or extra-intestinal symptoms, depending on the predominant site of the disease. Up to 30% of children with Crohn's disease may have growth failure and it is an important presenting complaint in children with undiagnosed Crohn's disease (Caprilli *et al.*, 2006). Anaemia must also raise the suspicion of inflammatory bowel disease (IBD). Chronic diarrhoea is the most common presenting complaint, with abdominal pain and weight loss frequently observed too (Bouma and Strober, 2003). Extra-intestinal manifestations most commonly involve the joints, but disorders of the skin, eyes and liver are all recognised. They are more common in patients with colonic or perianal Crohn's – up to a third of patients will have one extra-intestinal manifestation (e.g. pyoderma gangrenosum (necrotic tissue with ulceration), uveitis (inflammation of the eye), spondylarthropathy (joint diseases in the vertebral column) and primary sclerosing cholangitis (disease of the bile ducts)) (Rutgeerts *et al.*, 2006). Patients may also present with complications secondary to malabsorption such as renal stones, gallstones and osteopenia.

Once a patient is suspected of having Crohn's disease, a series of laboratory, endoscopic and radiological investigations are carried out following a detailed history and physical examination. As the disease can affect multiple sites of the gastrointestinal tract, imaging and endoscopic investigations must be carried out based on an individual assessment of each patient. Colonoscopy with ileoscopy is often the first-line procedure (Bouma and Strober, 2003). In children, use of upper gastrointestinal endoscopy is far more common, with evidence of granulomatous disease in the upper gastrointestinal tract being detected in around a quarter of patients (Carroll, 1998; Van Assch *et al.*, 2010). Imaging modalities at diagnosis can be as limited as a plain abdominal radiograph, but often computed tomography and magnetic resonance imaging are used. It is important to consider radiation exposure in this group of patients who, because of the chronicity and unpredictability of their disease, will often undergo multiple imaging throughout their disease course. Van Assche and colleagues described macroscopic and microscopic criteria in order to establish a diagnosis (Van Assche *et al.*, 2010). The European Crohn's and Colitis Organisation suggests the diagnosis should be made by a defined set of findings comprised of the clinical, radiological and histological evidence. The Montreal phenotype classification has risen to prominence and is the internationally regarded standard for Crohn's disease (Odes *et al.*, 2007).

Medical management

Treatment is aimed at disease remission, as cure is not currently possible. As with investigations, management must be individualised depending on site and severity of disease. Medical management will almost always involve steroid use to induce remission and at various courses of disease relapse, but it is not acceptable for steroids to be used to maintain remission (Mowat *et al.*, 2011). Thiopurines such as azathioprine and 6-mecaptopurine are widely used in long-term management; methotrexate is used less commonly. In recent years use of biological therapies has increased greatly and has changed the way we manage the disease. Both infliximab and adalumimab are licensed by the National Institute for Health and Care Excellence for patients with severe active Crohn's disease who have not responded to conventional therapy or who are intolerant or have contraindications to conventional therapy (NICE, 2012). There are many other important considerations including iron replacement and bone protection. A large amount of research is currently in progress and it is likely that management regimens will be updated multiple times in the coming years.

Surgical management

Surgical management should be carefully considered and undertaken only by colorectal surgeons who are core members of the IBD team (IBD Standards Group, 2009). Common indications for surgery are fistulae and fibrotic strictures. The majority of patients will undergo surgery at some point in their disease course, and many will have recurrent disease following surgery (Caprilli *et al.*, 2006; Sachar, 1990). As decision-making is complex, it is increasingly carried out in the context of a multidisciplinary meeting (Mowat *et al.*, 2011). Screening for colorectal cancer is also an important consideration in managing patients with Crohn's colitis, and the British Society of Gastroenterology lay out clear guidelines regarding when to perform colonoscopy (Stone *et al.*, 2003). Surveillance usually starts 10 years from diagnosis.

Role of multidisciplinary team

The UK IBD Standards recommend the input of a number of named allied professionals in the multidisciplinary management of patients with Crohn's disease in addition to the paediatrician, specialist surgeon and gastroenterologist running a transition to adult service. These include a specialist psychologist, a rheumatologist, a dermatologist and a dietetics support team.

Smoking cessation (older adolescents) and good nutrition are important therapeutic considerations and are part of the UK IBD Standards. In particular, enteral nutrition in children often forms a large part of the therapeutic strategy involved in inducing remission rates (IBD Standards Group, 2009). The psychological impact is large, and specific consideration to psychological support must be given. Multidisciplinary team working is of huge importance in this complex, chronic and heterogeneous condition and will be discussed in detail elsewhere (*see* also Chapter 6).

CHALLENGES IN MANAGING YOUNG PATIENTS WITH CROHN'S DISEASE

It is easiest to illustrate the clinical challenges faced by medical professionals by using several case-based discussions. These case histories illustrate many of the issues young patients with Crohn's disease face which present both clinical and psychological challenges in management; delay in diagnosis, early surgery, no transition clinics, steroid dependence, poor university performance, rectovaginal fistulae (direct connection between the rectum and vagina) and concerns regarding fertility.

Case Study 1

CH was aged 13 when she presented to the general paediatric department of her local hospital. She had a short history of colicky generalised abdominal pain, loose stools and blood-stained motions following a viral upper respiratory tract infection. A barium meal and follow-through X-ray showed evidence of terminal ileal Crohn's disease and she was started on systemic steroids. Two years after diagnosis she underwent an ileocaecal resection and was commenced on post-operative prophylactic treatment with azathioprine. At the age of 18, while away at university, the combination of stress and poor diet contributed to her relapsing and she was recommenced on an elemental diet and systemic steroids. Missing much time from university she eventually underwent a subtotal colectomy and ileostomy at the age of 20, followed by a complete proctectomy and permanent ileostomy 1 year later because of ongoing problems with a rectovaginal fistula. She had a stable course for the next 10 years on azathioprine and is now on no treatment and is hoping to start a family.

Case Study 2

Similar concerns are highlighted in the case history of ZL, who presented to an adult gastroenterologist at the age of 18 having been unwell for more than 1 year and struggling to complete her university degree course. She developed a viral gastroenteritis bug while skiing at the age of 17, a bug that affected many of her family but, unlike everyone else, her symptoms did not settle. She complained of abdominal bloating, initially constipation turning to watery diarrhoea, right iliac fossa pain, feeling tired all the time and substantial weight loss. She was only using Complan for nutrition. She had had bouts of erythema nodosum and mouth ulcers and presented with very raised inflammatory markers (erythrocyte sedimentation rate, C-reactive protein). A colonoscopy showed her to have severe Crohn's colitis and although systemic steroids helped her, a repeat examination (to determine maintenance treatment) showed her to still have very active disease. She was maintained on infliximab (intravenous biological agent) for nearly 2 years before having surgery to resect a long terminal ileal stricture. After quite a stormy post-operative course she is stable on home-injected (subcutaneous) Humira.

Case Study 3

Another similar case history is that of CJ. She presented to a paediatric gastroenterologist aged 15 with a 6-month history of weight loss, abdominal pain and diarrhoea. She was anaemic with raised inflammatory markers. A colonoscopy showed a stricture (narrowing) at the hepatic flexure and active disease all the way around the colon. She suffered multiple relapses over the next 2 years and was managed on a combination of mesalazine, elemental diet and systemic steroids, missing much time from school and failing to attain her desired academic achievements. She was handed over to the adult service without any 'transitioning' aged 18 but in a relatively stable condition. She was started on azathioprine but developed a severe reaction to this. One year later because of dependence on steroids she had a subtotal colectomy and ileostomy but with no post-operative prophylaxis. Within 1 year she had had a further relapse, treated with systemic steroids. She developed an ischiorectal abscess 1 year later, as well as involvement of her vulva, and a later magnetic resonance imaging scan showed her to have gross pelvic disease (multiple abscesses and fistula). After an examination under anaesthetic and insertion of setons (to help drain infection and aid healing) she eventually had a proctectomy and refashioning of her ileostomy. She had some problems with cutaneous fistulae on her anterior abdominal wall but is now on maintenance infliximab. She has just married and is hoping to start a family in the near future.

These cases highlight the complex issues facing young patients with Crohn's disease. All three young women had significant time off from either school or university impacting on educational achievement. They had complicated disease with at least two of them having pelvic abscesses or fistulae which may well impact on their future fertility and all three of them had to have semi-emergency surgery, with two of them having little time to plan for the consequences of having a stoma for life.

FOCUS GROUP DISCUSSION

As health professionals working within the field of IBD, it is imperative to constantly reassess the service that is delivered through national, local and departmental guidelines. At the core of any service are the patients who can help professionals mould their service but who are often not consulted. Gaining an insight into a patient's experience, not only of the patient's disease and medical management but also his or her quality of life, is invaluable to any service improvement plans. It also reminds health professionals that these diseases are life-changing and have a huge impact on patients and their families.

The assessment of health-related quality of life plays an increasingly important role in the day-to-day management of those with a chronic disease such as IBD. As 'well-being' is so much more complex than clinical remission and mucosal healing, there have been many health-related quality-of-life measures designed for Crohn's disease in an attempt to quantify overall health.

Patient-reported outcome measures allow the patient to provide his or her viewpoint (Van Assche *et al.*, 2010). Much of the work has been focused on adults with IBD, and there is little known about the impact on adolescents (Bouma and Strober, 2003). Questionnaires such as the IMPACT III, designed to measure health-related quality of life in paediatric patients, has been found to be a useful and reproducible tool (Lichtenstein *et al.*, 2006; Stone *et al.*, 2003). Although IMPACT III has good retest reliability, it is well known that key quality-of-life issues can be under-represented, as the emphasis of what determines quality of life is personal to each patient. In order to provide good-quality care, we must gain insight into what impacts most on our patients' overall well-being. As health providers, we are acutely aware that patient populations show regional variation in disease incidence and health needs, and so a patient's concerns and life goals will also differ depending on his or her postcode.

The benefit of focus groups has long been established. They are a form of qualitative research (Van Assche *et al.*, 2010) that allows the opinions and attitudes of a population to be voiced in their own words. Through direct interaction they can provide a very candid insight into the attitudes and concerns of adolescents with Crohn's disease – information that may have been left untapped by questionnaires. Patients can identify new areas of concern, rather than focusing on issues that the healthcare professionals assume are important. A recent publication from the Mayo Clinic described its positive experience of holding a large number of focus groups in patients with IBD (Hanauer, 2006).

Focus groups can have a positive effect on psychological health themselves by allowing the patient to have a voice and be able to contribute to the understanding of his or her disease, giving the patient a sense of empowerment and providing a supportive environment that encourages patients to address sensitive issues (Henderson *et al.*, 2011). In preparation for the Standards of Care for IBD, in 2004/05 the UK National Association for Colitis and Crohn's Disease ran two focus groups in order to improve services. This gave a detailed account of the experience IBD patients have of health services and how they feel they could be improved. Of course outcomes from focus groups cannot be assumed to have generalisability to the greater population and must be used as an additional research method along with national consensus.

Our team carried out a focus group in order to gauge the experience, attitudes and concerns of our local adolescent population with IBD. This was held as an evening session within a District General Hospital, and involved a gastroenterology registrar and IBD specialist nurse as moderators and a gastroenterology consultant who acted as an observer only. Patients were invited to participate by phone. The group size was six, with one male and five females, and ages ranged from 16 to 29 years. The session was an hour long and was loosely structured around questions asked by the moderator, although the emphasis was on listening to the group members and asking questions prompted by the topic of conversation. Every member of the group was encouraged to voice an opinion, but with no expectation that they had to speak.

In preparation for the focus group, a few key areas were identified that had been reviewed within the UK IBD Standards (Lichtenstein *et al.*, 2006). The purpose was to put the onus on the group to have a discussion on these pertinent issues among themselves. The focus group involved six young people with a mean age of 22 years; the group was facilitated by a doctor and an IBD nurse, with ground rules of confidentiality established and the aim of the session explained. Three topics were discussed, as time was limited, but there are many areas identified that warranted further discussion; these three topics were (1) employment, (2) attitudes and (3) care from the health professionals. The use of headings was used to explore the group's perspective on employment, attitudes towards their disease and how the service provider could make improvements.

Group perspective on employment
The group were asked how their friends and family react to their diagnosis. Generally the response was positive, but there was a consensus that friends and family didn't really know much about the disease, which could lead to difficulties when they have symptoms.

> 'It is hard to explain what the disease is.'

> 'Sometimes I think people think I am exaggerating the condition to get sympathy, because I look well.'

> 'My friends and family were great.'

The group talked about employers without any prompting, and the response was mixed:

> 'I loved my job, and they were so supportive, but I had to give it up because the stress made my colitis worse.'

> 'I have had no problems, they give me the time off I need for appointments, or if I'm unwell.'

> 'My boss makes me take leave to attend appointments, and we can only have so many sick days a year, so sometimes I drag myself into work because I don't want to get into trouble.'

Some of the group were well informed of their rights and how to access information on employment and sick leave rights, but others were not and would be reluctant to investigate this for fear of stigmatisation by their employer:

'It is more stressful when I get back, because no one covers the work for me, so I just have to catch up when I get back.'

Some group members touched on experience with education – university and sitting exams:

'they were understanding, I knew if I didn't feel well they were take that into account.'

On the topic of employment the emerging themes were:

'worried about their sick record'

'concerns how colleagues perceive their illness in relation to work capacity and not pulling their weight'

'becoming unemployed'

'annual leave was to be used for hospital appointments'

'work was not often covered in periods of absence'

'sick leave was unpaid and that at times of illness they felt that they had to almost show their employers how ill they were to justify having time off.'

This mirrors the findings of Crohn's and Colitis UK in their 2010–11 study Career Aspirations to Reality (Stone *et al.*, 2003) where it was cited that two in five respondents to the survey said that they worry about their colleagues thinking they do not pull their weight at work because of their IBD symptoms. A quarter said that they worry about being discriminated against in the workplace and one-third fear losing their jobs as a result of having IBD.

Health professionals need to improve to support our patients at a local and a national level to facilitate young people to secure and progress within their chosen career. The United Kingdom has the Equality Act 2010 (IBD Standards Group, 2009) and other countries share similar legislation that employers and patients are legally required to adhere to. Long-term conditions (Hanauer, 2006) have an impact on individuals and their families, but also, in states that receive universal benefits, the burden on the economy can be huge. To keep people in employment reduces the financial burden on the economy, which is of benefit to the state.

More information needs to be readily available to employers about these diseases, which will, with reasonable adjustments to working patterns, allow patients to achieve the optimum from their workforce. Communication and information are key factors to understanding these diseases from patients to politicians, all of whom need to be aware of the impact that chronic conditions have on society. By working together, employers, healthcare professionals and policymakers can help people with functional gastrointestinal disorders reach their full potential in the workplace.

Group perspective on attitudes towards their disease and others'

In order to initiate discussion, the group were asked, 'How do you feel about your diagnosis?' and some described relief:

> 'I knew I had Crohn's because my relative has it, but I had always been told it was nothing serious.'

> 'I was relieved that there was actually something there, because I think the doctors thought I was moaning over nothing.'

> 'My parents thought I was anorexic, I knew I wasn't but they were getting so upset because I was so ill, and the GP [general practitioner] couldn't tell me why.'

Some were more reflective of the long-term issues of a chronic disease:

> 'I wouldn't say I felt relief, I knew there was something wrong, and getting the diagnosis I knew it wasn't something I could take a tablet for and it would go away.'

When asked 'What are your concerns as a patient with IBD?' The long-term risk of cancer, issues of requiring surgery, and having a stoma were not mentioned by the group; instead, their immediate issues seemed to take precedence and were determined by how well controlled the Crohn's was.

> 'I constantly worry about where the toilet is.'

> 'I know where all the public toilets are in my town.'

> 'Sometimes the symptoms can be very mild, sometimes severe – you just don't know.'

The group's experience of attitudes towards them and the disease was very negative in that

> 'it is often hard to explain what the diseases are'.

> 'Their effects as can vary from mild to severe and debilitating at any time.'

> 'These are diseases that people find very personal and therefore difficult to approach.'

Overwhelmingly, the feedback was that people felt that they

> 'were over-exaggerating their disease and symptoms for a response or sympathy'.

A study recently published in the journal *Inflammatory Bowel Diseases* (Caprilli *et al.*, 2006) found that over 80% of study participants with IBD reported experiencing some social stigma about having IBD. Stigma has been found to affect many different groups, including people with chronic illnesses such as HIV, psoriasis, epilepsy and mental illnesses. It also highlighted that the majority of IBD patients report some perceived stigmatisation. Another study (Rutgeerts *et al.*, 2006) suggested that perceived stigma is a significant predictor of poorer outcomes in patients with IBD and therefore there is a need to address and correct popular misconceptions of these diseases.

Education is the key factor where information is disseminated to lift stigma about IBD. Crohn's and Colitis UK has an information service as well as information leaflets, in order that the correct information is given out to patients, relatives and employers. Celebrities also endorse this charity, which tries to raise the profile of these diseases for the public so that there is a greater understanding of how they affect not only on the individual but also his or her family and employers. As health professionals we can sustain our patients by writing letters of support, providing education sessions for people to empower themselves and supporting the national charity of Crohn's and Colitis UK.

Patients' experience of health services

We were keen to find out how patients viewed their interaction with health services. Again an open question was asked: *'What was your experience of the healthcare in and around your diagnosis?'* This seemed to provoke the most discussion, as the whole group had experienced a delay in diagnosis, which is unfortunately common in patients with IBD. Four out of the group had decided to access private healthcare to get a secondary care opinion. There was a negative attitude to primary care:

> *'My GP didn't seem to have a clue what it was.'*

> *'He kept telling me it was stress.'*

Attitudes to secondary care were mixed and depended on how quickly the diagnosis was made and how effective treatment was. Lack of time with the consultant was mentioned repeatedly, and information on the disease has been lacking:

> *'They just want you in and out.'*

> *'You don't get enough time with the doctor.'*

There were positive comments too:

> *'Dr x was brilliant, I was on infliximab within a few weeks and felt so much better.'*

'I feel very confident being looked after by Dr y.'

One member of the group had a negative experience when trying to transfer healthcare to another region for a university move:

'They told me I couldn't have Humira, therefore I had to leave and come back home.'

'I had to wait 4 months to see a specialist.'

There was a positive attitude to IBD specialist nurses with a feeling that they were given time and clear explanation of their disease. They also commented positively on the nursing staff who administered biological therapy, about how they listened to their concerns:

'(IBD nurse) has been great.'

'she is the only one who has explained to me what the disease is.'

There are some key points that highlight areas that need improvement in the patient experience of health services. Educating GPs about IBD seems important and providing quick access to secondary care appointments if the GP has concerns. Time pressure is a huge problem in secondary care; certainly the implementation of a specialist nurse has been overwhelmingly positive and joint clinics with a consultant and nurse can hopefully address the feeling among patients that there was a lack of explanation about the disease.

The overall consensus on the topic of service provider by the group was that they had a received positive experience from the hospital setting once they had a confirmed diagnosis. Delays in diagnosis and management from the initial presentation with their GP, to being referred and investigations undertaken by a gastroenterologist, were reported. Comments noted were:

'I was fobbed off by my GP.'

'visited numerous GPs'.

Also noted was that four out of the six people resorted to going privately to receive a diagnosis. Once an IBD had been confirmed, again the consensus was that they received

'a clear action plan and information albeit limited about Inflammatory Bowel Disease but enough to build upon as well as direction to join Crohn's and Colitis UK for further information'.

An invaluable tool in the care of patients with IBD is the implementation of the IBD helpline. This allows access to advice quickly from specialist nurses.

The value of specialist nursing posts in caring for patients with long-term conditions is well recognised by the Royal College of Nursing (RCN, 2010). Audit work within the IBD specialty (Mowat *et al.*, 2011) has illustrated the quality indicators provided by an IBD nurse specialist and the advantages of the service the nurse can provide, not only as a service provider but also as a support mechanism for those who have IBD. Through audit (RCN, 2012), the numbers of IBD nurses have been increased nationally but they are not at the target numbers as yet, although numbers are increasing annually.

QUALITY-OF-LIFE MEASURES

(*See* also 'assessment resources' Part III, 3.1.) Over the last 3 decades both the financial and psychological burden of chronic diseases has driven clinicians and scientists to develop many quality-of-life indices. Since the World Health Organization defined health as 'complete physical, mental and social well-being and not merely the absence of disease and infirmity' (WHO,1946), hundreds of generic and disease specific tools have been tried and tested; few have managed to encompass all that is pertinent to a patient's 'quality of life'. Many such measures have been designed specifically to use in clinical trials – to show the benefit of one drug over another (Guyatt *et al.*, 1989) and because of this have tended to focus too much on disease activity.

Studies of health-related quality of life in adolescents with Crohn's disease and its impact on psychological aspects of well-being, as well as effects on family life, have increased over the last decade. The IMPACT III questionnaire is the most commonly employed disease-specific measure used in paediatric IBD (Otley *et al.*, 2002). As stated earlier, IMPACT III has good retest reliability but it is well known that key quality-of-life issues can be under-represented. In order to address this deficit some investigators have chosen to look at the individual factors that affect daily life in adolescents with Crohn's disease.

Some investigators have looked at the mechanisms that patients use to help them manage chronic ill health, and such 'coping mechanisms or strategies' can predict those who may have a better outcome, particularly after surgery (Karwowski *et al.*, 2009). Similar themes emerge as successful coping strategies such as exercise (keeping fit), education and self-management, and being positive (positive outlook and predictive cognitive control). Exploring patients' attitude to illness particularly ambivalence to having Crohn's disease and other conflicting views (including or excluding parents) is also important in managing young patients with Crohn's disease.

The European Federation of Crohn's and Ulcerative Colitis Associations has comprehensively surveyed patients with Crohn's disease across 27 different European countries and concluded that patients have a mixed experience at diagnosis, they often have to use emergency services to get diagnosed, they have high hospital admission rates, they have high usage of corticosteroids, they experience poor communication about their illness (not asked probing questions), they have a high proportion of relationship difficulties (secondary to their illness), they are chronically fatigued and they suffer discrimination in the work place (Wilson *et al.*, 1994). These findings are very similar to our focus group's concerns. They suggest that working in partnership with our patients and lobbying governments will lead to a better outcome for our patients.

The UK IBD Standards have forced healthcare decision-makers to adopt a multidisciplinary approach to care of patients with Crohn's disease. More emphasis is placed on a multidisciplinary team discussion of complex patients, especially adolescents, and their access to psychologists and the growth of 'transition clinics' to ease the transfer of care of young patients with this chronic disease to the adult service. These forums for discussion of clinical care should include a 'map' of the likely clinical course of the disease and early and appropriate intervention with disease modifying treatments to minimise long-term complications and their consequent effect on health and well-being.

SUMMARY

Quality of life in adolescents with Crohn's disease is poorly addressed in current clinical practice. There is much variation across the services available to young patients diagnosed with this disabling and currently incurable disease. Focus group discussions remain one of the best tools to investigate the concerns and issues facing young patients with Crohn's disease. The concerns of these young patients can then be used to model services in individual departments. The service needs to be continually evaluated to make sure it is meeting the needs of all its young patients with Crohn's disease.

Education is also a vital tool in improving the long-term consequences of young people with Crohn's disease. Improving awareness among the general population about Crohn's disease will lessen the burden and stigma young patients often feel when diagnosed. Working with schools, colleges, universities and employers will raise the profile of this disabling disease and allow patients to attain their full educational potential and thus allow them to enter employment of their choice. Studies have previously shown such patients can achieve as good results as their peers but fail to gain equivalent employment (Mayberry *et al.*, 1992) and it has been shown that employers lack understanding regarding Crohn's disease (Moody *et al.*, 1992). Thus, only a comprehensive service, adopting national IBD Standards, incorporating regular focus group discussions and community-wide education programmes can improve the long-term consequences of adolescents with Crohn's disease.

REFERENCES

Bamias G, Nyce MR, De La Rue SA, *et al.* New concepts in the pathophysiology of inflammatory bowel disease. *Ann Intern Med.* 2005; 143(12): 895–904.
Bouma G, Strober W. The immunological and genetic basis of inflammatory bowel disease. *Nat Rev Immunol.* 2003; 3(7): 521–33.
Caprilli R, Gassull MA, Escher JC, *et al.* European Crohn's and Colitis Organisation. European

evidence based consensus on the diagnosis and management of Crohn's disease: special situations. *Gut.* 2006; **55**(Suppl. 1): i36–58.

Carroll K. Crohn's disease: new imaging techniques. *Baillières Clin Gastroenterol.* 1998; **12**(1): 35–72.

Crohn BB. Regional ileitis: a pathological and clinical entity. *J Am Med Assoc.* 1932; **99**: 1323–9.

Guyatt G, Mitchell A, Irvine EJ. A new measure of health status for clinical trials in inflammatory bowel disease. *Gastroenterology.* 1989; **96**(3): 804–10.

Hanauer SB. Inflammatory bowel disease: epidemiology, pathogenesis, and therapeutic opportunities. *Inflamm Bowel Dis.* 2006; **12**(Suppl. 1): S3–9.

Henderson P, Hansen R, Cameron FL, *et al.* Rising incidence of pediatric inflammatory bowel disease in Scotland. *Inflamm Bowel Dis.* 2011; **18**(6): 999–1005.

IBD Standards Group. *Crohn's and Colitis UK publication Quality Care: service standards for the healthcare of people who have inflammatory bowel disease (IBD).* Brighton: Oyster Healthcare Communications; 2009. Available at: www.bsg.org.uk/attachments/160_IBDstandards.pdf

Karwowski CA, Keljo D, Szigethy E. Strategies to improve quality of life in adolescents with inflammatory bowel disease. *Inflamm Bowel Dis.* 2009; **15**(11): 1755–64.

Lichtenstein GR, Feagan BG, Cohen RD, *et al.* Serious infections and mortality in association with therapies for Crohn's disease: TREAT Registry. *Clin Gastroenterol Hepatol.* 2006; **4**(5): 621–30.

Mayberry MK, Probert C, Srivastava E, *et al.* Perceived discrimination in education and employment by people with Crohn's disease: a case control study of educational achievement and employment. *Gut.* 1992; **33**(3): 312–14.

Moody GA, Probert CSJ, Jayanthi V, *et al.* The attitude of employers to people with inflammatory bowel disease. *Soc Sci Med.* 1992; **34**(4): 459–60.

Mowat C, Cole A, Windsor A, *et al.* Guidelines for the management of inflammatory bowel disease in adults. *Gut.* 2011; **60**(5): 571–607.

National Institute for Clinical Excellence (NICE). *Crohn's Disease: management in adults, children and young people. Clinical guidelines CG152.* London: NICE; 2012. Available at: http://guidance.nice.org.uk/cg152

Odes S, Vardi H, Friger M, *et al.* Effect of phenotype on health care costs in Crohn's disease: a European study using the Montreal classification. *J Crohns Colitis.* 2007; **1**(2): 87–96.

Otley A, Smith C, Nicholas D, *et al.* The IMPACT questionnaire: a valid measure of health-related quality of life in pediatric inflammatory bowel disease. *J Pediatr Gastroenterol Nutr.* 2002; **35**(4): 557–63.

Royal College of Nursing (RCN). *Specialist Nurses: changing lives, saving money.* London: RCN; 2010. Available at: www.rcn.org.uk/__data/assets/pdf_file/0008/302489/003581.pdf (accessed 30 July 2013).

Royal College of Nursing (RCN). *Inflammatory Bowel Disease Nursing: results of an audit exploring the roles, responsibilities and activity of nurses with specialist/advanced roles.* London: RCN; 2012. Available at: www.rcn.org.uk/__data/assets/pdf_file/0008/433736/004197.pdf (accessed 30 July 2013).

Rutgeerts P, Van Asscghe G, Vermeire S. Review article: infliximab therapy for inflammatory bowel disease – seven years on. *Aliment Pharmacol Ther.* 2006; **23**(4): 451–63.

Sachar DB. The problem of postoperative recurrence of Crohn's disease. *Dev Gastroenterol.* 1990; **11**: 107–114.

Stone MA, Mayberry JF, Baker R. Prevalence and management of inflammatory bowel disease: a cross-sectional study from central England. *Eur J Gastroenterol Hepatol.* 2003; **15**(12): 1275–80.

Van Assche G, Dignass A, Panes J, *et al.* The second European evidence-based consensus on the diagnosis and management of Crohn's disease: definitions and diagnosis. *J Crohns Colitis.* 2010; **4**(1): 7–27.

WHO, World Health Organization. Preamble to the Constitution of the World Health

Organization as adopted by the International Health Conference, New York, 19–22 June, 1946; signed on 22 July 1946 by the representatives of 61 States (Official Records of the World Health Organization, no. 2, p. 100) and entered into force on 7 April 1948. Available at: www.who.int/about/definition/en/print.html

Wilson JD, Braunwald E, Isselbacher KJ, *et al. Harrison's Principles of Internal Medicine.* New York, NY: McGraw-Hill; 1994.

CHAPTER 13

Transition from artificial enteral tube nutrition to oral eating: tube-weaning feeding therapy

Clarissa Martin

INTRODUCTION

Gastrointestinal disorders, such as those that manifest in malabsorption or poor digestion, may require medical intervention and the use of enteral or parenteral nutrition to ensure that these children thrive (Duggan *et al.*, 2008). Medical conditions requiring intervention to ensure adequate nutrition through tube-feeding include disorders beyond those characterised as gastrointestinal. These include disorders of the neuromuscular and cardiopulmonary systems. Tube-feeds are also prescribed for premature babies and those who fail to thrive.

Parenteral nutrition through the bloodstream has become ubiquitous in the treatment of critically ill children and in the management of extremely premature newborns (Moreno-Villares *et al.*, 1998). Some premature infants initially under parenteral nutrition schedules will also require prolonged enteral tube-feeding (Quigley and Iglesias, 2008). Enteral tube nutrition delivered by either gastrostomy or a nasogastric tube is also indicated for infants and toddlers who have a functioning gastrointestinal tract but cannot ingest enough nutrients orally because they are unable or unwilling to take oral feeds (August *et al.*, 2002). Children with neurodevelopmental disabilities such as cerebral palsy, spina bifida, or congenital disorders of the metabolism frequently have associated gastrointestinal problems (Sullivan, 2008). Problems such as oesophageal and foregut dysmotility may cause several further conditions, such as dysphagia and delayed gastric emptying. Gastro-oesophageal reflux disease is also common and often requires surgical intervention. Oral motor dysfunction leading to feeding difficulties, risk of aspiration and prolonged feeding times are also common presenting problems. Furthermore, functional constipation may also be present, but the lack of oral intake of solid food may not present initially within this population.

One of the common co-morbidities with gastrointestinal disorders is that of reflux, dysphagia and behavioural problems during feeding. Schwarz *et al.* (2001) found that gastro-oesophageal reflux, with or without aspiration, were present in 56%, oropharyngeal dysphagia in the 27%, and aversive feeding behaviours in 18% of children with gastrointestinal problems. Treatment recommendations included medical therapy for gastro-oesophageal reflux for 25%, fundoplication plus gastrostomy tube for 23% and oral supplements to 22%. Schwarz and co-authors concluded that in children with developmental disabilities required tailored medical and psychological treatment to significantly improve their nutritional status. Not all authors advocate a multidisciplinary approach. It is widely accepted that some medical disorders will result in long-term artificial feeding to ensure survival. One such condition is extreme short bowel syndrome, where the individual does not have the biological capability to absorb nutrients. The systematic literature review by Olieman *et al.* (2010) of published data from 1966 to 2007 on feeding and nutritional strategies implemented on children who had received a diagnosis of short bowel syndrome recommends that enteral nutrition be initiated as soon as possible after bowel resection to promote intestinal adaptation. Several surgical interventions are then required to lengthen the bowel after it has been determined that the current length is insufficient for survival. Once the length of the bowel has been corrected, a psychological intervention may be required to initiate oral feeding. In other conditions, best practice would include concomitant behavioural, dietetic and medical support throughout the progression of the disorder.

The number of enteral-fed infants and children with nasogastric, gastrostomy or jejunostomy tubes has increased significantly in the last 20 years (Daveluy *et al.*, 2006). Although these non-oral methods of feeding are helping children to survive, they inevitably interfere with crucial stages of development. Oral feeding experiences are required for optimal oral motor function. Prolonged tube-feeding in the preschool years can disrupt natural feeding experiences (Byron, 2011). Research consensus establishes that tube-feeding provides a temporary means of improving nutritional status and growth until a child can be nourished by oral means (e.g. Schauster and Dwyer, 1996).

Children who are tube-fed should be exposed to oral-tactile stimulation with food. For example, Olieman *et al.* (2010) recommended that children with short bowel syndrome who are tube-fed should receive small volumes of bottle-feeding to stimulate the suck and swallow reflexes so that solid food can be introduced later. The wisdom is to stimulate oral motor activity and to avoid the development of feeding aversion behaviours. It is common in children who have suffered prolonged periods of tube-feeds to display developmental and behavioural feeding problems when weaning from tube-dependence (Schauster and Dwyer, 1996).

Working with children who are under enteral tube-feeding nutrition is common practice for multidisciplinary teams (MDTs) at gastroenterology clinics. In this chapter we will revisit basic concepts such as methods and types of tube-feeding and consider the impact that having a child who is tube-fed may have on the child's family. Aspects of tube-weaning feeding therapy process will also be offered.

ENTERAL TUBE NUTRITION: BASIC CONCEPTS

Enteral feeding is the delivery of a nutritional formula directly to the gastrointestinal tract (Forcielli *et al.*, 2008). The tube may be inserted through the nose (nasogastric) or directly into the stomach through a surgically placed button (gastrostomy). Enteral nutrition mimics the normal gastrointestinal response following the ingestion of a meal, with the exception of the oral phase. It is required when children cannot take nutrients orally and are at risk of malnutrition. In a child with oral feeding resistance whose growth falters, gastric tube-feedings may be essential to the delivery of basic nutritional requirements (Dellert *et al.*, 1993).

BOX 13.1 Gastroenterological conditions where tube-feeding is indicated

- Failure to thrive
- Inappropriate caloric intake
- Gastro-oesophageal reflux
- Short bowel syndrome
- Crohn's disease
- Intestinal pseudo-obstruction
- Delayed gastric emptying
- Malabsorption of nutrients

(Di Lorenzo *et al.*, 1995; Ferry *et al.*, 1983; Israel and Hassall, 1995; Vanderhoof and Langnas, 1997)

BOX 13.2 Common complications of tube-feeding

- Diarrhoea
- Nausea and vomiting
- Constipation
- Malabsorption
- Bacterial contamination
- Perforation
- Tube occlusion and dislodgement
- Pulmonary aspiration

Methods and types of tube-feeding

There are several variables to consider when establishing the method of delivery for enteral nutrition: the position of the tube within the gastrointestinal tract and the frequency and duration of the feeding pattern (*see* Box 13.3). Tubes are classified depending on their position within the gastrointestinal system (*see* Box 13.4). In cases where children require tube-feeding for a short period of time, usually no longer than 6 weeks, to allow the gastrointestinal system to recover from insult, a nasogastric tube may be indicated. For children requiring nutritional support for a longer duration, a surgically placed gastrostomy may be performed under general anaesthesia. The guiding principle for placing a gastrostomy tube is to ensure that the scarring to the oesophagus that is associated with long-term nasogastric feeding does not occur. Advantages, disadvantages and risks for nasogastric and gastrostomy tubes are provided by doctors as specialised paediatric medical teams are responsible for inserting all tubes. Families may be trained by health professionals in the further care of the tube and adjacent areas, as well as to be responsible for providing tube-feeds with prescribed formula when discharged from hospital to the community and home care.

BOX 13.3 Methods of enteral nutrition

The method of delivery of enteral nutrition will depend on:

- the route of administration (gastric, duodenal or jejunal)
- characteristics of the feeding tube (small- versus large-bore catheter)
- the desired feeding pattern (bolus, intermittent, cyclic or continuous)
- the cost and availability of equipment (by gravity or syringe, or by infusion pump).

BOX 13.4 Types of tube-feeding and tube

Types of enteral tube-feeding

- *Nasogastric tube* or NG: a plastic tube inserted from the nose to the stomach.
- *Nasoduodenal tube*: from the nose to the duodenum (the first or upper part of the small intestine, immediately below the stomach).
- *Nasojejunal tube*: from the nose to the jejunum (the next or middle part of the small intestine, and before the much longer ileum).
- *Gastrostomy tube* or GT: requires a surgical operation to open the skin through the abdominal wall to insert the tube directly into the stomach.
- *Jejunostomy tube* or JT: requires a surgical operation to open the skin, through the abdominal wall and directly into the jejunum.

Types of gastrostomy tube
- *Percutaneous endoscopy gastrostomy* or PEG: inserted under endoscopy control that avoids a full surgical procedure.
- *Malecot*: inserted through surgery and in place for 3–4 months. After this time a MIC-KEY button is recommended.
- *MIC-KEY*: the exterior of the tube sits against the skin.

Note, images of various tube types are shown in Part III (*see* pp. 366–7).

Part of the paediatric gastroenterology MDT's duties is to establish the appropriate feeding pattern tailored to a particular child's needs. Dietitians may prescribe continuous feeds or regular 'bolus' feeds through a syringe. The type of feeding selected (e.g. bolus or continuous) should be individualised for each child. It is recommended to use a combination of oral and tube-feeding when possible and to fit this management within the routine family meal schedule.

The common nutrient composition of enteral formulas contains a combination of carbohydrates, lipids, proteins, water, micronutrients and fibre. It is common in clinical practice for the paediatric gastroenterologist and dietetians to discuss formula with families. Several factors such as the child's age and medical condition require consideration before a feeding regimen can be devised (*see* Box 13.5).

BOX 13.5 Factors for formula selection
- *Child's age*: formula content (calories, protein, vitamin and mineral) are tailored to meet the needs of the child at various ages (premature, infant, toddler and child).
- *Medical diagnosis*: some children with specific chronic conditions (e.g. diabetes) require specific formulas.
- *Allergies*: some children suffer allergies or sensitivities to specific proteins (e.g. milk or soy) and they also need specific formulas.
- *Volume tolerance*: some formulas are more calorically dense than others.
- *Absorption capabilities*: some formulas are more easily digested than others.

Multidisciplinary approach
Before nutritional supplementation of any kind is implemented, the nutritional status of the patient should be assessed, the target goals defined, and the risks and benefits explained to both the parents and, if age-appropriate, the child (Nightingale and Woodward, 2006). An MDT approach to the care and assessment of children who receive enteral tube-feeding nutrition is present in the literature (e.g. Martin *et al.*, 2008). MDT intervention is common in the clinical practice and recommended by the British Association of Parenteral and Enteral Nutrition (Elia *et al.*, 2001) and guidelines on paediatric tube-feeding (NHS,

2003). It is also important that professionals have a time frame in place for the duration of supplementation or replacement. A plan should be devised at the point of intervention for the removal of the support and transition to oral feeding. Policies of waiting and observing are not appropriate and may hinder the development. Children on enteral support are at greater risk of being ostracised from mealtimes and social gatherings with food at its heart. Periodic assessment of oral feeding is necessary even if long-term enteral support is necessary. Long-term tube-feeding can develop into tube dependency following recovery from all medical conditions. Therefore, earliest-possible transition to oral feeding must be advocated in all cases under advisement and negotiation of all members of the MDT.

Tube-feeding at home

Home enteral nutrition therapy has been established as part of the management of infants and children with chronic disease and/or feeding problems (Howard *et al.*, 1995). The main indications for home enteral nutrition are conditions leading to failure to thrive – for example, cerebral palsy, cystic fibrosis, malignancies, various major congenital malformations and metabolic disorders (Fereday *et al.*, 2009; Wright, 2004).

Enteral tube-feeding provided at home has increased at a rate of up to 20% per year in the United Kingdom (BANS, 2008). In Britain, children constitute 40% of the patients receiving home enteral nutrition therapy, compared with 5%–20% in the United States (Elia, 1994). This indicates that there is variation in medical decision-making surrounding the need or ability to insert feeding tubes. A steady increase in the proportion of children receiving nasogastric rather than gastrostomy feeding in the United Kingdom has also been reported. One potential explanation could be regarding inequalities in distribution of gastroenterological services throughout the UK geography, as some areas do not have specialist paediatric surgical or gastroenterology services for gastrostomy tube placement (BANS, 2008).

Scientific developments regarding nutritional formula composition, tube design and material improvement, as well as advances in surgical procedures, have made it possible for home enteral nutrition therapy to be safer for children with chronic medical conditions (e.g. short bowel syndrome). The literature also highlights the importance of taking into consideration individual patient profiles when establishing this approach for children. For example, Pedrón-Giner *et al.* (2012) described the profile of this type of paediatric patient on enteral tube support. Results indicated that 28% of their patients were under 1 year old. The main indications for home enteral nutrition treatment were for oncological diseases (29.9%) followed by digestive problems (27.6%). Nutrients were delivered through nasogastric tube in the majority of the children (71.7%), with overnight enteral nutrition the preferred infusion regimen (51%). They indicated the need to design a appropriate individualised and tailored strategy for home enteral nutrition intervention.

Families of children who are tube-fed must be trained and supervised by health professionals for them to feel confident in the management of their children's needs. This may place increased responsibility and pressure on primary caregivers (Tucker *et al.*, 2009). Indeed, while this group of children benefit from technological advances that improve their health, their families experience constraints of diary-intensive feeding routines that seem incompatible with social needs of the family and full-time employment. Hazel (2006) completed a review of the literature regarding parents' experiences of long-term tube-feeding in children. Results of this study indicated that parents found the decision of inserting a tube in their children stressful. They also reported feeling pressured by health professionals to make a quick decision to insert the tube when they had not processed all of the new medical information presented. They also expressed the need for receiving consistent and accurate information from doctors and nurses. However, once the enteral tube nutrition was established they acknowledged a positive impact on their children's lives. Calderón *et al.* (2011) conducted a prospective observational study of primary caregivers of paediatric patients with nasogastric and gastrostomy tube-feeding that required home enteral nutrition intervention. They found that psychological distress and anxiety showed a positive correlation with caregivers' feelings of burden. They highlighted the important role that psychological factors play and the potential impact on the emotional well-being of caregivers of children who need home enteral nutrition therapy.

Emotional and social impact of enteral tube-feeding on families

Families experience angst when their children suffer a life-threatening condition or when they have gone through an extended period of difficult feeding. In this scenario, enteral feeding nutrition may be welcomed and experienced as a relief for parents. Enteral feeding ensures their child survives and develops, protecting the child from malnutrition and decreasing potential risks such as aspiration (*see* Box 13.6).

BOX 13.6 Summary example for parents – minimum care needs for percutaneous endoscopic gastrostomy (PEG)

- Check for any redness, swelling, granulation tissue or skin problems around the PEG tube
- Prevent infections
- Wash the skin around PEG tube with soap and water
- Safely rotate the bolster to fully clean the PEG tube site with warm water
- Dry the area especially the skin around the PEG tube
- Correctly tape the feeding tube to the child's stomach
- Flush the tube before and after each feeding and medication session
- Report if your child suffers pain, diarrhoea, vomiting or fever

(Guenter and Silkroski, 2001)

Engaging families to participate in decisions related to the care of their tube-fed child and helping them to understand treatment options and choices should be part of routine clinical practice (Sidey and Torbet, 1995). Aspects related to tube-feeding management, such as introducing and maintaining a correct body position, may be of little relevance to health professionals but constitute a major trauma for children, as well as for their parents. Therefore, the child's allocated specialist nurse on paediatric wards commonly conducts the training and educating of parents on tube-feeding care. However, it has been reported that parents receive different levels of training depending on services (Culverwell, 2005).

BOX 13.7 Summary of common problems that parents of tube-fed children have to face

- To understand and manage tube-feeds equipment (gravity feeds, syringes, and so forth) and its care
- To be familiar with practicalities such as formula supplements, milk storage, stoma care, and so forth
- To familiarise with infection and emergency procedures (e.g. in cases of percutaneous endoscopic gastrostomy, accidental removal)
- To gather information about local and national suppliers
- To be familiar with specific social and economical support they may be entitled to because of their child's condition (e.g. disability living allowance)
- To coordinate all medical appointments their child may require
- To participate in continuous risk assessment when discharged to community and home care

---

The development of international guidelines and standard formal training procedures for parents on enteral tube nutrition is paramount. Furthermore, it must be acknowledged that parents must learn new skills for tube management. This must be adapted somewhat to the family home. However, these practical issues are often overlooked. Often parents perceive applying for all entitled social support for their child's disability condition (*see* Box 13.7) takes precedence, so that they are financially solvent to deal with their child's additional needs. On discharge form hospitals, parents are typically required to collect enteral tube-feeding equipment and feeds on a daily basis until arrangements for home delivery of supplies can be made.

These essential and often overwhelming parental pressures are not acknowledged, with the focus entirely on training procedural elements of tube-feeding. The management of care for a child with enteral tube-feeding involves a range of professionals; therefore, it is common to allocate a key health professional to coordinate multiagency approaches when planned discharged is established. The role of this key worker may be filled by a paediatric community nurse, dietetic services or speech and language therapy. The designated worker is the first point of contact for information and support for families, as well as to provide information, support and training to school staff to manage the child's feeding requirements (Townsley and Robinson, 2000). Routine follow-up home visits are common in the care of tube-fed children.

Once children are discharged home, parents have to incorporate the care of their tube-fed child within their own family routines. This may include attendance at medical appointments that are incompatible with the parents' work and other family commitments. It is understandable, therefore, that these demands serve as additional sources of stress for the parents. The literature has identified the severity of the child's illness, the constant caretaking demands placed on parents and the level of social support parents receive as main contributory stress factors for these families (e.g. Fereday et al., 2009; Pedersen et al., 2004).

At some point of their child's tube-feeding, parents are going to question the permanence of the artificial tube. Benoit et al. (2001) retrospectively reviewed a sample of 325 medical records of all patients from birth to 36 months of age who had an enteral tube, with the aim to identify factors that predict removal of the tubes within 12 months of insertion. They found that the main difference between children whose tubes were removed and those whose tubes were not was related to the medical diagnosis. In their sample, no children with cerebral palsy had their tube removed. In comparison, 33% of the children who had been diagnosed with cancer and had gone into remission had their tube removed.

Guidelines indicating prescription of enteral feeds do not include recommendations, suggestions or specific plan indications for the future potential removal of feeding tubes. Surprisingly, they are not recognised as being in need of study. Recent research literature identifies the need to pay attention to the whole process, including both starting enteral tube nutrition and ending it (e.g. Gottrand and Sullivan, 2010). Tube-feeding should be seen as an added indication of the child's disability rather than as a constant necessity. The idea of having artificial feeds 'forever' may create further stress for parents and remove all hope. To feed and nurture their own children is a core parenting task and parents may experience tube-feeding as a personal failure (Spalding and McKeever, 1998). There are sociocultural rules that associate the strong emotional connection between feelings of inadequacy and the inability to feed their child. Research has found that these families, especially mothers, struggle to negotiate their and their child's identities as well as their own parenting roles (e.g. Craig and Scambler, 2006). However, the psychological implications of home enteral tube-feeds for families and carers have received little attention in the research literature, as the majority of studies had been mainly focused on medical and nutritional outcomes (Rouse et al., 2002). Some researchers (e.g. Fereday et al., 2009; Townsley and Robinson, 2000) have emphasised the need to pay attention to the voices of these families and to use their experiences to raise public awareness as well as to develop the services that may be required to support them.

BOX 13.8 Families of children with enteral tube-feeding

Families of children with enteral tube-feeding would benefit from:

- a mandatory multiagency coordinated approach
- the development of national and international guidelines for enteral feeding that include psychological aspects of care
- standardised hospital paediatric staff training in how to interact with and understand the role of carers
- national guidelines for training parents and carers on management of tube-feeds
- the development of standard, regularly updated information packs available for parents
- being provided with a list of available community resources and services at the time of discharge planning
- the development of community paediatric services as minimum standard accessible services
- wider information about suppliers.

(Culverwell, 2005; Limbrick, 2001; Townsley and Robinson, 2000)

Parents are also encouraged by health professionals to include their child with enteral tube nutrition within the family meals and their eating-related social activities. However, parents report experiencing distress and feeling stigmatised when being with their tube-fed child in social situations (e.g. going to restaurants, family meals, or feeding their child in a public place) (Craig and Scambler, 2006). Participating in family meals provides important learning experience for children who are tube-fed. This may be seen as paramount to supporting the tube-fed child in developing oral feeding skills and all the social and emotional aspects that are included in the learning of human eating behaviour. Behavioural feeding problems are common in children who are tube-fed, which could be ameliorated or tempered by inclusion within social mealtimes. Parents should be made aware of, and trained to deal with, the myriad negative factors associated with eating as a consequence of being tube-fed.

FACTORS TO CONSIDER IN CHILDREN WHO ARE TUBE-FED

Initially enteral tube nutrition may be a priority to help children to survive and grow. It may even improve quality of life of those who suffer severe medical conditions in the short- to medium-term. However, it must be acknowledged that the intervention impacts on the whole family system and child's individual development (*see* Box 13.9). Research evidence has shown that physiological, anatomical, social and behavioural factors all contribute to successful oral feeding in infants and children (Lipsitt *et al.*, 1985; Satter, 1999). Therefore, a number of factors must be considered to eliminate oral feeding problems in children who have suffered long-term enteral tube nutrition. These factors include the characteristics of the illness that initially impeded oral eating experiences and its associated medical complications, as well as the age and stage of development of the child at the time of the insertion of the tube (Mason *et al.*, 2005). Minimum levels of physiological and biological requirements are required for oral eating. Development of musculoskeletal tone and functional swallowing skills are essential. Feeding and swallowing are activities that occur in the upper aerodigestive tract and are orchestrated by a complex specific arrangement under the control of the brain and cranial nerves, as detailed in Chapter 2 (Arvedson, 2006).

BOX 13.9 Tube-feeding impact
- Reducing the development of oral autonomy
- Limiting the child's learning to eat autonomously
- Impairing speech and language, social and motor development
- Contributing to oral hypersensitivity, hyperactive gag reflex, frequent gagging and immature bite–chew–swallow sequence
- Contributing to active food refusal and may create food fears or phobia
- Creating a strong defence against any contact with fluids and pureed or solid food contributing to burden to the family
- Producing social and financial constraints and stress on families

---

Early experiences of the gastrointestinal system

Children who are tube-fed are generally exposed to a single nutritional formula. Therefore, it is common for them to miss the opportunity for their gastrointestinal system to practise and accommodate to a diverse range and variety of food and eating experiences. For example, for children who are under pump feedings, the liquid formula arrives and departs from the stomach slowly; therefore, they do not experience the same stomach movements as children consuming large amounts of food in mealtime arrangements. Stomach movements or noises associated with hunger sensation and appetite awareness are not experienced. Learning must occur to associate these gastric perceptions once tube-feeds are removed. Furthermore, tube-feeds are prescribed to provide nutrients to the infant and follow a regimen that may not relate to biopsychosocial patterns of children's appetite. Inevitably the tube-fed child learns to be passive to food and eating (Delaney and Averdson, 2008).

Critical periods for the development of oral feeding and eating

A child's development is a complex process where physical, cognitive and experiential influences are intertwined (Byron, 2011). Theory and research on a child's development emphasises the notion of achieving milestones; however, it is important to take into account that the time frames that the literature suggests are representatives of an average (Dovey and Martin, 2011). It has also has been indicated in the early literature that critical periods in infancy exist within which normal nutritive feeding patterns develop (Illingworth and Lister, 1964; Handen *et al.*, 1986). For example, tongue mobility improves with the presentation of pureed foods at 4–6 months of age. Furthermore, oral eating requires active effort by the infant, who must developed timing and coordination for sucking, swallowing and breathing at the breast or bottle. Following this developmental approach, some authors (e.g. Abad-Sinden and Sutphen, 2003; Olieman *et al.*, 2010; Vanderhoof and Langnas, 1997) have recommended that the introduction of solid food for children with gastroenterological conditions (e.g. short bowel syndrome) should be initiated usually between 4 and 6 months of age, in order to avoid significant problems with feeding aversion behaviour that may develop if this important milestone is missed.

Adequate growth, defined by weight gain in early infancy and for the first few years of life, is the primary measure of successful feeding (Dunbar *et al.*, 1991). Infants and children who are deprived of oral feedings for prolonged periods and who are tube-fed for months or years from birth can experience great difficulty in re-establishing oral feeding when they have sufficiently recovered from their initial medical problems (Geertsma *et al.*, 1985) and may be at a disadvantage in comparison with their peers. The disadvantage stems from missing the developmental transition from reflexive to voluntary, independent feeding (Linscheid and Rasnake, 1992). For this group of children, hypersensitivity or defensiveness, resistance to presented food, and delayed oral motor skills are common presenting behavioural problems (Blackman and Nelson, 1987). Oral hypersensitivity, laryngeal incompetence, nasal regurgitation, a lack of pharyngeal coordination, irritation caused by nasogastric tube-feedings, or a combination of these factors are well documented as physical and behavioural causes of feeding dysfunction in infants who have been tube-fed (e.g. Vogel *et al.*, 1986).

Distressing and traumatic experiences

Enteral tube nutrition may be initiated as a consequence of medical conditions that have caused pain and physical discomfort. Unfortunately, it is common for this group of children to also have been exposed to aversive but necessary medical treatments (e.g. intubation, tube insertion and other life-maintaining procedures). Moreover, the constant feelings of nausea, pain and vomiting in association with feeding, and oral sensory deprivation due to nasogastric tube-feedings, are also common features of children who have been tube-fed (Arvedson and Brodsky, 2001). For example, in the case of children who suffer gastro-oesophageal reflux disease, tube-feedings may have produced or exacerbated irritation and pain. Gradually these feelings are associated with mealtimes. Resultant aversive and avoidant responses to food lead to feeding problems. It has been estimated to that 40% of infants who have had oesophageal surgery (Di Scipio *et al.*, 1978) and 4% of those with gastro-oesophageal reflux disease, who do not have a neurological or craniofacial problem, or a history of oesophageal surgery (Dellert *et al.*, 1993), present with significant resistance to feeding.

BOX 13.10 Summary of oral-feeding development that tube-fed children may miss

From birth to 3–5 months
- Oral experiences related to skin/tactile stimulation
- Gag reflex strong at birth
- Gag reflex accommodates to hand–mouth experiences
- Development of suck–swallow–breath pattern coordination

From 6 to 12 months
- Longer sequences of suck–swallow–breath pattern
- By 7 months gag reflex is similar to that of adults
- Self-feeding skills
- Lateral and diagonal rotary tongue movements
- Tongue, lip and cheek coordination
- Use of jaws and tongue to mash food

From 12 to 18 months
- Lateral and diagonal rotary tongue movements developed
- Tongue, lip and cheek coordination improved
- Active lips during chewing
- Controlled bite
- Chewing missing vertical and rotary movements

(Adapted from Dovey and Martin, 2011)

Research reports indicate that aversive experiences surrounding feeding result in avoidant responses to eating to escape from the anticipated pain, discomfort or intense anxiety (e.g. Arts-Rodas and Benoit, 1998; Hyman, 1994). Some infants and young children who had undergone traumatic and distressing experiences involving the mouth, nose, throat and oesophagus have also been reported as refusing to eat. These children express severe distress before feeding and exhibit behaviours resembling phobic responses seen in posttraumatic stress conditions (Di Scipio *et al.*, 1978; Griffen, 1979). Sometimes families and children find themselves trapped in a vicious circle where children's resistance to eat orally may often be severe enough to require enteral feeding for nutritional support (Dellert *et al.*, 1993) and in some cases may also involve a conditioned dysphagia. Therefore, it can be extrapolated from this data that a cyclical dependence can develop. The child needs the tube for a medical condition. They then develop a conditioned aversion to food because of the tube. The child is then deemed to require the tube to remain to sustain them. All professionals should be aware of the potential of this cycle and attempt to break it with tailored intervention when possible.

TRANSITION FROM ENTERAL TUBE NUTRITION TO ORAL EATING

Establishing normal eating behaviour in children who have required enteral tube nutrition is clinically challenging. The recognised role an intertwined biological, medical, developmental, behavioural, emotional and social milieu must be fully understood (e.g. Byars *et al.*, 2003; Bernard-Bonnin, 2006; Martin *et al.*, 2008; Rommel *et al.*, 2003).

Clinical consensus appears to be that the transition from tube- to oral feeding should be established as soon as tube-feeding is no longer necessary. In the cases where children refuse to eat orally, tube-weaning therapy is required. To prepare for this transition to oral eating, children under enteral feeding should be required to engage in basic oral activities and stimulation when the tube is first placed. This should be considered paramount for the future development of their feeding skills. Oral motor stimulation programmes, as well as exercises that facilitate positive emotional and behavioural association of food and eating while they are on enteral tube-feed regimens, should be developed and tailored for the child.

Some children under enteral tube nutrition are capable of eating orally and may have even successfully done so prior to the tube being fitted. At the other end of the spectrum other children may aspirate, but in all the cases they would benefit from building positive oral and tactile stimulation associated with feeding within the boundaries of safety (*see* Box 13.11). Furthermore, some authors have highlighted the importance of early exposure to flavours to facilitate further food variety acceptance (Mennella, 1998).

BOX 13.11 Examples of sensory stimulation while being in enteral tube nutrition

- Incorporate oral activities that the child would be performing naturally accordingly to his or her stage of development (e.g. exploring toys with mouth, licking sweets for tasting)
- Facilitate pleasant touch with soft textures around the mouth area (e.g. playing to make tickles around the mouth with a feather)
- Facilitate the exploration of textures such as spoons, own hands, and so forth
- Massage the face and oral area of the child while listening to music
- Facilitate oral experiences while tube-feeding
- Facilitate the exposition to different tastes and flavours
- Facilitate messy play experiences
- Help the child to associate those experiences with positive emotions, feelings and behaviours in a relaxed and playful environment

- Facilitate same experiences during play activities and/or incorporate play during feeding
- Stop if the child starts showing distress signs, to help the child to relax as a priority for future positive associations

Considerations before tube–weaning therapy

Transition from enteral tube nutrition to oral eating is a process that should be considered on an individual basis. Factors such as the child's age and medical condition, child and family readiness, parents' characteristics should all be examined prior to engaging in the weaning process. Consensus regarding the need for the evaluation of minimum criteria to be established and achieved by the child, family and professionals is required before tube-weaning therapy is advised and implemented (e.g. Blackman and Nelson, 1985; Martin and Dovey, 2011; Schauster and Dwyer, 1996).

Medical stability

Tube-weaning therapy generally involves a reduction in enteral feeding nutrition to facilitate the hunger sensation and the development of the biological drive to eat orally. It is important for this process that the child's overall health is at its optimum and the medical condition remains stable (Blackman and Nelson, 1985). Medical stability is a minimum criterion for tube weaning therapy (Dunbar *et al.*, 1991). The presence of medical complications is a critical factor that may interfere with the tube-weaning therapy. It is worth considering that prematurely focusing on tube-weaning therapy may worsen the child's initial medical condition.

Safety swallowing process and swallowing capacities

Many children with medical conditions aspirate foods or liquids or are at increased risk of aspiration. Assessing the child's capabilities for a safe swallow is a paramount requirement for tube weaning therapy. Special attention should be placed on observation of the child's ability to handle his or her own saliva; the presence of frequent coughing and/or choking while eating and drinking, periods of a wheezing following meals indicative of fluid on the lungs/trachea, and recurrent/persistent bouts of chest infection, are all poor signs for a successful tube-weaning outcome. Exploration of the child's breathing pattern to identify changes during eating and drinking may aid in assessing the potential risk for airway obstructions (Delaney and Arvedson, 2008). In short, an endoscopic assessment for a safe swallow should be a minimum requirement prior to starting a tube-weaning.

Developmental status

Some authors have advocated for a developmental approach for tube-weaning (*see* Box 13.12). It is believed that the child's functional, experiential and cognitive level is going to be a contributing factor for tube-weaning success. It may determine the level of developmentally appropriate feeding interactions the child may achieve and provide an immediate target to achieve and possible point to reflect, reassess and alter goals according to outcome. The assessment of the child's developmental status should also include evaluation of the gross motor status (e.g. head, neck and trunk support), as well as observation of the sensory–motor system to identify potential sensitivities/defensiveness and the child's quality of oral motor skills (e.g. chewing, tongue movements and oral motor control) (Dovey *et al.*, 2013; McIntosh *et al.*, 1999).

BOX 13.12 Developmental approach for tube-weaning
- To provide guidance on nutrition
- To promote a positive feeding relationship between caregiver and child
- To determine child and family readiness
- To initiate a behavioural feeding plan

(Schauster and Dwyer 1996)

Parent and child's readiness

The transition from enteral tube nutrition to oral feeding is a process that requires commitment from the family. It is going to be a dynamic procedure that includes a reciprocal interchange between parents and child. This will require parents to recognise and to respond to infant cues during feeding (Satter, 1999) and to manage the child's difficult reactive and adaptive behaviour. Therefore, it is important to take into consideration parents' psychological individual characteristics such as anxiety and depression, as well as their individual skills (Blissett *et al.*, 2006; Martin *et al.*, 2013). To identify added psychosocial stressors is also significant, as it can lead to difficulties to facilitate a calm and successful feeding process. Parents can provide the opportunity and the encouragement for children to progress in their oral feeding; however, children also have to be ready for this process. The assessment of children's readiness for transition to oral eating should be conducted on an individual basis and it would require the child to show a minimum interest in interacting with food items and feeding (*see* Box 13.13).

In the clinical practice, both family and child's readiness are assessed when considering tube-weaning therapy. Readiness is not well documented within the literature; although some authors have identified tube-weaning readiness as requirement prior admission to hospital based tube-weaning therapy (e.g. Tarbell and Allaire, 2002).

BOX 13.13 Checklist example – assessment of readiness for inpatient tube-weaning therapy

- Parental clinical interview
- MDT meeting: (medical condition stabilised, safety of swallowing assessed, growth pattern allows flexibility for minor weight loss, nutritional requirements known)
- Summary of psychological feeding intervention completed at outpatient setting
- Direct assessment of child's observed feeding behaviour completed 2 weeks before admission
- Paediatric assessment scale for severe feeding problems
- Child psychotherapeutic sessions for residual paediatric traumatic stress symptoms 2 weeks before inpatient intervention
- Child shows ability or capability to eat and drink to a minimum baseline that allows intensive intervention for tube-weaning
- Feeding behaviour observed and a minimum baseline agreed
- Child and family willing to participate and consent signed
- Medical team support network on admission agreed

First steps: multidisciplinary team assessment

The importance of the MDT's approach in relation to the prescription of enteral feeding nutrition has been consistently referenced throughout this book. An MDT is also paramount for tube-weaning therapy because of the recognised multifactoral aspects of establishing oral eating behavior in children who have been tube-fed. Examples of MDT assessment and management for tube-weaning therapy are found in the literature (e.g. Martin *et al.*, 2008; Harding *et al.*, 2010). Ideally, a group of professionals with wide expertise in the field would work together collaboratively. In real-world clinical practice this will depend on the resources available in the child's geographical area of residence. Very often professionals work in isolation because of the unequal distribution of services. This may lead to delays in diagnosis and intervention (Culverwell, 2005). All too often, the onus is on the parent to collect, retain and deliver information gathered at disparate services, rather than health professionals operate as a single MDT. This behaviour is not indicative of a functioning MDT; rather, it is simply poor communication between different departments. A copied letter sent to other interested services is also not an MDT. An MDT in the tube-weaning process is the frank and open discussion among professionals in a single location working together to transition the child from tube dependency to oral eating. Lack of coordination may actually undermine successful transition, as detailed in Chapter 3. Unless a unified and single message is delivered to the family by the MDT, then any discrepancies, no matter how small, will unduly question the competency of professionals, leaving the parent to decide which individual within the MDT is the best person to follow.

The literature identifies that the following professionals should to be involved in tube-weaning.

Doctors

Enteral tube nutrition is a medical prescription. One of the requirements for tube-weaning therapy is for the child to present as medically stable. Doctors from different specialties of medicine may be involved through this process. The child's general practitioner and/or paediatrician may be involved if the child's tube-weaning process takes place within the community. If the child suffers a particular medical condition and the tube-weaning therapy is expected to be implemented at outpatient and/or inpatient acute hospital services, then the consultant specialist (e.g. gastroenterologist, respiratory) at the hospital may lead the process by setting and monitoring safe weight targets (either gain or loss) and prescribed medication for the particular illnesses.

Dietitians

Before initiating tube-weaning therapy, an evaluation of child's nutritional status is required and the design of the pattern for discontinuing enteral feeds is established by paediatric dietitians. They identify and monitor the child's nutritional needs and diet before, during and after the tube-weaning therapy process, supervising the child's caloric intake, nutritional status, nutrients and fluid intake.

Speech and language therapists, speech pathologists

Specialist dysphagia speech and language therapists evaluate the child's ability to swallow and identify if it is safe or not, identifying potential aspiration risks. Oral development includes the acquisition of skills that are not only motor based but also sensory based. Speech and language therapists explore the child's oral structure, oral functioning, oral motor skills and the child's oral-sensory status, identifying tolerance to textures and flavours. The mastery of oral abilities allow children to eat a variety of foods and its impairment may be subtle but enough to thwart the tube-weaning process.

Occupational therapists

Children who are tube-fed are at risk of developing sensory difficulties. It is common for them to lack exposure to early sensory experience in tastes, smell, touch of textures, and so forth, mainly when their tube-feeds have started at an early age. It is important to identify the child's sensory profile (Dunn, 1999; Dunn and Daniels, 2002) and sensory modulation abilities, as this may contribute to the child's food and feeding avoidance. This area of expertise is usually under the remit of the occupational therapist. This may be complemented by direct behavioural assessment measures on oral sensitivity by another professional (Dovey et al., 2013).

Psychologists

In relation to tube-weaning therapy, the psychologist assesses and manages the child's behaviour at mealtimes and with food. The intervention proper is usually under the control of this professional group. Therefore, the account-ability, but not necessarily the responsibility, for an effective outcome rests with this profession. In some countries, applied behaviour analysts cover these aspects, while in other countries generic psychologists or clinical psychologists are required. Irrespective of the designation of the psychologists, some form of accountability for outcome is necessary. Indeed, a minimum repertoire of behaviours is required for making mealtimes and eating possible. These include coming to the table, accepting to be seated in a suitable chair at the table, remaining seated during mealtimes, being willing to accept food offered, to consume it orally and be able to follow adult instruction (McGrath *et al.*, 2009); these are all necessary behavioural cusps to mealtimes. Assessment of a child who has not eaten orally will also include a more in-depth functional analysis of the child's behaviour to identify potential controlling environmental vari-ables and behavioural patterns of avoidance that will help to micromanage the new feeding situation and modify the child's behaviour when teaching new eating skills (Byars *et al.*, 2003).

Several child and family factors need consideration to determine the feasibility of tube-weaning therapy; although familial factors have not been extensively studied, assessments are common in clinical practice. Evaluation of the child's developmental status and cognitive abilities may be required to identify effective and structured approaches (Schwarz *et al.*, 2001), as well as to set an individualised baseline that facilitates the selection of specific beha-vioural techniques. Furthermore, the assessment of children with complex feeding disorders involves more aspects than clinical observation of the child's feeding patterns (Arvedson, 2008). Research indicates that special considera-tion should be paid to parental emotional status. The role of parental anxiety within this context has been well documented (e.g. Blackman and Nelson, 1985) and has been found to be a key element mediating tube-weaning ther-apy outcomes (Harding *et al.*, 2010).

TUBE-WEANING FEEDING THERAPY

The process of weaning children from enteral nutrition therapy to oral eat-ing is a difficult challenge for health professionals, children and their families to undergo an individual journey. Some children may withdraw from tube-feeding quickly and with little support, while other children with multiple co-morbidities associated with, or developed as a consequence of, enteral tube nutrition may require extensive professional support and tube-weaning therapy.

Currently, there is no consensus in the literature regarding definition of terms within tube-feeding. Most papers refer to single clinics and posit that their approach is the best on the grounds of cost-effectiveness, methodology recommended, or identification of the appropriate setting (inpatient vs. outpatient; rapid vs. slow weaning) for helping children to withdraw from tube-feeds. Moreover, there are no guidelines or central recommendations for best practice for tube-weaning. Although research studies acknowledge the difficulties associated with this process, to date the literature related to the initiation or restitution of oral eating after a long period of enteral tube nutrition is limited (Dunbar *et al.*, 1991; Harding *et al.*, 2010). Agreement can only be reached that tube-weaning is not an easy task, as children with feeding difficulties are not a heterogeneous group and a variety of interventions may be required. For the purpose of this chapter, the definition of tube-weaning feeding therapy will be the process of supporting children to withdraw from enteral tube nutrition towards oral eating through the application of health therapies. Within the chapter will be a summary of the process (what one could do) the settings (where this could be done) and the therapies (how it may be achieved).

The process

Within this chapter it has been explained what considerations have been assessed before starting tube-weaning therapy (*see* Box 13.14). The majority of the evidence-based practice and literature findings indicate an application of a combination of appetite manipulation, behavioural management and parental training approaches once tube weaning therapy has been prescribed (Martin and Dovey, 2011; Martin *et al.*, 2008). In the clinical practice, the advised method is to create a supportive team around the child that includes family and professionals working together simultaneously to achieve goals.

Appetite manipulation is achieved through decreasing enteral tube-feeds. Dietitians may develop specific individualised programmes for progressively reducing tube-feeds (*see* example in Part III 3.5b). It is considered by many to be a crucial part of the tube-weaning intervention and needs to be carefully considered in the planning of the treatment (Byars *et al.*, 2003). Dietitians also monitor the percentage of daily calories and fluids received artificially and may make adjustments to balance daytime hunger against the child's weight loss and hydration status. Concomitant to the feed reduction, a specifically planned and developmentally appropriate diet that compensates for nutritional needs and is tailored to the child's capacity is developed for oral eating.

BOX 13.14 Stages of tube-weaning therapy

Before

- Medical stability
- Safe swallowing
- Oral motor skills and sensory motor development
- Parent and child readiness
- Minimum mealtime behaviours
- MDT assessment

During
- Appetite manipulation
- Behavioural intervention
- Parent training
- Other therapies

After
- Establishing follow-up visit regimen
- Monitoring growth patterns
- Parental support for behavioural management

It is common for children who start eating orally after a period of being tube-fed to present behavioural problems of differing frequency and intensity during the tube-weaning therapy process. Behavioural intervention and treatment designed to help children to decrease their oral feeding resistance, to increase the variety and quantity of food consumed and to progress on their diet have been widely described in the literature of children with feeding disorders (Byars *et al.*, 2003; Piazza *et al.*, 2003). Initially, therapists apply direct behavioural techniques, while simultaneously parents are trained on behavioural and nutritional principles and observe their application by the professional to aid in managing their child's resistant behaviour during mealtimes (*see* Box 13.15). Once parents have mastered behavioural intervention skills (determined to be 90% consistency), triadic sessions with the therapist managing their child's behaviour at mealtimes can take place. The objective is to gradually fade out or thin the therapist's involvement so that the parent takes control of the child's feeding (Byars *et al.*, 2003; Martin *et al.*, 2008).

BOX 13.15 Parent training
- Parents learn behavioural techniques through didactic and direct observation sessions
- Parents may practise using role-play approaches
- Parents continue rehearsal until therapist achieves stable outcomes on the child's oral eating intake
- Parents feed their child under the therapist's support
- Parents feed their child without the presence of the therapist

(Martin and Dovey, 2011)

The setting

Tube-weaning therapy may take place at acute hospital and/or specialised feeding disorder units using inpatient facilities or through outpatient appointment visits. In other cases, this therapy can be conducted at home or at schools supported by community-based services. Limiting therapy to a single approach is not currently supported by evidence – in fact, the small amount of evidence would suggest that many methods of tube-weaning are effective. A one-size-fits-all policy for tube-weaning is indicative of an attempt to curtail the offering of services for tube-weaning, rather than base the process on evidence. It would appear the only common factor between services is the involvement of the different professionals and their level of effective communication. It is important that the setting is adapted to local circumstances and availability rather than follow a prescriptive model of necessity.

Historically, inpatient and outpatient day interventions are considered the main settings for tube-weaning therapy and many programmes describe treatments conducted in both locations (Byars *et al.*, 2003; Cornwell, 2010; Martin *et al.*, 2008;). However, research findings have been primarily based on single case studies and case design (Gutentag and Hammer, 2000) with a scarcity of appropriately controlled studies. The same pattern is repeated regarding studies on the effectiveness of long-term ambulatory feeding intervention programmes (Luiselli, 2000). One exception is the appropriately controlled study provided by Benoit *et al.*, (2001). These authors compared behavioural therapy with nutritional intervention and found that the behavioural treatment was more effective.

Retrospective outpatient multidisciplinary interventions have also been reported. Davis *et al.* (2009) reviewed nine children receiving total enteral tube nutrition through gastrostomy who had been treated by an MDT within an outpatient-based protocol that included the administration of pain management and hunger provocation medication. They reported that eight of the nine children treated were able to maintain their weight and were eating orally during follow-up sessions. Wright *et al.* (2011) studied children treated by their MDT tube-weaning clinic over a period of 5 years. They described in detail their clinical management protocol and reported that 78% of those children were on normal oral diets after a median of 1.7 years of follow-up. They concluded that for them the key element in the withdrawal process had been the management of parental anxiety.

Intensive day treatments have also been illustrated. This approach requires the child and his or her family to stay all day within the premises of the specific feeding treatment unit, being able to return home at night. Tarbell and Allaire (2002) described an MDT intervention in a paediatric day treatment setting. After 2–3 weeks of intervention their results indicated that 72% of the children treated were completely weaned from their artificial feeds. They concluded that children's internal motivation and immersion in oral eating alongside parental education on normal feeding behaviour was paramount to the success of their programme. Successful tube-weaning interventions conducted in an inpatient setting share similar management steps and outcomes. Typically, they implement treatment programmes that include several significant components. These include both appetite regulation and behavioural intervention (e.g. Blackman and Nelson, 1987; Byars *et al.*, 2003).

There are also examples of established interdisciplinary teams offering tube-weaning feeding therapy in inpatient settings. The Kennedy Krieger Institute (Greer *et al.*, 2008) and the Munroe-Meyer Institute (Piazza *et al.*, 2003) both have long-standing feeding disorder programmes. The effectiveness of tube-weaning therapy in inpatient settings has been established with strong treatment effects. Kinderman *et al.* (2008) treated 10 children following a five-step protocol. Follow-up results after discharge from hospital indicated that 8 of those 10 children had been completely weaned from tube-feeds and were continuing to eat orally and gain weight. Cornwell *et al.* (2010) studied inpatient treatment that combined treatments from dietetic, speech and therapy, occupational therapy and psychology disciplines to manage tube-dependency. Their results indicated that at the end of the intervention, 42.5% of children from their sample were meeting their nutritional needs through oral eating. Silverman *et al.* (2013) completed a retrospective study of 77 children with gastrostomy tube dependence who were under an inpatient tube-weaning intensive protocol. Their study described the long-term effects of behavioural strategies to wean children from artificial feeds. They concluded that inpatient intensive behavioural interventions are highly effective for transitioning children from tube-feed dependence to oral eating. Summary of inpatient intervention approaches with their advantages and disadvantages as well as examples of cases can also be found elsewhere (see Martin and Dovey, 2011).

Reports on home- and school-based tube-weaning feeding therapy interventions are rare in the literature: Gutentag and Hammer (2000) tube-weaned a 3-year-old medically fragile child at home using behavioural approaches and results were then generalised to the school setting. McKirdy *et al.* (2008) completed a successful transition to oral eating with two children who had been long-term tube-fed through a school-based intervention programme. They adapted the Schauster and Dwyer (1996) protocol to the school environment. These data indicate that it is not the location or environment of the tube-wean that is important; rather, it is the methods employed that determine success. Therefore, it is suggested that a child can be weaned in multiple locations and the only consideration that will determine potential effectiveness of the various interventions is generalisation between environments. No matter where the wean is undertaken, it is important that generalisation between different environments is maintained.

The therapies

It is common for children who are in the process of being weaned from artificial tube-feeds to be in contact with several different professionals providing specific therapeutic interventions. These therapies may be in place before, during and/or after the tube-weaning. As a reference guide, the most frequent therapies applied to tube-weaning feeding intervention may be physical therapy, nutritional therapy, oral motor and speech therapy, oral sensory and/or sensory integration therapy, play therapy and psychological therapy (emotional and behavioural).

Physical therapy

Minimal body ability such as stability and coordination of the trunk and shoulders are required as a foundation for the development of oral motor skills necessary for eating. Advanced chewing for eating solid food also requires a more secure trunk and neck development, as well as sophisticated muscle control. For example, an extended trunk and neck position may contribute to extra tongue extension interfering with swallowing (Kumin and Bahr, 1999). An upright position during mealtimes is important for all children. Those with reduced motor control will require individualised and specific physical programmes to facilitate its development prior to tube-weaning therapeutic intervention.

Nutritional therapy

Children who have been on long-term tube nutrition are going to require very careful monitoring of their nutritional and caloric needs during the whole weaning process. Specific menus created in discussion with the child (if appropriate) and the child's family will include friendly and developmentally appropriate food presentation, target familial preferences and provide a variety of textures. Caloric-based supplements in liquid or powder form may be added to the child's food during or between mealtimes. The amount of these caloric supplements can be decreased proportional to the increase in the child's ability to eat a wider variety of food items and textures. During the tube-weaning process, some parents also benefit from nutritional counselling and advice (Borowitz *et al.*, 2002).

Oral motor and speech therapy

Mastering oral motor skills is required for eating and drinking and children who are tube fed require support to develop their oral motor abilities. Oral motor development is a complex process and it is an important foundation for feeding, as well as for speech and language skills. A variety of activities may be designed to stimulate the oral area and support coordination of oral structure: blowing candles, making soap bubbles, imitating sound and tongue position, massages of the external oral area and face, playing Mr Tongue (Love and Reilly, 1995). Behavioural protocols for teaching children how to chew are also present in the literature (Dovey *et al.*, 2013).

Oral sensory and/or sensory integration therapy

Intervention aiming to improve sensory motor abilities of children who are tube-fed may include activities that allow them to play with and explore food items in a relaxed atmosphere (cooking, baking, etc.), to orally explore toys for younger children, and so forth. Systematic desensitisation procedures may also applied to children with complex sensory sensitivity issues (Dovey and Martin, 2012). Tailored diets accommodating sensory sensitivities can also be devised to match the unique sensory processing needs of a child (Wilbarger, 1995).

Play therapy

For children, to play is one of natural ways to learn about the world and to work through their anxieties. Play is essential to healthy development (Ginsburg, 2007). Play elements may be found in other therapy approaches. Play specialists may recommend that parents allow children to play with and explore feeding utensils or to play with food items, so that children become familiar with them and their anxiety is reduced. Some play activities have been now integrated within computer-based programs – for example, those developed by Lo *et al.* (2007). These authors developed the Playful Tray to reinforce active participation of children with the eating process.

Psychological therapy

Behavioural approaches and specific intervention protocols to help children to develop oral eating behaviour have been extensively documented (e.g. Linscheid, 2006; Rommel *et al.*, 2003). Sharp *et al.* (2010) completed a systematic review of the literature on treatment intervention for paediatric feeding disorders including 48 single case studies that reported outcomes for 96 children. They found that all studies revisited included behavioural intervention. Results indicated that behavioural intervention was associated with significant improvements in feeding behaviour. Behavioural interventions may vary from application of positive reinforcement techniques to more elaborate behavioural protocols that may include specialist shaping, fading, escape extinction procedures, and so forth (Piazza *et al.*, 2003; Williams *et al.*, 2007).

To date, no appropriately randomised controlled trial evidence is available for any other form of psychological intervention for children requiring tubeweaning. Any programme that operates outside of the limited evidence available is currently not offering an evidence-based intervention. Unfortunately, there are many such interventions currently circulating and health professionals should be wary in advocating or allowing their clients to engage with those programmes without consultation.

SUMMARY

When children cannot take nutrients orally and are at risk of malnutrition, medics prescribe tube nutrition with enteral formulas that contain all required nutrients for children to survive and thrive. There is no doubt that this group of children benefit from these interventions to improve their health. However, the care of a child who is tube-fed increases responsibility and pressure on the primary caregivers. Intensive tube-feeding routines seem incompatible with social family needs and full-time employment. More research regarding the impact that having a child who is tube-fed has on the emotional and social aspects of the whole family system is necessary.

There are many factors to take into account in children who are tube-fed and these have to be carefully considered when recommending tube-weaning feeding therapy. Earliest-possible transition to oral feeding under advice and supervision of health professionals must be advocated in all cases where oral feeding proves to be safe. There are cases where tube-weaning feeding therapy may require specialist treatment intervention. The setting where the tube-weaning feeding therapy is undertaken may vary (hospital, home, school, and so forth); however, generalisation between different environments has to be achieved.

Recent research literature identifies the need for paying attention to the whole process, including both starting enteral tube nutrition and ending it. The development of international guidelines for best practice for tube-weaning feeding therapy and standard formal training procedures for parents on enteral tube nutrition is paramount at this point in time.

REFERENCES

Abad-Sinden A, Sutphen J. Nutritional management of pediatric short bowel syndrome. *Pract Gastroenterol*. 2003; **12**: 28–48.

Arts-Rodas D, Benoit D. Feeding problems in infancy and early childhood: identification and management. *Pediatr Child Health*. 1998; **3**(1): 21–7.

Arvedson JC. Assessment of pediatric dysphagia and feeding disorders: clinical and instrumental approaches. *Dev Disabil Res Rev*. 2008; **14**(2): 118–27.

Arvedson JC. Swallowing and feeding in infants and young children. *GI Motility Online*. 2006. Available at: www.nature.com/gimo/contents/pt1/full/gimo17.html (accessed 12 March 2012).

Arvedson JC, Brodsky L. *Pediatric Swallowing and Feeding: assessment and management*. New York, NY: Cengage Delmar Learning; 2001.

August D, Teitelbaum D, Albina J, *et al*. ASPEN Board of Directors and the Clinical Guidelines Task Force. Guidelines for the use of parenteral and enteral nutrition in adult and pediatric patients. *JPEN J Parenter Enteral Nutr*. 2002; **26**(1 Suppl.): SA1–138.

Benoit D, Wang EE, Zlotkin SH. Characteristics and outcomes of children with enterostomy feeding tubes: a study of 325 children. *Paediatr Child Health*. 2001; **6**(3): 132–7.

Bernard-Bonnin AC. Feeding problems of infants and toddlers. *Can Fam Physician*. 2006; **52**(10): 1247–51.

Blackman JA, Nelson CL. Reinstituting oral feedings in children fed by gastrostomy tube. *Clin Pediatr*.1985; **24**(8): 434–8.

Blackman JA, Nelson CL. Rapid Introduction of oral feedings to tube-fed patients. *J Dev Behav Pediatr*. 1987; **8**(2): 63–7.

Blissett J, Meyer C, Haycraft E. Maternal and paternal controlling feeding practices with male and female children. *Appetite*. 2006; **47**(2): 212–19.

Borowitz D, Baker RD, Stallings V. Consensus report on nutrition for pediatric patients with cystic fibrosis. *J Pediatr Gastroenterol Nutr*. 2002; **35**(3): 246–59.

British Artificial Nutrition Survey (BANS). *Annual BANS Report, 2008: artificial nutrition support in the UK 2000–2007*. Redditch, Worcestershire: British Association for Parenteral and Enteral Nutrition (BAPEN); 2008. Available at: www.bapen.org.uk/pdfs/bans_reports/bans_report_08.pdf (accessed 12 March 2012).

Byars KC, Burklow KA, Ferguson K, *et al*. Multicomponent behavioral program for oral aversion in children dependent on gastrostomy feedings. *J Pediatr Gastroenterol Nutr*. 2003; **37**(4): 473–80.

Byron M. Interventions with children who are tube fed. In: Southall A, Martin C, editors. *Feeding Problems in Children: a practical guide*. Oxford, UK: Radcliffe Publishing; 2011. Chapter 11, pp. 213–23.

Calderón C, Gómez-López L, Martínez-Costa C, *et al.* Feeling of burden, psychological distress, and anxiety among primary caregivers of children with home enteral nutrition. *J Pediatr Psychol.* 2011; **36**(2): 188–95.

Cornwell SL. *Pediatric Feeding Disorders: a controlled comparison of multidisciplinary inpatient and outpatient treatment of gastrostomy tube dependent children* [dissertation]. Denton: University of North Texas; 2010.

Craig GM, Scambler G. Negotiating mothering against the odds: gastrostomy tube feeding, stigma, governmentality and disabled children. *Soc Sci Med.* 2006; **62**(5): 1115–25.

Culverwell T. The parent's perspective. *Proc Nutr Soc.* 2005; **64**(3): 339–43.

Daveluy W, Guimber D, Uhlen S, *et al.* Dramatic changes in home-based enteral nutrition practices in children during an 11-year period. *J Pediatr Gastroenterol Nutr.* 2006; **43**(2): 240–4.

Davis AM, Bruce AS, Mangiaracina C, *et al.* Moving from tube to oral feeding in medically fragile nonverbal toddlers. *J Paediatr Gastroenterol Nutr.* 2009; **49**(2): 233–6.

Delaney AL, Arvedson JC. Development of swallowing and feeding: prenatal through first year of life. *Dev Disabil Res Rev.* 2008; **14**(2): 105–17.

Dellert SF, Hyams JS, Treem WR, *et al.* Feeding resistance and gastroesophageal reflux in infancy. *J Pediatr Gastroenterol Nutr.* 1993; **17**(1): 66–71.

Di Lorenzo C, Flores AF, Buie T, *et al.* Intestinal motility and jejunal feeding in children with chronic intestinal pseudo-obstruction. *Gastroenterology.* 1995; **108**(5): 1379–85.

Di Scipio WJ, Kaslon K, Ruben RJ. Traumatically acquired conditioned dysphagia in children. *Ann Otol Rhinol Laryngol.* 1978; **87**(4 Pt. 1): 509–14.

Dovey TM, Alridge V, Martin C. Measuring oral sensitivity in clinical practice: a quick and reliable behavioural method. *Dysphagia.* 2013; **28**(4): 501–10.

Dovey TM, Martin C. Developmental, cognitive and regulatory aspects of feeding disorders. In: Southall A, Martin C, editors. *Feeding Problems in Children: a practical guide.* Oxford, UK: Radcliffe Publishing; 2011. Chapter 5, pp. 94–110.

Dovey TM, Martin C. A parent-led contingent reward desensitisation intervention for children with a feeding problem resulting from sensory defensiveness. *Infant Child Adolesc Nutr.* 2012; **4**(6): 384–93.

Duggan C, Watkins JB, Walker A, editors. *Nutrition in Pediatrics: basic science and clinical applications.* Hamilton, ON: BC Decker; 2008.

Dunbar SB, Jarvis AH, Breyer M. The transition from nonoral to oral feeding in children. *Am J Occup Ther.* 1991; **45**(5): 402–8.

Dunn W. *The Sensory Profile: user's manual.* San Antonio, TX: Psychological Corporation; 1999.

Dunn W, Daniels DB. Initial development of the Infant/Toddler Sensory Profile. *J Early Interv.* 2002; **25**(1): 27–41.

Elia M. Home enteral nutrition: general aspects and a comparison between the United States and Britain. *Nutrition.* 1994; **10**(2): 115–23.

Elia M, Russell C, Stratton R. *Trends in Artificial Nutrition Support in the UK during 1996– 2000. A report by the British Artificial Nutrition Survey a committee of the British Association for Parenteral and Enteral Nutrition.* Berkshire: BAPEN; 2001.

Fereday J, Thomas C, Forrest A, *et al.* Food for thought: investigating parents' perspectives of the impact of their child's home enteral nutrition (HEN). *Neonat Paediatr Child Health Nurs.* 2009; **12**: 9–14.

Ferry GD, Selby M, Pietro TJ. Clinical response to short-term nasogastric feeding in infants with gastroesophageal reflux and growth failure. *J Pediatr Gastroenterol Nutr.* 1983; **2**(1): 57–61.

Forcielli ML, Richardson D, Folkman J, *et al.* Better living through chemistry, constant monitoring, and prompt interventions: 26 years on home parenteral nutrition without major complications. *Nutrition.* 2008; **24**(1):103–7.

Geertsma AM, Hyams JS, Pelletier JM, *et al.* Feeding resistance after parenteral hyperalimentation. *Am J Dis Child.* 1985; **139**(3): 255–6.

Ginsburg KR. The importance of play in promoting healthy child development and maintaining strong parent-child bonds. *Pediatrics.* 2007; **119**(1): 182–91.

Gottrand F, Sullivan PB. Gastrostomy tube feeding: when to start, what to feed and how to stop. *Eur J Clin Nutr.* 2010; **64**(1): S17–21.

Greer AJ, Gulotta CS, Masler EA, *et al.* Caregiver stress and outcomes of children with pediatric feeding disorders treated in an intensive interdisciplinary program. *J Pediatr Psychol.* 2008; **33**(6): 612–20.

Griffen KM. Swallowing training for dysphagic patients. *Arch Phys Med Rehabil.* 1979; **55**(10): 467–70.

Guenter P, Silkroski M. *Tube Feeding: practical guidelines and nursing protocols.* Gaithersburg, MD: Aspen Publications; 2001.

Gutentag S, Hammer D. Shaping oral feeding in a gastronomy tube-dependent child in natural settings. *Behav Modif.* 2000; **24**(3): 395–410.

Handen BL, Mandell F, Russo DC. Feeding induction in children who refuse to eat. *Am J Dis Child.* 1986; **140**(1): 52–4.

Harding C, Faiman A, Wright J. Evaluation of an intensive desensitisation, oral tolerance therapy and hunger provocation program for children who have had prolonged periods of tube feeds. *Int J Evid Based Healthc.* 2010; **8**(4): 268–76.

Hazel R. The psychosocial impact on parents of tube feeding their child. *Paediatr Nurs.* 2006; **18**(4): 19–22.

Howard L, Ament M, Fleming CR, *et al.* Current use and clinical outcome of home parenteral and enteral nutrition therapies in the United States. *Gastroenterology.* 1995; **109**(2): 355–65.

Hyman PE. Gastroesophageal reflux: one reason why baby won't eat. *J Pediatr.* 1994; **125**(6 Pt. 2): 103–9.

Illingworth RS, Lister J. The critical or sensitive period, with special reference to certain feeding problems in infants and children. *J Pediatr.* 1964; **65**: 839–48.

Israel DM, Hassall E. Prolonged use of gastrostomy for enteral hyperalimentation in children with Crohn's disease. *Am J Gastroenterol.* 1995; **90**(7): 1084–8.

Kinderman A, Kneepkens CMF, Stok A, *et al.* Discontinuation of tube feeding in young children by hunger provocation. *J Pediatr Gastroenterol Nutr.* 2008; **47**(1): 87–91.

Kumin L, Bahr DC. Patterns of feeding, eating and drinking in young children with Down syndrome with oral motor concerns. *Down Syndrome Quarterly.* 1999; **4**(2): 1–8.

Limbrick P. *The Team around the Child: multi-agency service co-ordination for children with complex needs and their families.* Worcester: Interconnections; 2001.

Linscheid TR. Behavioural treatments for pediatric feeding disorders. *Behav Modif.* 2006; **30**(1): 6–23.

Linscheid TR, Rasnake LK. *Handbook of Clinical Child Psychology.* New York, NY: Wiley; 1992.

Lipsitt L, Crook C, Booth C. The transitional infant: behavioural development and feeding. *Am J Clin Nutr.* 1985; **41**(2 Suppl.): 485–96.

Lo J-L, Lin T-Y, Chu H-H, *et al.* Playful Tray: adopting UbiComp and persuasive techniques into play-based occupational therapy for reducing poor eating behaviour in young children. *Lect Notes Comput Sci.* 2007; **4717**: 38–55.

Love E, Reilly S. *Time for Talking: speaking and listening activities for lower primary students.* Pearson Learning: Good Year Books; Australia,1995.

Luiselli JK. Cueing, demand fading, and positive reinforcement to establish self-feeding and oral consumption in a child with chronic food refusal. *Behav Modif.* 2000; **24**(3): 348–58.

Martin CI, Dovey TM. Intensive intervention for childhood feeding disorders. In: Southall A, Martin C. *Feeding Problems in Children: a practical guide.* Oxford, UK: Radcliffe Publishing; 2011. Chapter 15, pp. 277–93.

Martin CI, Dovey TM, Coulthard H, *et al.* Maternal stress and problem-solving skills in a sample of children with nonorganic feeding disorders. *Infant Ment Health J.* 2013; **34**(3): 202–10.

Martin CI, Southall A, Shea E, Marr A. The importance of a multifaceted approach in the assessment and treatment of childhood feeding disorders. *Clin Case Stud.* 2008; **7**: 79–9.

Mason SJ, Harris G, Blissett J. Tube feeding in infancy: implications for the development of normal eating and drinking skills. *Dysphagia.* 2005; **20**(1): 46–61.

McGrath A, Bruce AS, Hyman P, *et al.* Moving from tube to oral feeding in medically fragile nonverbal toddlers. *J Pediatr Gastroenterol Nutr.* 2009; **49**(2): 233–6.

McIntosh DN, Miller LJ, Shyu V, *et al.* Overview of the Short Sensory Profile (SSP). In: Dunn W, editor. *The Sensory Profile: examiner's manual.* San Antonio, TX: Psychological Corporation; 1999. pp. 59–73.

McKirdy L, Sheppard J, Osborne M, *et al.* Transition from tube to oral feeding in the school setting. *Lang Speech Hear Serv Sch.* 2008; **39**(2): 249–60.

Mennella JA. Development of the Chemical Senses and the Programming of Flavor Preference. Physiologic/immunologic responses to dietary nutrients: role of elemental and hydrolysate formulas in management of the pediatric patient. *Report of the 107th Conference on Pediatric Research.* 1998; **9**: 201–8.

Moreno-Villares J, Galiano Segovia MJ, Marín Ferrer M. [Changes in feeding behavior of patients who had received enteral nutrition during the 1st year of life] [Spanish]. *Nutr Hosp.* 1998; **13**(2): 90–4.

National Health Service (NHS). *Nasogastric and gastrostomy tube feeding for children being cared for in the community Nursing & Midwifery Practice Development Unit (now part of NHS Quality Improvement Scotland).* London: NICE; 2003. Available at: www.cen.scot.nhs.uk/files/12j-nastrogastric-and-gastronomy-tube-feeding-for-children-being-cared-for-in-the-community.pdf (accessed 14 January 2014).

Nightingale J, Woodward JM; Small Bowel and Nutrition Committee of the British Society of Gastroenterology. Guidelines for management of patients with a short bowel. *Gut.* 2006; **55**(Suppl. 4): iv1–12.

Olieman JF, Penning C, Ijsselstijn H, *et al.* Enteral nutrition in children with short-bowel syndrome: current evidence and recommendations for the clinician. *J Am Diet Assoc.* 2010; **110**(3): 420–6.

Pedersen SD, Parsons HG, Dewey D. Stress levels experienced by the parents of enterally fed children. *Child Care Health Dev.* 2004; **30**(5): 507–13.

Pedrón-Giner C, Calderón C, Martínez-Zazo A, *et al.* Home enteral nutrition in children; a 10 year experience with 304 pediatric patients. *Nutr Hosp.* 2012; **27**(5): 1444–50.

Piazza C, Fisher W, Brown K, *et al.* Functional analysis of inappropriate mealtime behaviours. *J Appl Behav Anal.* 2003; **36**(2): 187–204.

Quigley S, Iglesias J. Enteral tubes: care and management. In: Brodsky D. *Primary Care of the Premature Infant.* Philadelphia: Elsevier Health Sciences; 2008. Chapter 4E, pp. 109–21.

Rommel N, DeMeyer A, Feenstra L, *et al.* The complexity of feeding problems in 700 infants and young children presenting to a tertiary care institution. *J Pediatr Gastroenterol Nutr.* 2003; **37**(1): 75–84.

Rouse L, Herrington P, Assey J, *et al.* Feeding problems, gastrostomy and families: a qualitative pilot study. *Br J Learn Disabil.* 2002; **30**(3): 122–8.

Satter E. The feeding relationship. In: Kessler DB, Dawson P, editors. *Failure to Thrive and Pediatric Nutrition: a transdisciplinary approach.* Baltimore, MD: Brookes; 1999. pp. 121–45.

Schauster H, Dwyer J. Transition from tube feeding to feedings by mouth in children: preventing eating dysfunction. *J Am Diet Assoc.* 1996; **96**(3): 277–81.

Schwarz SM, Corredor J, Fisher-Medina J, *et al.* Diagnosis and treatment of feeding disorders in children with developmental disabilities. *Pediatrics.* 2001; **108**(3): 671–6.

Sharp WG, Jaquess DL, Morton JF, *et al.* Pediatric feeding disorders: a quantitative synthesis of treatment outcomes. *Clin Child Fam Psychol Rev.* 2010; **13**(4): 348–65.

Sidey A, Torbet S. Enteral feeding in community settings. *Paediatr Nurs.* 1995; **7**(6): 21–4.

Silverman AH, Kirby M, Clifford LM, *et al.* Nutritional and psychosocial outcomes of gastrostomy tube-dependent children completing an intensive inpatient behavioural treatment program. *J Pediatr Gastroenterol Nutr.* 2013; **57**(5): 668–72.

Spalding K, McKeever RN. Mothers' experiences caring for children with disabilities who require a gastrostomy tube. *J Pediatr Nurs.* 1998; **13**(4): 234–42.

Sullivan PB. Gastrointestinal disorders in children with neurodevelopmental disabilities. *Dev Disabil Res Rev.* 2008; **14**(2): 128–36.

Tarbell MC, Allaire JH. Children with feeding tube dependency: treating the whole child. *Infants Young Child.* 2002; **15**(1): 29–41.

Townsley R, Robinson C. *Food for Thought? Effective support for families caring for child who is tube fed.* Bristol: Norah Fry Research Centre; 2000.

Tucker CM, Butler AM, Loyuk IS, *et al.* Predictors of a health-promoting lifestyle and behaviours among low-income African American mothers and white mothers of chronically ill children. *J Natl Med Assoc.* 2009; **101**(2): 103–10.

Vanderhoof JA, Langnas AN. Short-bowel syndrome in children and adults. *Gastroenterology.* 1997; **113**(5): 1767–78.

Vogel J, Mulliken JB, Kaban LB. Macroglossia: a review of the condition and a new classification. *Plast Reconstr Surg.* 1986; **78**(6): 715–23.

Wilbarger P. The sensory diet: activity programs based upon sensory processing theory. *Sensory Integration Special Interest Section Quarterly.* 1995; **18**(2): 1–4.

Williams KE, Riegel E, Gibbons B, *et al.* Intensive behavioural treatment for severe feeding problems: a cost-effective alternative to tube-feeding? *J Dev Phys Disabil.* 2007; **19**: 227–35.

Wright C. Home enteral nutrition. *J Commun Nurs.* 2004; **18**(2): 8–13.

Wright CM, Smith KH, Morrison J. Withdrawing feeds from children on long term enteral feeding: factors associated with success and failure. *Arch Dis Child.* 2011; **96**(5): 433–9.

CHAPTER 14

On learning from the experts …

Taigh Giles and Angela Southall

INTRODUCTION

Why have we written this chapter?

From decades of clinical and research experience we have learnt it is important to understand and value patients' experiences, to learn from patients and to include this learning in our programmes of training, assessment, treatment and support. We understand that it is important to do things *with* our patients, rather than *to* them. We have come also to appreciate that patients understand their experiences better than the professionals around them, and that if we are going to make a real difference to the lives of people with chronic conditions we need to find a way of harnessing this experience and helping everyone make the most of it. We 'know' all of these things but do not yet know exactly how to do them.

Taigh and I have written this chapter so that Taigh can share her experiences and hopefully help readers to understand more about what it is like to be a child growing up with an undiagnosed gastrointestinal problem and all of the difficulties – medical, psychological and social – that this has led to for her. Her mother, Tracey, has also contributed, sharing her thoughts and experiences.

We acknowledge that many hopes, beliefs and prejudices impinge on how we approach children like Taigh and how we think about them and their families. We hope to also explore some of these issues, in the hope that they will help us understand more about how we work together, professional and patient, and how we might do this better.

This chapter explores some of the basic beliefs about medicine and why it is that we find it so hard to put the patient experience central to what we do. It also considers some of the ideas that are working their way through the health system that might make a difference to other families like Taigh's and help them to have a different kind of experience in the future.

A PERSONAL STORY

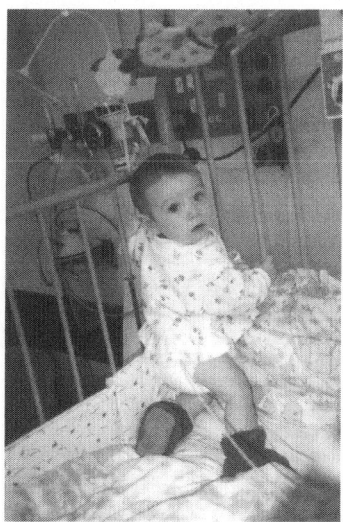

FIGURE 14.1 Welcome to my world: Taigh at 9 months old, weighing just 9 lbs

Taigh's story

I was born on the 21st of May 1992, a lovely sunny day, weighing 8 lbs 10½ oz. By the time I was 5 months old I weighed 5 lbs – that's less than my birth weight. I was skin and bones. This was due to me constantly being sick. My weight dropped, as I wasn't keeping anything down. Mum was told to put me on solids at 3 months to try to get my weight up. But it still didn't help, as I kept on bringing it back up. The doctors didn't know what was wrong with me, so I was fed by tube ...

I moved around different hospitals but nobody seemed to come up with the actual problem. Doctors would peer through the hospital window just to check I was still alive – they didn't know what else to do with me. Nobody understood what was going on. Doctors began to discuss surgery. In the end, this wasn't done because at 9 months old and weighing only 9 lbs, I started walking and gravity seemed to help the food stay down. I was then discharged without a diagnosis.

From here is where the real problem started. Up until I was about 6 months old I was being sick up to 100 times a day. This gradually reduced to about four or five times a day by about 8 months. My family had to adapt our home because of this, by leaving a bucket by my bed at night and removing all the carpets. I didn't always know when it was coming ... I could be sick anywhere or at any time, whether this be walking to school or at the dinner table. Mostly I used to be sick during or after eating. Eventually I began to associate the food with my sickness, and I decided, 'if I don't eat that, then I won't be sick'. This was now a phobia, not just an unknown medical condition.

Throughout her childhood, Taigh continued to be sick, day and night, several times a day. Finally, at 17 years of age, she was diagnosed with acid reflux. By this time she had a damaged oesophagus, major gut dysfunction, damaged sinuses and a severe food phobia.

THE BELIEF SYSTEM REGARDING MEDICINE

There is a powerful 'dominant story' within Western culture about the authority and infallibility of science. This authority is embodied in medicine, which is generally held to have its roots firmly embedded in scientific theory and practice. Several authors have questioned the accuracy of this belief in recent years (Bentall, 2003; Southall, 2007, 2009), most notably in relation to psychiatry. Nevertheless, over time these beliefs have become hegemonic; that is, they have come to be so much a part of our way of thinking that they are seen as unchallengeable and govern the way we think about things – whether consciously or unconsciously.

How we deal with conflicting beliefs

The notion of medicine as infallible is incompatible with real-life medicine as experienced by both doctors and patients. Therefore, it is often the case that encounters within the medical system challenge this belief and give rise to a conflict between expectation and experience. This leads to something known in the psychological literature as *cognitive dissonance* (*see* Box 14.1). The dominant belief systems that govern our thinking about medicine also give rise to a number of conceptions regarding illness, especially those regarding *whose fault it is* when someone gets ill. In the event of the illness becoming chronic, or diagnosis proving elusive, the anxiety generated by this dilemma can become acute. When medicine fails to find an answer, both doctor and patient can find themselves feeling like failures (Cardillo, 2004): the doctor has failed to find 'the answer' and the patient has failed to get better. The behaviours that follow can be seen as a response to this mutual sense of failure and the need for both doctor and patient to defend against it.

The conviction that illnesses can be prevented and controlled by doctors is often accompanied by a belief that those who develop them are somehow responsible (Cardillo, 2004). This attributional bias is explained in psychological theory by the 'Just World' hypothesis (Lerner and Miller, 1978) and reflects a process in which attributions of blame tend to be made about the victim when something bad happens to him or her. It helps us make sense of a world in which horrible things can happen to us. It makes us feel better to imagine that when these things happen to others, they are somehow complicit in the events. Importantly, these processes occur automatically, rather than being the result of conscious processes: we remain unaware of our own attribution bias and our own efforts to adjust our thinking.

Parents often experience feeling 'blamed', not being believed and, sometimes, of being thought to be harming their child. Tracey, Taigh's mother, was

BOX 14.1 Cognitive dissonance at work

The notion of cognitive dissonance has been extensively researched and written about since its initial formulation by Leon Festinger in 1957. To summarise, it is the sense of acute unease that we experience when we hold two differing and conflicting views. What we do is we act immediately to reduce this dissonance so that we feel 'normal' again.

For example, if a doctor cannot find the source of the patient's illness, he or she may choose to believe that the patient is not really ill at all, or that the patient is fabricating the illness. Conversely, the patient may choose to believe that the doctor cannot find out what is wrong with him or her because the doctor is a poor doctor. As the situation continues, each becomes more and more entrenched in his or her views in order to help alleviate his or her own feelings of guilt and blame and to reduce cognitive dissonance.

suspected of not feeding her and expressed to me her relief when Taigh was admitted to hospital, 'because they would see for themselves what was happening'. Later, Taigh would go on to describe her feelings of being 'judged' as a young adult 'because of my history and the fact that I have a thick file'. The same thought processes are at work here: a history of repeated investigations, consultations and episodes of treatment is incongruous with a model of an infallible medical system, so it must, instead, say something about the client. These anxieties, beliefs and stereotypes contribute towards us not hearing what the child and family are really saying and not truly understanding their experience. This was a major problem for Taigh: although she tried hard to help herself, she simply could not. When she tried to tell doctors what was

When I looked at food I didn't see it as food, but something that made me ill. I ended up despising food, and breakfast lunch and dinner were chores for me. When I whittled my diet down to the eight foods I knew I could eat without being sick I felt safe: these foods didn't make me sick but everything else did. I developed a fear of food, which became worse and worse and turned into a phobia. The smell, sight or even thought of food would make me panic, cry, feel – or actually be – sick. I couldn't eat in the same room as my family and my life became quite difficult. The thought of eating a different food became unbearable.

I went to the doctors to try to explain what I was feeling. But as I wasn't under- or overweight they would say to me, 'Try something new every day'. I came to despise these words. Doctors didn't understand – nobody really understood. Only I know what I felt when I saw a bit of food.

People would describe me as a fussy eater. I was not a fussy eater. Fussy eaters simply don't eat something because they don't want to. But me, I wanted to eat: I just couldn't. I didn't choose not to; it was like a kind of mental block.

happening to her and how difficult it was for her to eat, they did not respond in a way that was helpful to her.

Taigh continued to see doctors in the hope that someone would listen to her and understand the 'mental block' she experienced when faced with food: no one did. In the meantime, she tried to lead a life that was as close as possible to normal. She went to school every day but would be sent home day after day because of her vomiting. Her teachers were at a loss to know what to do. Taigh's mother, Tracey, told me of a time when Taigh's head teacher decided that she should 'try school dinners', in an attempt to normalise her eating. Not surprisingly, this did not help her, although it may have helped the staff at school to appreciate the extent of her difficulties. Tracey told me, 'after a week, I got called in and she wasn't allowed to stay dinners any more'.

Taigh continued to be sick throughout the day and night, although the frequency of her sickness decreased over time. Her mother described her being sick up to four times a night, 'every night for years'. Like all of us, Taigh experienced vomiting as aversive and, in order to avoid this aversive experience, she tried to cut out the foods she associated with being sick. Her association of sickness with eating developed into a food phobia and to a strong reliance on a group of only eight foods that she 'trusted' would not make her sick. She stuck to this 'safe' food group and did not venture outside it. As she became older, these experiences and subsequent eating behaviours marked her out as different.

THE ISSUE OF DIFFERENCE

Childhood is characterised by the developing importance of peer relationships and by the need to 'fit in' with peers. This becomes especially acute during adolescence. As Cardillo (2004) points out, 'To live with a chronic illness or disability, especially as a child or adolescent, is to experience oneself as different' (p. 8). At secondary school, Taigh began to develop more of an awareness of 'being different' to her peers, something her mother noticed had begun to make school very hard for her.

> At the age of 11 I realised how different my problem was making me and how it was taking over my whole life. From the age of 11–16 I visited my general practitioner regularly for help. When I would say, 'I have a phobia of food' people would laugh or ignore it. But anyone with a phobia would understand. Some people have a phobia of buttons or the colour red, so why couldn't I have a phobia about food?
>
> I noticed how much I couldn't do – for example, going to a friend's house was a nightmare. Unless their mum knew my mum, having dinner there was so stressful. Searching through the freezer looking for something I could eat. Pulling out a bag of sausages, I would be relieved, but then I would realise they had herbs in them ('green bits' as I called them). This would fill me with sadness, so in the end I wouldn't go round to people's houses, or go out to birthday meals or

little parties. I was embarrassed and it was holding me back ... I didn't eat with my family, as I didn't like sitting around food for that long. When I did, I ate my food as quickly as I could so that I could leave. Another reason I didn't like eating with them was because I couldn't eat what they were eating, and how different my plate of food looked. Also, what I ate determined how many plates I needed. If something from one food could pass over to the other, I would need separate plates. But sometimes if I had a large plate I could put the food far enough apart on the same plate.

What Taigh describes here is an exacerbation of her problem that will be very familiar to psychologists who specialise in feeding problems. Her problem with eating has at its source a conditioned response in which an aversive association has been formed between food and sickness. Her reliance on a limited 'safe' subgroup of foods is typical, as is the fear of contamination of one food by another – hence the need to keep the food items separate on her plate, or even on different plates entirely. She is acutely sensitive to certain smells and tastes and can distinguish between brands of foods, leading to the 'brand loyalty' that children who have this problem often exhibit. Not only the vomiting but also now her behaviour around food makes Taigh objectively different from her peers. Her *food phobia* limits her exposure not only to new foods but also to new situations and experiences.

Social factors

Throughout all of this time, Taigh describes having had friends. These were not just playmates but individuals who accepted Taigh as she was and even joined her at mealtimes, eating her 'safe' foods alongside her: 'Of course, I had my friends who understood and would eat bacon and chips with me.' We know that children learn to perceive themselves through their interactions with others and that peer relationships, in particular, play an important part in this (Cardillo, 2004; Clarke and Kirton, 2003). Taigh's friends will have been a significant

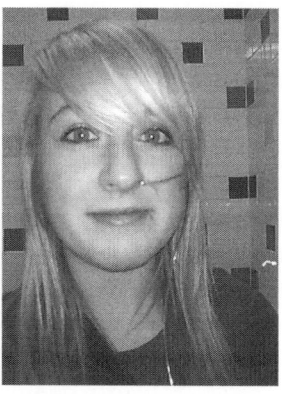

FIGURE 14.2 Taigh as a young adult

influence on her self-perception and on her ability to maintain a positive self-concept, despite her huge difficulties. This will have helped temper her sense of being different.

The turning point

The turning point for Taigh came when she was 16 years old and her grand-father came across a newspaper article about another girl, like Taigh, who had been treated by a doctor who specialised in eating. Taigh's family arranged a private consultation with him and, for the first time, she felt someone under-stood her and could help: 'I left so happy and excited that finally after all these years, I was going to be normal like everyone else.' However, when she attended her next appointment she saw a different doctor and found herself in the all-too-familiar situation where she felt her problem was dismissed. This was simply too much for her and, as her mother puts it, 'Taigh had a meltdown in the room.' Later, and with her emotions more under control, she wrote a letter. This letter is repeated in full. It's an important letter, because, as Taigh puts it, *this is the letter that changed my life.*

Taigh's letter

8th November 2008

I have been living with strange eating habits my whole life and have wanted to sort it out for years. When I was younger I didn't swallow, and was in hospital for a long time. Nothing ever got sorted out properly. So I have been living on chips, sausages, Yorkshire puddings, pancakes, bacon, bread, ice cream / sweets my whole life. It's not that I don't want to try other things. It's that I physically can't. I don't like the look of food, the smell and the thought of what it might taste like repulses me. I find it so incredibly hard to try new foods, as I can't even get to the stage of touching it. If I can get to the stage of getting it near my mouth, I heave and feel sick. I am 16 now and food has become a phobia.

I have been to doctors many times and explained to them. I have been told a range of different things such as 'your not underweight, there is nothing we can do', 'you're just doing it for attention', 'you will grow out of it' and the worst 'try something new everyday'. Why can't they just understand me? Do they not want to help me?

Finally we found out about you, and people you have helped in the past, from a newspaper article. We booked a private appointment to see you, which cost £160 which is a lot of money. In the appointment with you, you told me exactly what I wanted to hear. You understood what I was saying, believed every word, which is not how doctors have been my whole life and was completely on my side. You told me how you were going to help me, and that my eating difficulties would get sorted. I left so happy and excited that finally after all these years, I was going to be normal, like everyone else.

We had an appointment. Every day I was more excited for it all to be sorted. When I got there, waiting in the waiting room I was thinking about when I would be able to go out for meals with my friends and have a proper meal, not eating sausage and chips from the kids menu. I got called in and I saw a different doctor. He was asking me questions about my eating difficulties. I was explaining and thought he understood. He then told me that your idea of how you were going to help me was not necessary and I was going to have a barium mill [sic].

He explained to me that it was a powdery liquid that I would have to swallow. He stood up and walked out the room to collect something and I burst into tears. He just didn't understand what I was saying. When he came back into the room, I said to him that I wouldn't be able to swallow the barium mill [sic]. He replied saying, 'In life you have to just make yourself do things. You need to grow up as your becoming a young adult'. There was nothing I could say that was going to make him understand.

I felt like I had hit a brick wall. Everything I had been hopeful of came crashing down. I wasn't going to be helped. Nobody wanted to help me. Once again, I wasn't being believed.

When the letter came through, we read it and it made everything worse. The notes he took where completely wrong. He hadn't taken into account what I was saying, but instead written his own thoughts of what was wrong. This isn't fair, as I thought he was going to listen and understand and want to help me.

This upset everyone, me especially. My mum wrote a letter to you explaining what had happened. Still we have had no reply. It's as if everyone has given up on me. I don't think its fair that I have been given this hope and for it to have been snatched away from me, leaving me how I was before. I know what I am eating is ruining my body. Will cut me short of life and I have been told it could make me infertile. I just want you to help me, as I want this so much.

Please get back to me

Taigh Giles

What happened next ...

Taigh got a call back within 2 days of sending her letter and was invited back to the clinic for an appointment to see the doctor who had originally seen her. She described feeling an incredible relief that she had been heard at last. After having some overnight tests she was finally, at 17 years of age, diagnosed with acid reflux.

I had some tests run, and it was clarified that I have severe acid reflux, that was worse every time I ate. I also have a damaged oesophagus from where the acid has been coming up so much. I was put on some tablets to help decrease the acid, and also some tablets to give me the vitamins and minerals that I don't get in my diet. Even from being on these tablets I felt a little better. I didn't have a

> feeling in my stomach that I've always had, something I just thought was normal, and the smells of foods started to smell a bit different – although I wouldn't say nicer, it was definitely different. This wasn't enough change to sort me out completely.

Taigh was referred to a psychologist and a speech and language therapist, who, together, helped her to begin to overcome her food phobia.

THE LONG, HARD ROAD TO RECOVERY

The development of feeding skills is highly complex and involves the interaction of many disparate elements, ranging from anatomical, neurophsyiological and medical factors to those that are social, relational, environmental and cultural (*see* Chapter 13). Feeding development is a learned process that relies heavily on oral sensation, motor development and opportunities for experimentation (Stevenson and Allaire, 1991). For all of these reasons, starting out on a programme to improve her eating was always going to be hard work for Taigh.

> Something I had to learn before I could eat normally was how to actually eat the foods. I missed the stage in life where you naturally learn to chew food. And I grew up not chewing my food properly, if at all. I used to cut my sausage up into bits and just swallow them whole. When I ate chips I would suck them and then swallow down. I only used my teeth for biting into things, not chewing. So this is where my speech and language therapist came in and taught me the different techniques of chewing. I worked on this a lot, until eventually I could do it naturally most of the time.

What Taigh is describing is common in children who have been tube-fed and who have not experienced the various stages of weaning and finger feeding that infants typically go through. Also, like many of these children she did not recognise the sensation of hunger, and neither could she identify being full (and so, ironically, she could overeat and make herself sick). She describes having very little knowledge about different types of food and varying textures. All of these issues would have to be addressed as part of her treatment.

> I had appointments with the psychologist every other week, and we would talk about the types of food I found harder, and the foods that I would like to eventually be able to eat. Something I said I wanted to eat straight away was pizza. Pizza is so sociable and it would really make my life a bit easier to be able to share pizza with my friends. But pizza is very complex, so the foods we decided to start with were strawberries, lettuce and plain pasta.

> We came up with a strategy to help me overcome the fear of particular foods. First of all I would become comfortable with being around the food, and then move on to touching it and finding out about the texture, cutting it up and finding out what it was like inside, smelling it, and eventually licking it, or putting a tiny bit in my mouth. I think to get to this stage it took about 2 months. So it proved that it was going to be a very long process. But I was willing to put all my time and effort in.

The psychologist who treated Taigh took a graded desensitisation approach, in which Taigh was supported through a range of psychological techniques to gradually approach different foods, starting with what were the easiest for her and progressing, at her pace, to those that were more difficult. She broke down the process of tasting each new food into tiny steps, even before Taigh put the food anywhere near her mouth; the whole process was one of 'look, touch, smell, lick and taste'.

Interestingly, Tracey described this as 'a mutual learning process', which suggests that the therapists were learning just as much as Taigh. She added that Taigh liked seeing them 'because they actually listened to her'. Taigh was able to begin to add new foods to her diet, including strawberries, lettuce and pasta. She told me, 'it doesn't sound much for over a year's work, but for me it was an amazing success'. The impact of these small steps on Taigh's life was phenomenal, and this serves as a reminder of the many factors that are part of the eating experience for us and that we take for granted.

> After about a year and half that went so quickly, I was really proud of what I had achieved. My chewing techniques improved and I was feeling better after eating.
>
> I had become more comfortable around food, and my understanding of food had become a bit better. I could be in my kitchen while my mum was preparing dinner without freaking out, and I would try to eat a bit more with my family. I would go out to meals with my friends, even if it meant eating a plate of chips or dough balls when at PizzaExpress.

Gradually things began to get better.

Then something changed. Taigh reached 18 years of age and was told she would have to transfer from the children's service, as she was now an adult. The treatment she had been receiving to help her to eat would no longer be available. She would have to continue by herself, using the strategies she had learnt. This wasn't easy for her.

> It took me a while to get my head into gear and to do this by myself, and I would go up and down. Some days I would feel really motivated, and other days I would be upset and think, 'I'm never going to change.'

Taigh also tried other types of help, including hypnotherapy, in an attempt to try to change her responses to different kinds of food. Nothing worked. She describes trying to convince herself that she was thinking more positively about things, and then realising that this wasn't the case. Finally, she realised that the only way she had managed to get any results was to go back to the strategy that she had used previously – the 'look, smell, touch, lick and eat' approach. She continues to try to use this. It's hard for her. She no longer has the support and encouragement of the psychologist and the speech and language therapist who helped her so much in the past. Taigh described to me how frightening it is to be given a message that there is no help, 'and you're on your own'. As her mother, Tracey, puts it, Taigh had 'fallen out of the system'.

WHAT CAN WE LEARN FROM TAIGH?

Hindsight is a wonderful thing in healthcare, as well as in other areas of life. Looking back on Taigh's experience, there are many things that could have been done differently and better. Healthcare professionals looking in would most probably ask themselves why it took such a long time for the problem underlying Taigh's sickness to be identified. Others will wonder about the professional 'mix' in the hospital where she was being monitored and ask themselves why there was not more knowledge about feeding problems.

Tracey told me of her anticipation that things must be different for parents and children now, some 20 years on from her own experiences with Taigh. She believes parents have access to more information, thanks to the Internet, and are less likely to be left 'in limbo', not knowing what is happening to their child. She is a passionate and persuasive proponent of early intervention.

Taigh's story helps us to understand and appreciate how her physical health problem (gastro-oesophageal reflux disease) and the problems associated with it led her to experience eating as aversive and to develop a conditioned food-avoidance. Taigh was left to cope with the physical, social and emotional consequences of both of these sets of problems as best she could. Her story is punctuated by frequent 'cries for help' and repeated experiences of her distress being dismissed. This was so much a part of her lived experience that she talked to me of 'becoming suicidal', had something not changed to give her hope.

In trying to learn from Taigh and Tracey's experiences, it is important to focus not only on what was difficult for them but also on what helped. Tracey was advised to stop breastfeeding Taigh and went through a series of alternatives – none of which worked – to try to stop Taigh being sick. Taigh vomited so much throughout this time that Tracy told me she had to get used to holding

Taigh facing away from her, so that she wouldn't be continually covered in vomit. Thankfully, Taigh was not Tracey's first child, so she had already experienced 'successfully' feeding a child whose eating had progressed normally. It is not difficult to imagine a different scenario, in which an anxious mother might have blamed herself for not being able to feed her child, and a mother and child whose relationship and ability to form a positive and secure attachment might have been compromised by the medicalisation of the feeding experience. Taigh's long hospitalisation would have presented further challenges to their relationship. This does not seem to have been the case for Tracey and Taigh. We don't know what kinds of things helped them both to survive the early years: that would be another study. However, it seems likely that Taigh and Tracey had managed to develop a positive, secure relationship prior to Taigh's admission to hospital and that Taigh had become securely attached to her mother. Once established, this attachment endured over time, exerting a protective influence and helping them both to survive their many setbacks.

When I asked Tracey what she thought had kept Taigh going through this difficult time, she told me without any hesitation, 'she's always been a real character!' She went on to describe a child who was always full of energy and was determined to achieve whatever she set out to. Even at the worst of times when Taigh was in hospital, tiny and physically frail, her mother describes her as having been incredibly active and sociable. For Tracey, this meant there was always hope: her daughter was a survivor. She commented, 'Taigh's a very strong person – I think that's been her coping mechanism.'

There were two other things Tracey mentioned. First, she told me that Taigh had always 'had things she was good at' and that this helped balance out her negative experiences. Second, Taigh always had friends. Both of these things seem to have helped Taigh develop and maintain a positive self-concept. We know that these factors are important for all children, and the literature suggests they are especially important for those with a chronic condition (e.g. Cardillo, 2004).

THE IMPORTANCE OF FORMULATION

One of the most striking things about Taigh's story is the way professionals within the medical system became 'stuck'. It is worth returning to some of the fundamental ideas and processes that underpin medicine in order to try to understand this. The medical model can be seen to have precluded Taigh's own wish to be helped to eat like other children, because for any 'treatment' to be initiated there first has to be a diagnosis. This was the first sticking point in Taigh's story. It raises an important issue for us as professionals working within the medical system. What do we do when we *don't know what's happening*?

BOX 14.2 The analogy of the hit-and-run driver

What do you do when you see someone knocked down by a hit-and-run driver?
    You can do one of the things:
1. you can chase the car
2. you can run away and try to get help
3. you can pick the person up and try to help him or her.

(The third option doesn't stop you looking for the culprit, by the way.)[12]

Dealing with uncertainty

'Not knowing' is something that is particularly difficult for human beings, and we often fill this gap, unconsciously, with 'false certainty' (Southall, 2007). For medics, 'not knowing' can be particularly challenging, as the concept, especially after one's best efforts have been spent, is incompatible with the notion of 'expertness'. As has been already noted, this expert status is implicit within medicine and medical training, and it is also attributed to medical doctors by their patients and by society in general and helps them deal with their own anxieties about illness. The diagnostic system both shapes *and is shaped by* these beliefs. The ensuing wisdom is that something is 'real' because it has a diagnostic label and, conversely, if it doesn't, then it's not. What psychologists bring to this is important. What we do when we don't know what's happening medically, is we do what we always do: we formulate the problem properly.

Formulation

For a great many years clinical psychologists have used the process of psychological formulation to summarise their clients' difficulties and identify ensuing pathways of help. Formulation differs from diagnosis in a number of important ways and is in keeping with the argument that medicine should have an emphasis on patients' narratives of their own experiences of illness (Kleinman, 1998), what Zook (1994) refers to as 'ontological health', rather than that exemplified by the biomedical model. Formulation allows us to develop a shared understanding with the client of the problem or problems *in the present* and a shared plan of how the client can address the problem using the unique resources he or she has (*see* Box 14.3).

---

12 The third option is what most psychologists would advocate!

BOX 14.3 A basic behavioural formulation of Taigh's food phobia

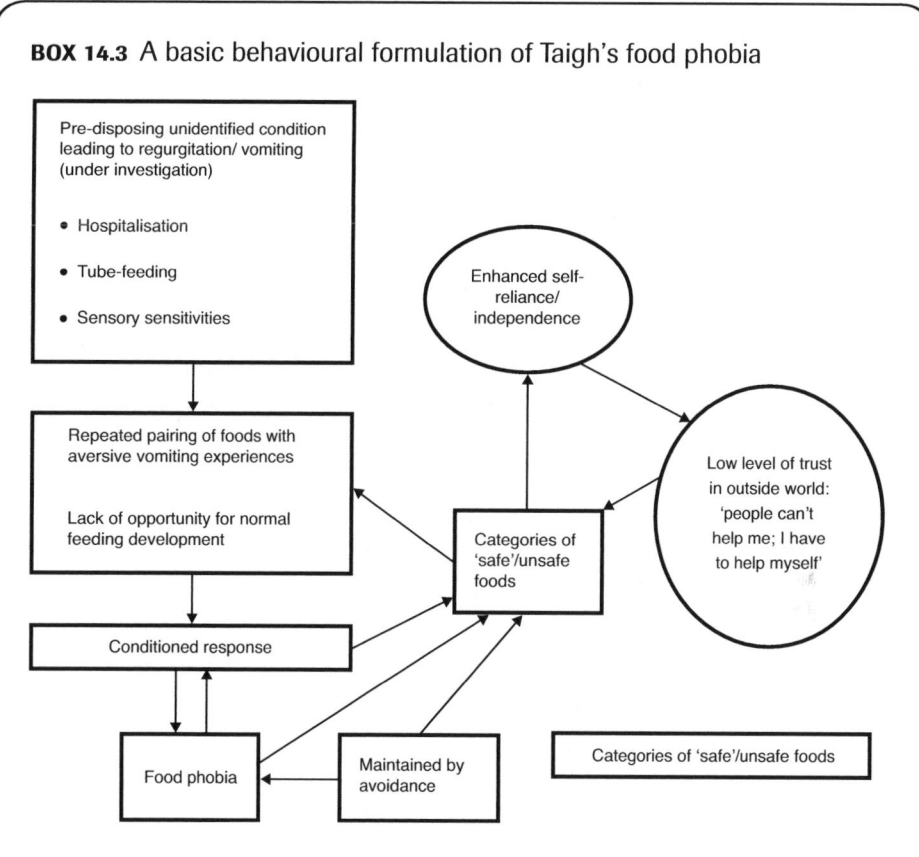

Formulation suggests a treatment plan that addresses the avoidance and conditioned response elements of Taigh's difficulties, enabling exposure to new foods through graded exposure and helping her to create new, positive associations for different foods and for the eating experience as a whole.

Taigh's early experiences have contributed to an enhanced self-reliance that can be harnessed to help motivate her in her treatment programme. Her story suggests that social reinforcement would be effective; therefore, incorporating social settings in her programme will be important.

The exacerbation cycle (*see* Box 14.4) shows how Taigh's eating problem was being maintained by food avoidance.

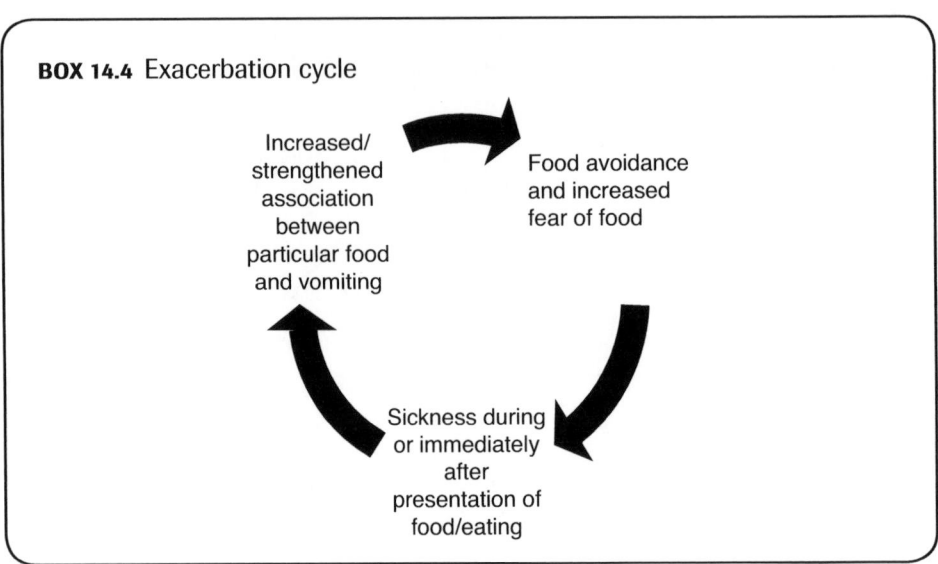

BOX 14.4 Exacerbation cycle

Increased/strengthened association between particular food and vomiting

Food avoidance and increased fear of food

Sickness during or immediately after presentation of food/eating

BOX 14.5 Diagnosis vs. formulation

	Diagnosis	Formulation
Format	Descriptive label	Explanatory hypothesis
Focus	Shared features	Unique characteristics
Process	Structured examination	Interactive interview
Use of theory	Theory neutral	Informed by theory
Predicts	Course of illness	Responses to illness
Treatment	Identifies treatment	Informs psychological intervention(s)

Chronic conditions or those of unknown origin challenge us to focus on helping people manage their condition, rather than 'curing' it. This is not simply 'coping', which carries with it connotations of passivity, but includes working to prevent or reduce the physical, psychological and social sequelae of the condition, by whatever means are most helpful to the individual him or herself.

EXPERT PATIENTS

There is a well-established culture of acknowledging patients' expertise in managing their own care. In the United Kingdom, the development of a major initiative on expert patients was first set out in the government's White Paper *Saving Lives: Our Healthier Nation* (DoH, 2001) a formal commitment to which was contained in the *NHS Improvement Plan* of June 2004 (DoH, 2004). The 2001 initiative was greeted by a mixed response, with many health workers remaining sceptical. A MORI survey of health professionals soon afterwards found that 63% of doctors and 76% of pharmacists believed that, in the long term, better-informed patients would require more, not less, of their time.[13] Children seemed to be excluded from the agenda entirely, their only mention in the government's White Paper relating to 'mental health' rather than physical health problems.

However, this was not the first and only call for increased involvement of patients in their own care, and it came following the United Nations Convention on the Rights of the Child (1989), which heralded something of a cultural change within children's services. This change was accompanied by a growing emphasis on consulting with and empowering young people and on seeking their direct involvement, both in clinical services and in research.

The need to give a voice to children and young people with chronic conditions has since been reflected in a number of UK initiatives. The Health Experiences Research Group at the University of Oxford has been running a qualitative research project since 2000, collecting and analysing video and audio-recorded interviews with people about their experiences of illness. The views expressed are remarkably reminiscent of Taigh's, with repeated references to 'not being believed' or 'not being listened to'. One young person comments: 'It can be very upsetting to have physical symptoms that are not explained, or be given a diagnosis that has no clear treatment' (http://healthtalkonline.org/young-peoples-experiences).

The information collated by the Health Experiences Research Group has been used as a resource for people with health conditions to understand how others experience the condition they are living with and has led to opportunities for young people to share their stories through dedicated websites so that their experiences can help others.[14] The project was funded to research specific health conditions and by the end of 2012 had data on 60 different conditions. An associated study, Growing Up with Chronic Illness,[15] was undertaken at the University of Exeter, between 2010 and 2012 (Maslow *et al.*, 2011). Elsewhere in the United Kingdom, young people's groups have been set up to focus on the management of specific long-term conditions such as diabetes.

Contrary to the views expressed by healthcare professionals early on in the evolution of 'expert' programmes, research shows that participation in them can result in less and better use of health professional time. For example, studies at Stanford University show a reduction of visits to doctors of 42%–44% (Lorig *et al.*, 2001). Such outcomes have contributed to a changing attitude among doctors and to renewed pleas for service user engagement in expert patient programmes. Shaw and Baker (2004) concluded in the *British Medical Journal*:

> Doctors need to act on what they already know – that all patients are experts, however uninformed or misinformed they may be about health issues. Patients'

---

13 Cited by the *British Medical Journal*, 2004
14 healthtalkonline.org and youthhealthtalk.org
15 www.guci.org.uk

expertise is valuable because by understanding the patient's views and situation, the doctor is better equipped to identify a solution that will lead to a successful outcome, however defined. (p. 3)

Although a small number of expert patient courses are being run in the United Kingdom for children, these are not widespread. The fact that such initiatives are being considered separately to the Healthier Nation expert patient agenda suggests that there is an urgent need for a more holistic understanding of children's mental and physical health and well-being and for paediatric psychology to be at the forefront of developments.

Taigh's experiences tell us a great deal about what it is has been like for her to grow up with an unidentified, chronic gastrointestinal condition and how this has affected almost every aspect of her life. Professionals need to be able to listen to experiences like Taigh's if they want to understand more about what is important to young people with chronic conditions. So often, as we have seen, they do not listen. The added insight that we can gain from listening to Taigh and other young people like her aids our understanding and ability to adopt, together, the kinds of treatment regimen that are most helpful. It is also offers us an additional research dimension. As Britt (2013) wrote:

If researchers want to truly understand a condition they are investigating, there is no substitute for learning from those who have experienced or are experiencing the condition. Their insights are unique and different from those of even the most experienced and empathic staff. (p 6)

> I get a feeling of fear every day – even if it's just thinking about dinner later, or walking past someone in the street with a sandwich. What most people don't understand is how hard every single day is for me.
>
> A lot of people don't take me seriously and will wave food under my nose, but this is because they just don't understand. Just like my general practitioners – they didn't understand either.
>
> Incidents still happen where I am moving forwards but then something in my head changes, and I will cry and it will put me back to the beginning, but it makes me more determined to get further the next time I try. I have my family, friends and my boyfriend who support me a lot. I am realistic about it. I know I won't be eating like everybody else, but I can widen my diet, and I will be able to eat more foods.
>
> I want to raise awareness, as I don't want people to go through what I have gone through. Children need to be helped before they get to my age, as if it's caught early, it's easier to fix.

Taigh's experiences suggest that improvements are needed along the entire assessment, treatment and care pathway. Her story highlights the lack of understanding of the psychological processes that mediate chronic illnesses and their sequelae (which may become even more difficult and damaging than the original illness itself) as well as an absence of the necessary knowledge and skills that would enable the kinds of treatments she needed. These and other associated issues fall within the domain of the paediatric psychologist, whose specialist skills span the medical and psychological. The evidence embedded within Taigh's account of her difficulties suggests that urgent work is needed to enhance understanding of the child, family and professional system and to enhance communication. As every good paediatric psychologist knows, this is ongoing work, unique to each family and staff group and their particular circumstances. Other pressing needs include the requirement to address the transition between children's and adult services.

We already know from clinical and research evidence some of the ingredients of successful programmes of treatment. These include:

- a multisystemic framework for assessment and treatment, which includes home, education or vocational, social and relationship issues
- personalised treatment programmes that are shaped to the child or young person and his or her family
- a range of support programmes
- skilled interventions that can enhance self-efficacy
- a positive psychology focus.

A national paediatric psychology lead on children's chronic conditions would ensure the primacy of these factors as well as their quality assurance. The inclusion of children on the national 'expert patient' agenda would seem to be a 'must'. At the moment, we are failing children and young people like Taigh, who, while they are often successful socially, are disadvantaged in terms of their educational and vocational outcomes, because multisystemic factors are poorly understood and are not incorporated into health treatment and rehabilitation programmes. The result is that they are less likely to achieve the earning capacity of their peers who do not have chronic illnesses and have a higher likelihood of becoming dependent on state benefits (Maslow *et al.*, 2011). For the sake of their own independence and quality of life, and to help prevent entirely the kinds of health and economic dependencies that are currently reported, we need to rethink our approach. Narratives such as Taigh's can help us do this.

Living a good life

Taigh is a vivacious, bubbly, attractive young woman, with long shiny blonde hair, clear skin and big, blue eyes that sparkle with enthusiasm for life. It's hard to imagine she has had the experiences she has. When you meet her, it's almost impossible to see her as someone who, at one time, could not eat, did not even know how to chew and who experienced such despair. The last word belongs to her.

In the past 4 years I am now still nibbling at strawberries and I will eat a handful of plain pasta. My latest task has been cheese, and I have really come far with this. I will eat cheese on crackers, when I feel like it. And when I was on holiday I was eating a cheeseburger, but without the burger! It is basically a cheese roll, but I really liked it. My most recent breakthrough is pizza! I don't have the red sauce, but I have the base, cheese and bacon. I am now trying to get chicken into my diet.

I also cook for my boyfriend, things like spaghetti bolognaise, which I never used to even be able to be around – although eating it myself is a long way off. 'Wet' foods and foods that have a strong smell are a lot harder, but I am really proud of how far I have come, and I'm going to keep on going.

I am a qualified fitness instructor, and have my own small business going. I also teach horse riding, so I am very active and I am living a good life.

SUMMARY

A great many children suffer from chronic illnesses, a substantial proportion of whom have gastrointestinal illness. We already know that the incidence of mental health problems amongst the population of children and young people with chronic illness is much higher than in the general population and we have learned from Taigh how these difficulties may emerge. All of these factors make it imperative that there is a paediatric psychology lead on this issue, so that children can be included in a national drive for better outcomes for everyone with chronic conditions.

REFERENCES

Bentall RP. *Madness Explained: psychosis and human nature*. London: Penguin Books; 2003.

Britt D. Lay persons and professionals – partners in research. *Clin Psychol Forum*. 2013; **241**: 41–4.

Cardillo LW. *Constructing and Making Sense of Difference: narratives of the experience of growing up with a chronic illness or disability* [doctoral thesis]. Ohio: Ohio State University Press; 2004.

Clarke M, Kirton A. Patterns of interaction between children with physical disabilities using augmentative and alternative communication systems and their peers. *Child Lang Teach Ther*. 2003; **20**(3): 136–51.

Department of Health (DoH). *Saving Lives: our healthier nation*. London: Her Majesty's Stationery Office; 2001.

Department of Health (DoH). *The NHS Improvement Plan: putting people at the heart of public services*. London: DoH; 2004. Available at: http://webarchive.nationalarchives. gov.uk/20130107105354/www.dh.gov.uk/en/Publicationsandstatistics/Publications/ PublicationsPolicyAndGuidance/DH_4084476 (accessed 14 January 2014).

Festinger L. *A Theory of Cognitive Dissonance*. Stanford, CA: Stanford University Press; 1957.

Kleinman A. *The Illness Narratives: suffering, healing, and the human condition*. New York, NY: Basic Books; 1998.

Lerner MJ, Miller DT. Just world research and the attribution process: looking back and ahead. *Psychol Bull*. 1978; **85**(5): 1030–51.

Lorig KR, Ritter P, Stewart AL, *et al.* Chronic disease self-management program: a 2-year health status and health care utilization outcomes. *Med Care.* 2001; **39**(11): 1217–23.

Maslow GR, Haydon A, McRee AL, *et al.* Growing up with a chronic illness: social success, educational/vocational distress. *J Adolesc Health.* 2011; **49**(2): 206–12.

Shaw J, Baker M. 'Expert Patient' – dream or nightmare? *BMJ.* 2004; **328**(7442): 723–4.

Southall A. *ADHD Exposed and Explained.* Oxford, UK: Radcliffe Publishing; 2007.

Southall A. Enough's enough: conversations with myself and other practitioners. *Clin Child Psychol Psychiatry.* 2009; **14**(4): 481–94.

Stevenson RD, Allaire JH. The development of normal feeding and swallowing. *Pediatr Clin North Am.* 1991; **38**(6): 1439–53.

United Nations. *Convention on the Rights of the Child.* Geneva: United Nations; 1989. Available at: www.ohchr.org/en/professionalinterest/pages/crc.aspx (accessed 1 February 2014).

Zook EG. Embodied health and constitutive communication: towards an authentic conceptualisation of health communication. *Communication Yearbook.* 1994; **17**: 344–77.

Tools for clinical practice

INTRODUCTION

Among other things we have selected for this section some examples of tools used in clinical practice and provided by experienced clinicians. At the end of Part III we have included leaflets on tube-feeding product ranges.

3.0: The development of gastric systems in children

We start Part III with a summary of the unique characteristics of the anatomy and physiology of normal development and the maturation of the digestive system in infants provided by Dr Ghosal and Mr Martin.

3.1: Assessment resources

This section includes assessment measures commonly used in clinical practice that may be applied across the diverse paediatric gastroenterology conditions. This list has been compiled by Dr Maddux, Dr Deacy and Dr Lukens, leading members of the Assessment Working Group of the *Pediatric Gastroenterology Special Interest Group* of Division 54 (Society for Pediatric Psychology) of the American Psychological Association.

3.2: Children with toileting problems

We include here tools from a nurse-led constipation clinic at a district hospital that has been run by Mrs Mobberley, Advanced Nurse Practitioner, and other material provided by other associations. We also have included here the hand-outs of Chapter 8 provided by Dr Danda and Dr Hyman.

3.2a   A flow chart of an example of a multidisciplinary approach to the management of children with toileting problems

3.2b   An example of a clinical interview form for children with toileting problems

3.2c   The flow chart titled 'Idiopathic constipation in children policy' would help us to understand all the necessary steps to consider when managing children with this condition

3.2d   Medications indicated in child idiopathic constipation and for dis-impaction of faecal masses are illustrated in these specific tables

3.2e,f   Promoting continence and product awareness is an integral service of the charity Disabled Living, which produces free-to-download leaflets for children with toileting problems (available at: www. disabledliving.co.uk/Promocon/Publications)

3.2g   Handouts from Chapter 8

3.3: Notes on cyclical vomiting syndrome

The summary notes included here would help us to familiarise with this rare disorder. These notes compiled by Ms Martin expand on the introduction to cyclical vomiting syndrome included in Chapter 1.

3.4: Functional gastrointestinal disorders: a case example

This standard clinical letter describes all 'typical' symptoms and problems that adolescents with recurrent abdominal pain may exhibit. It has been developed by Ms Martin including and mixing common features previously found in several different cases that were seen in a paediatric gastroenterology clinic. It serves as an example to illustrate the impact of this condition on the quality of life of young people and their families. It also highlights common problems found in resource allocation and pathways of care as well as the clinical management of the condition.

3.5: Example of tube-weaning feeding therapy at inpatient setting

The co-editors of this book (Ms Martin and Dr Dovey) are happy sharing the following material from one of their cases that required tube-weaning feeding therapy at inpatient setting. This case was selected because it also illustrates how health professionals from gastroenterology clinics may be working in partnership with other specialist clinics, such as respiratory services.

3.5a An example of a behavioural assessment for tube-weaning feeding therapy. The protocol was developed for a 5-year-old child with cystic fibrosis who was very resistant to eating orally. After several years of outpatient intervention it was decided to admit the child to the hospital for tube-weaning feeding therapy (from a percutaneous endoscopic gastrostomy tube to oral eating).

3.5b An example of how the tube-feed reduction, caloric recount and food selected as targets for intervention were managed in this particular case.

3.5c These graphics show results of the inpatient tube-weaning therapy intervention.

3.5d The follow-up session recorded the child's eating at home and at school. The school report completed by Ms Emiliou (Assistant Psychologist at Midlands Psychology) is included here to illustrate how the intervention enabled generalising behaviour to several settings, normalising the child's eating behaviour.

3.0: The development of gastric systems in children

Shomik Ghosal and Adrian G Martin

THE DEVELOPMENT OF THE DIGESTIVE SYSTEM

The digestive system is made up of a series of organs within the gastrointestinal (GI) tract that have the task of transforming ingested food into nutrients that the human body uses. Through a complex endocrinological process, specialised organs containing unique cells secrete enzymes and hormones that facilitate the intake and absorption of nutrients, as well as the excretion of waste. The GI system is also part of the organism's host defence mechanism through the mucosal immune response. Development and functioning of the GI system is essential for function and growth. This section of Part III reviews the stages of the development of the GI tract from the gestational stages through human infancy.

INTRAUTERINE GESTATIONAL PERIOD

The human body is made up of cells that have undergone differentiation and have developed from a single origin, culminating in specialised organs and tissues, each of which has its own essential function. The development of the cell is encoded within the genome found within the deoxyribonucleic acid (DNA) situated in the nucleus of each cell. The genetic information within the cells is accessed, interpreted and used to produce the whole array of different cell types. Understanding of the mechanisms of this is considered to be instrumental in understanding the development of any complex structure within the body. The extent of the differentiation of any cell is controlled by the pattern of genes expressed from the vast congregation of genes within genomic DNA.

Summary of main intrauterine stages

Within a period of 9 months from conception to birth, the foetus develops into a complex organism capable of surviving independently. This development can be divided into three distinct stages. The current description will focus predominantly on the GI system.

First trimester: 0–12 weeks

GESTATIONAL STAGE, 0–4 WEEKS
- In this first stage, the combination of the sperm with the egg results in the zygote.
- The zygote then divides into a cluster of cells called a blastocyst.

- The inner group of cells within the blastocyst will differentiate and become the foetus.
- The outer group of cells will become the membranes that protect and nourish the growing foetus (amniotic sac and placenta).

EMBRYONIC STAGE, 4–8 WEEKS

- During this stage, the development of internal structures and organs begins. The gut develops from a single gut tube after week 4.
- By week 5 we see the gut subdivisions – foregut, midgut and hindgut.
- These will eventually become the oesophagus and stomach, the duodenum, jejunum, ileum and caesium, colon and rectum.
- By the end of the seventh week, all of the internal organs have begun to form and subdivisions within the larger organs are visible.

FOETAL STAGE, 8–12 WEEKS

- Beginning at week 7, the mouth and palate are formed, with the tooth buds developing within week 8.
- Between weeks 10 and 14 the foetus starts to swallow.
- The action of swallowing the amniotic fluid surrounding the developing child aids in the growth of the GI tract.
- The swallowing of amniotic fluid can be observed and measured from 11 weeks of gestation.
- The amount of amniotic fluid consumed varies from just a few millilitres to 450 millilitres per day by the end of the third trimester.
- The intake and swallowing of the amniotic fluid does not indicate that the child is gaining anything from the act beyond the initial coordination of the swallowing itself.
- The amniotic fluid passes through the immature gut without interaction and out of the child's anus.

Second trimester: 12–28 weeks

- From week 13, fine hair covers the entire body of the foetus. Eventually, some of this will develop into coarse and thick hair on the child's head.
- Within the second trimester, the head of the foetus accounts for almost half of its total size.
- Towards the end of the second trimester, air sacs begin to form in the lungs, all eye components are formed and rapid proliferation, specialisation and development of the brain begins.
- Within this trimester, the sucking reflex is formed and can be observed. Non-nutritive sucking – ability to latch and suck – has been shown to be fully developed between 20 and 24 weeks' gestation.
- The foetus does not gain any macro- or micronutrients from this behaviour. It is important to understand that although the foetus may be able to suck and swallow from an early age, the ability to integrate these skills into a functional act for intake does not appear to happen until much later in gestation.

- Children born before 37 weeks of gestation may not possess the ability to integrate these behaviours, despite being able to perform each in isolation.

Third trimester: 28–40 weeks
- Nutritive sucking starts from 30 weeks onwards. Therefore, for practical purposes the gut is not functional before this gestational age.
- Nutritive sucking refers to the swallowing and digestion of nutrients found in the amniotic fluid.
- The foetus is able to experience taste, as the composition of the amniotic fluid is dependent on the mother's diet.
- The gut is able to absorb nutrients from the swallowed fluid and undigested material is expelled appropriately.
- The foetus increases its body fat towards the end of the third trimester, in preparation for birth.

EMBRYOLOGY OF THE GASTROINTESTINAL TRACT
Although the gestational trimesters define the overall development of the foetus, the development of the GI tract is more appropriately divided into two major steps:
1. the formation of the gut tube
2. the formation of the individual organs.

Formation of the gut tube
The formation of the GI system polarises the embryo by forming an entry and exit canal. The tube is also split into an anterior and posterior axis. This derives from a single tube formed in week 4. During the fifth week of gestation, the two separate portions of the GI tract form the foregut, the midgut and the hindgut.

Foregut
The foregut is simply a single GI tract that lies behind the heart. This later divides in order to form the trachea, the oesophagus, the respiratory tract and the stomach. The foregut can also be divided into two further regions: cranial and caudal.

The *cranial* foregut, or pharyngeal gut, extends from the oropharyngeal membrane to (and includes) the respiratory diverticulum (lung bud). The derivatives of the pharyngeal gut include part of the mouth and tongue, pharynx, thyroid, parathyroid, thymus, lower respiratory tract and lungs. Development of the mouth comes from the pharyngeal gut and the stomodeum. After 4 weeks the lung bud appears – this will eventually become the lungs.

The *caudal* foregut starts after the respiratory diverticulum and extends to the hepatocystic diverticulum. Derivatives of the caudal foregut include the oesophagus, stomach, proximal duodenum, liver, gall bladder, hepatic ducts, bile ducts and pancreas. At 5 weeks the oesophagus begins lengthening and the stomach begins to take shape as a dilation of the foregut. In the fifth week, the stomach rotates 90°, making the dorsal side the left side. Also in this week the liver and pancreas begin to develop. Following rotation and throughout the sixth week, the left side of the stomach grows faster than the right, accounting for the greater and lesser curvatures of the stomach. In the seventh week, further growth occurs, moving the distal foregut to the right side.

Midgut

The midgut develops from weeks 5 to 10. The midgut can be divided into two regions: the cranial and caudal limbs. Derivations of the *cranial* limb include the distal duodenum, jejunum and proximal ileum, whereas the derivations of the *caudal* limb include the distal ileum, caecum, appendix ascending colon and two-thirds of the transverse colon. The length of the midgut grows at a faster rate than the embryo; this results in the gut forming a 'loop' with the omphaloenteric duct at the apex. In the sixth week the omphaloenteric duct closes and the midgut rotates 90°. In the tenth week the midgut returns to the abdomen and rotates even further. Once the midgut has returned to the abdomen the three intestinal segments are fixed to the posterior abdominal wall through the shortening of some segments of the mesentery. This fixation reduces the freedom of motion of bowel, avoiding complications such as intestinal infarction.

Hindgut

The hindgut develops between weeks 5 and 7. The hindgut runs from the junction with the midgut to the cloacal membrane; it is the distal segment of the primitive gut. The distal end of the hindgut is called the cloaca. Derivations of the hindgut include the distal third of the transverse colon, descending colon, rectum and anal canal as well as the urinary bladder and the proximal urethra.

Beginning in the fifth week the mesoderm develops into the urorectal septum. The formation of the urorectal septum results in the division of the cloaca; the cloaca divides into a ventral primitive urogenital sinus and a dorsal primitive anorectal canal. In the seventh week the cloacal membrane breaks down. In the site of the former cloacal membrane, ectoderm becomes the epithelium of the anal canal.

The formation of the individual organs

The divisions of the GI tract occur at early stages of development. There are regions of the embryo that become liver or intestines before the gastrulation process is completed (Montgomery, 2008). The oesophagus can be identified as a distinct structure at early stages of the embryo developing in maturity between 12 and 16 weeks of gestation (Montgomery *et al.*, 1999). Human gastric lipase is an enzyme that aids in fat digestion and it shows expression at 11 weeks of gestation. The stomach of the foetus grows progressively from the thirteenth to the thirty-ninth week of gestation. At the fourteenth week, characteristic features such as curvature, body and the pylorus can be identified (Montgomery *et al.*, 1999).

Genetic pathways have been identified in the complex process of the development of the liver. At about the fourth week of gestation, the liver diverticulum emerges from the most caudal portion of the foregut (Montgomery, 2008). The human liver primordium that emerges from the endoderm is formed by two parts, cranial and caudal. The caudal portion gives rise to the gall bladder and the extrahepatic bile (Shiojiri, 1997).

The formation of the pancreas is initiated by the emergence of dorsal and ventral pancreatic parts on the opposite sides of the foregut. These two parts come together at the seventh week of gestation as the tube gut grows and rotates (Grand *et al.*, 1976). At around 20 weeks' of gestation enzyme activity is detected in the exocrine pancreas and secretion begins immediately after activity is detected (McClean *et al.*, 1993).

By week 12, different types of enteroendocrine cells are also recognised and organogenesis of the human intestine is completed by the thirteenth week of gestation (Moxey and Trier, 1978). By the end of the first trimester, the absorptive epithelial cells in the foetus are similar to those of the adult human intestine (Trier and Moxey, 1979).

NEWBORN BABIES AND INFANTS
Before birth
Prior to birth the GI tract is sterile; however, within a few hours of birth a plethora of microorganisms begin by populating the mouth and eventually encompassing the whole length of the tract. There are several factors such as the mode of delivery, maternal microbiota or infant's diet that determine which microorganisms the infant is exposed to. After birth the intestinal lumen begins interaction with a new environment that is very complex and it contains nutrients in various concentrations (Sanderson, 2008).

After birth
The GI tract is prepared to cope with the shift from nutrition via the placenta to oral nutrition after birth. In order to prepare for this the GI tract grows and matures very rapidly in the weeks before birth. The level of development of the GI tract of each individual infant is a good indicator of whether or not the infant will be able to meet nutritional needs on his or her own (Neu and Douglas-Escobar, 2008). Therefore, preterm babies are less able to deal with oral nutrition than term babies.

The infant must be born with the ability to coordinate the swallowing process and sucking activities (Neu and Douglas-Escobar, 2008). When milk enters the stomach, the fundic smooth muscle relaxes. Generally newborn term babies feed every 2–4 hours. This would fit with data showing gastric residue of between 48% and 70% at the end of 1 hour in normal infants (Heyman, 1998; Seibert *et al.*, 1983). For most newborns the first bowel movement occurs within 48 hours of birth.

BOX 3.0.1 Important aspects of the gastrointestinal tract that require development at birth

- Suck–swallow coordination
- Gastro-oesophageal sphincter tone
- Gastric emptying
- Intestinal motility

(Neu and Douglas-Escobar, 2008)

Preterm infants

Several organ systems develop between weeks 34 and 37. A premature infant is defined as one that is less than 37 weeks' gestation and has not yet reached an appropriate level of foetal development that allows for survival outside of the womb. Premature infants are at greater risk of short- and long-term conditions. The standards of practice for postnatal nutrition in premature neonates is one designed to mimic in utero foetal growth rates as the preterm gut is essentially a foetal gut.

BOX 3.0.2 A comparison of premature and full-term infants

Preterm infants may require tube-feeding, as they may not be able to coordinate sucking activities during the swallowing process and this may result in aspiration of gastric contents into the lungs. In addition, in comparison with full-term infants, they typically show:

- poor oesophageal motility
- slower gastric empting
- poor bowel motility patterns
- limited gastric acid secretion.

Neonatal period

Immediately after the foetus has been born there are a number of morphological changes and extensive growth in the GI tract. The oesophagus displays a rapid cell proliferation and an increase in the mucus of glands. Meanwhile, the stomach shows an increase in acid secretion capacity. The intestine also shows tissue growth and epithelial cell differentiations (Xu, 1996).

There is a close interplay between all the major cell types lining the intestine, the nutrients and the microbes, which all constitute the intestinal ecosystem (Neu and Douglas-Escobar, 2008).

The baby microflora is affected by:

- mode of birth delivery
- dietary intake.

> **BOX 3.0.3** Intestinal cells
>
> Functions: nutrient absorption, bacterial mucosal cross-talk and innate barrier
> Types:
> - *Goblet cells* (mucus secretory cells)
> - *Paneth cells* (defending epithelial cell renewal through secreting antimicrobial peptides)
> - *M cells* (play a major role in specific immunity to antigens).
>
> (Neu and Douglas-Escobar, 2008)

Mode of birth delivery

During normal vaginal delivery, the baby comes into contact with the mother's vaginal and faecal flora; this results in the colonisation of the sterile GI tract with *Enterococcus* and *Escherichia coli*. In contrast, an infant who is delivered by caesarean section will be exposed to different types of microbes such as *Streptococcus* and *Clostridium*. Since there are no pre-existing microbes to compete with, the sterile GI tract is quickly colonised (Favier *et al.*, 2002, 2003).

Breast milk

Breastfeeding an infant fulfils two purposes: nutrition and immunological protection. Growth factors found in breast milk have been found to improve enzyme activity, which has an effect on the development of the intestinal epithelium (Siafakas *et al.*, 1999). Breast milk contains numerous components that are known to have protective effects, such as immunoglobulin, oligosaccharides and different types of white blood cells (Neu and Douglas-Escobar, 2008). There is a large range of antibacterial, antiviral and antifungal antibodies contained within the mother's milk. This range is representative of on the antigenic range of the mother's intestine and respiratory tract. The mother's milk is also colonised by bacteria, which play a positive role by acting as a natural probiotic (Duggan *et al.*, 2008). In all breastfed infants, bifidobacteria become dominant and faecal samples from breastfed infants also include lactobacilli and streptococci (Harmsen *et al.*, 2000).

Formula milk

Formula-fed babies develop different bacterial colonies in the intestine and the immunological benefits of breast milk are lacking. In most formula-fed infants, similar amounts of *Bacteroides* and bifidobacteria (approximately 40%) can be found in the infants' intestine. Faecal samples from formula-fed infants also contain staphylococci, *E. coli* and clostridia (Harmsen *et al.*, 2000). However, adequate nutrition can be achieved with formula milk and digestive processes are handled in the same way as for breast milk.

INFANCY

During the period of infancy there is great change in the intake of nutrients from liquid foods to solids. The pH of an infant's stomach decreases throughout infancy as feeding changes from milk to solids, which require more acid and gastric pepsin. Nevertheless, the acidity of the environment decreases the further down the GI tract (Berseth *et al.*, 2006).

The infant's stomach is a well-oxygenated area, as air is swallowed along with the food. This results in aerobic bacteria using up the available oxygen. The large intestines become colonised with anaerobic bacteria (Parracho *et al.*, 2007; Pender *et al.*, 2006). The intestines contain a protective mucus layer that is made up of glycoproteins; these glycoproteins can serve as attachments for colonies of microbes. These microbes are normally found at the surface of the mucus entrance (Neu *et al.*, 2007). It is in the intestine where most of the microflora of the GI tract resides. Microbes exit this tract through the anus on the faeces.

The development of teeth from 6 months of age onwards triggers a new phase when the infant is able to chew and swallow solid foods. The GI tract, with its swallowing mechanisms and digestive processes, continues to mature and undergo transformation so that the child is able to handle solid foods. The infant is then gradually weaned to solid foods, which then make up the major part of nutrient intake over 1 year of age.

ANATOMY OF THE DIGESTIVE SYSTEM

The human digestive system has evolved into a complex series of organs and glands adapted specifically to processing food. It consists of the GI tract, which is a long tube that extends from the mouth all the way to the anus. The rest of the digestive organs, such as the liver and pancreas, produce and store chemicals associated with digestion.

Anatomy and function of the gastrointestinal tract
The mouth

Structurally, the mouth is made up of the lips, the tongue, the teeth and the salivary glands. The lips are mainly made up of flexible muscle tissue. The front teeth are called the incisors (used for cutting) and have a flat front and a thin and long top. These are followed by the canines, which end at a point. Incisors are followed by the premolars, which have an irregular bicuspid shape and, lastly, the molars, which have a flat cusp (used for chewing). Children grow 20 deciduous teeth, whereas adults have 32 permanent teeth. The tongue, situated on the floor of the mouth, is made up of four intrinsic and four extrinsic muscles, which move it and change its shape to aid chewing and swallowing. Three main salivary glands produce liquid saliva to aid chewing, swallowing and digestion. The parotid gland, which is the largest, is found wrapped around the ramus of the mandible. The submandibular glands are located underneath the lower jaws and lastly the sublingual gland, which can be found underneath the tongue.

The mouth is where ingestion and digestion begins. Food enters the oral cavity, where it is chewed by the teeth and mixed up with saliva. The salivary glands react in a reflex action by secreting saliva to the flavour of foods. The purpose of saliva is to lubricate the food, allowing it to be swallowed. It also contains enzymes, particularly amylase, which is capable of breaking down starch. With tongue movements, there is formation of a soft rounded mass of food known as the bolus.

The pharynx

The pharynx is the part situated at the back of the mouth and nasal cavity. Anatomically, the pharynx can be divided into three sections: (1) the nasopharynx, located above the soft palate behind the nasal cavity; (2) the oropharynx, located behind the oral cavity; and (3) the laryngopharynx, which is the part of the throat, which connects to the oesophagus.

The pharynx receives the bolus and is responsible for initiating the swallowing action once the bolus is pushed against the palate. This action is initiated by touch receptors located in the pharynx. It is at this time when the epiglottis moves over the trachea to prevent food particles from entering the lungs. The bolus eventually empties into the oesophagus.

The oesophagus

The oesophagus is a hollow muscular tube in the thorax that connects the pharynx to the stomach. The oesophagus has two distinct sphincters: the upper oesophageal sphincter (UES) and the lower oesophageal sphincter (LES). The UES is under *voluntary* control and the LES is under *involuntary* control.

The oesophagus transports masticated food to the stomach by a series of wave-like contractions of smooth muscle, known as peristalsis. The oesophagus is also able to perform antiperistalsis – the action of vomiting. There is a muscular ring (the LES) at the bottom of the oesophagus, which squeezes shut in order to prevent fluids flowing back out of the stomach.

The stomach

The stomach is located in the abdomen and leads to the small intestine. The stomach is a hollow, distensible organ. It contains two smooth muscle valves: the LES at the top and the pyloric sphincter at the bottom. Nerve plexuses located around it regulate secretary and muscular activity. The stomach can be divided into four separate parts: the upper part is the cardia; then the fundus; the main body of the stomach is known as the corpus; and then the pylorus, which connects to the small intestine.

The main function of the stomach is to act as a reservoir for food and to continue the process of digestion. Food remains in the stomach for about 2–6 hours and is mixed with digestive acid and various enzymes designed to aid in the breakdown of proteins. The stomach wall is lined with a layer of mucus, which makes the stomach impermeable to its own acid juices. The digested bolus of food is called chyme; the chyme is then released slowly through the pyloric sphincter into the duodenum.

Anatomy of the lower gastrointestinal tract organs
Small intestine
The small intestine is situated in the abdomen and is the longest organ in the human body. Its name comes from its diameter rather than its length, since its diameter is significantly smaller than the large intestine. It can be divided into three distinct parts: (1) the duodenum, the first section leading from the stomach; (2) the jejunum or midsection; and (3) the ileum, which is the final section leading into the large intestine.

The structure of the small intestine provides an excellent lining for absorption of digested material, due to its large surface area. It is covered by millions of finger-like projections called villi. The small intestine is surrounded by a network of capillaries that absorb the products of carbohydrate and protein digestion. In the duodenum, chemical degradation of small amounts of food takes place, enzymes together with emulsifying bile are released. Digestion in the small intestine is due to small intestinal secretions, as well as those from the pancreas and liver bile. The digestion and absorption process continues throughout the jejunum and the ileum.

Large intestine
The large intestine forms an upside down U over the coiled small intestine. It begins at the lower right part of the abdomen and it ends at the lower left side. It is structurally divided into three parts: cecum, colon and rectum. Lastly, the anal canal connects the rectum to the exterior, which is controlled by the involuntary internal anal sphincter and the voluntary external anal sphincter.

The large intestine mainly reabsorbs fluids and some vitamins. It also compacts and produces faeces out of undigested food and fibres. The faeces are stored in the colon for excretion. The cecum is mainly a transition area and allows for the chyme (partially digested food) to travel from the small intestine. The colon is the last area where water is reabsorbed; bacteria in the colon aid in the digestion of remaining food products and faeces are formed. When faeces reach the rectum, the body experiences the urge to defecate. Finally, the faeces are excreted through the anus.

Pancreas, liver and gall bladder
Pancreas
The pancreas, located in the upper abdomen, is made up of several parts; from right to left they are the head, which lies on top of the duodenum; the uncinate process; the neck; the body; and lastly, the tail, which lies in contact with the spleen. The pancreatic duct joins the common bile duct, together entering the duodenum.

The pancreas has two main digestive functions: the first is to produce enzymes to aid in the digestion process in the duodenum; the second is to release insulin directly to the blood stream to control blood sugar levels. It also releases sodium bicarbonate directly into the intestine in order to control the acid levels.

Liver

The liver is the largest gland in the body. It is located to the right of the stomach and over the gall bladder and it fills the majority of the abdominal cavity. Nutrients absorbed from the intestine are processed by the liver before going through the bloodstream to the rest of the body.

The liver acts as a large reservoir for blood. With regard to digestion, it performs several key functions. The liver secretes bile to the gall bladder, metabolises carbohydrates, proteins and fats (the main nutrients from digestion) and, lastly, it also stores vitamins. It secretes bile, which acts almost like a detergent, promoting enzyme action in the intestines by emulsifying fats.

Gall bladder

Bile is a watery greenish fluid secreted via the hepatic and cystic ducts to the gall bladder for storage. The gall bladder continually stores the bile secreted by the liver until gastric emptying (the opening of the pyloric sphincter and release of chyme from the stomach into the intestines). The presence of the acidic contents in the intestine triggers the gall bladder to release its stored fluids into the duodenum through the common bile duct.

BRAIN–GUT INTERACTION

The gut is the only organ that contains a nervous system of its own, the enteric nervous system, which mediates its functions and with an ability to intervene autonomously from the brain or spinal cord. The enteric nervous system is organised into two networks: the myenteric plexus (intermuscular) and the submucosal plexus. These networks of neurons, neurotransmitters and proteins interchange messages between neurons and constitute 'the brain of the gut' (Wood, 1999). This network is embedded in the wall of the digestive tract located in the sheaths of tissue lining the oesophagus, stomach, small intestine and colon. It controls motility, regulation of fluid exchange, exocrine and endocrine secretions (gastric and pancreatic), defence actions of the GI tract wall, enteric network reflex activity, neuropeptide release, microcirculation of the gut and it is also involved in the response to enterotoxins and in the regulation of immune and inflammatory processes (Furness, 2007; Goyal and Hirano, 1996). Links between the nervous system and the digestive system have been well established in the neurogastroenterology literature (e.g. Whitehead *et al.*, 1990: Grundy *et al.*, 2006).

The gut also has endocrine, immunologic, sensory and motor functions in addition to digestion. Furthermore, the gut contains 100 million neurons, neurotransmitters like serotonin, dopamine, glutamate, norephinephrine and nitric oxide as well as neuropeptides and enkephalins (a member of the endorphins family) and it is a rich source of benzodiazepines (Riordan and Williams, 2010). Each aspect of digestion has a complex interaction with the rest of the body. Every cell has a vestige interest in the availability of immediate energy and must coordinate its functions accordingly. The principle mechanism of interaction between the gut and the rest of the body is through the endocrine system and hormonal signalling. Each section of the digestive system has a vaguely independent hormone associated with it. Therefore, the rest of the body that requires to coordinate with available energy can know exactly in which region the food currently resides. Interested readers in the endocrinological signalling of the GI tract are referred to Harrold *et al.* (2011).

The bidirectional 'communication system' between the gut and the brain with autonomic, neuro-endocrine and neuro-immune system involvement is denominated as 'the brain–gut axis' (Taché *et al.*, 1994). Neuroimaging techniques such as functional magnetic resonance, and positron emission tomography have confirmed the existence of this brain–gut axis (Derbyshire, 2003). When gut function is disturbed, the effects of this disturbance can be found in the mucosa or musculature of the gut. The effects manifest themselves as one of the functional GI disorders in which there are chronic and recurrent symptoms of the GI tract such as pain, nausea, vomiting, bloating, diarrhoea and constipation without detectable structural or biochemical abnormalities. Acute and chronic influences of psychological processes, such as stress and emotion, on the gut are increasingly acknowledged and understood as mediated by the brain–gut axis (Budavari and Olden, 2003). These stresses are likely to influence the symptomatology and morbidity of relevant functional GI disorders.

Physiology of the digestive system
The GI tract can be said to have four main functions:
1. **Ingestion**: swallowing food
2. **Digestion**: breakdown of food
3. **Absorption**: extraction of nutrients from the broken down food
4. **Excretion**: elimination of waste products.

All cells in the human body require nutrients to function. All nutrients enter the body in the form of food. However, food cannot directly reach the cells. The GI tract modifies the physical and chemical properties of the food and disposes of the remaining unusable waste. This process is called digestion. These modifications are dependent on the exocrine and endocrine secretions as well as the controlled movement of food through the digestive tract.

Ingestion
Once the food has been masticated, the bolus goes to the stomach through a complicated process known as swallowing which avoids the bolus from entering the windpipe. The initiation of swallowing is voluntary and starts by food

being forced into the laryngopharynx with the tongue. The rest of the swallowing process is a reflex, with the epiglottis closing off the trachea. If food however, does enter the trachea the choking reflex activates and coughing will expel the bolus. The bolus is moved through the oesophagus to the stomach by peristalsis aided by gravity.

Digestion

Digestion can be defined as the process by which food is broken down into nutrients, which can be utilised by the cells in the body. Digestion can be classified into three distinct phases: (1) the cephalic phase, where the nervous system is stimulated by the senses of taste and smell preparing the body for eating; (2) the gastric phase, where the passage of food into the stomach directly stimulates the secretion of gastric juices as well as pH regulators; (3) the intestinal phase, where sympathetic and parasympathetic reflexes regulate the digestion and passage of partially digestive food through the intestines.

Absorption

Once the food has been broken down its nutrient building blocks such as glucose from carbohydrate, amino acids from protein and fatty acids from fats, these nutrients need to be absorbed. This process takes place mainly in the small intestine where it is covered by many folds containing microvilli, which greatly increase the surface area. Water and fat-soluble vitamins are also absorbed from the small intestine.

Excretion

The undigested parts of food become waste products. Large amounts of water are reabsorbed in the small intestine and the remaining unusable part is compacted in the colon and excreted by a bowel movement.

SUMMARY

The digestive system consists of a series of organs within the GI tract that that have the task of transforming ingested food into nutrients that the human body uses. Therefore, a correct development and functioning of this system is essential for growth.

It is important to acknowledge the milestones of the development of the GI tract from the gestational stages through human infancy. Within a period of 9 months the foetus develops into a complex human body capable of surviving outside the mother's body. The GI tract has to adapt within a few hours of birth from a sterile uterus environment to one populated with microorganisms. The GI tract has to be prepared to cope with the shift to oral nutrition after birth and to accomplish this task it is required for the GI tract to mature rapidly in the weeks before birth.

REFERENCES

Berseth CL, Thureen PJ, Hay WW. Development of the gastrointestinal tract. *Neonatal Nutr Metab*. 2006; **2**: 67–73.

Budavari AI, Olden KW. Psychosocial aspects of functional gastrointestinal disorders. *Gastoenterol Clin North Am*. 2003; **32**(2): 477–506.

Derbyshire SWG. A systematic review of neuroimaging data during visceral stimulation. *Am J Gastroenterol*. 2003; **98**(1): 12–20.

Duggan C, Watkins JB, Walker WA, editors. *Nutrition in Pediatrics: basic science, clinical applications*. Ontario: BC Deker Publishers; 2008.

Favier CF, De Vos WM, Akkermans AD. Development of bacterial and bifidobacterial communities in feces of newborn babies. *Anaerobe*. 2003; **9**(5): 219–29.

Favier CF, Vaughan EE, De Vos WM, *et al*. Molecular monitoring of succession of bacterial communities in human neonates. *Appl Environ Microbiol*. 2002; **68**(1): 219–26.

Furness JB. *The Enteric Nervous System*. Oxford. Wiley-Blackwell; 2007.

Goyal RJ, Hirano I. The enteric nervous system. *N Engl J Med*. 1996; **334**(17): 1106–15.

Grand RJ, Watkins JB, Torti FM. Development of the human gastrointestinal tract: a review: *Gastroenterology*. 1976; **70**(5 Pt. 1): 790–810.

Grundy D, Al-chaer ED, Aziz Q, *et al*. Fundamentals of neurogastroenterology: basic science. *Gastroenterology*. 2006; **130**(5): 1391–411.

Harmsen HJ, Wildeboer-Veloo AC, Raangs GC, *et al*. Analysis of intestinal flora development in breast-fed and formula-fed infants by using molecular identification and detection methods. *J Pediatr Gastroenterol Nutr*. 2000; **30**(1): 61–7.

Harrold JA, Dovey TM, Blundell JE, *et al*. CNS regulation of appetite. *Neuropharmacology*. 2011; **63**(1): 3–17.

Heyman S. Gastric emptying in children. *J Nucl Med*. 1998; **39**(5): 865–9.

McClean P, Harding M, Coward WA, *et al*. Measurement of fat digestion in early life using a stable isotope breath test. *Arch Dis Child*. 1993; **69**(3): 366–70.

Montgomery RK. Gastrointestinal development: morphogenesis and molecular mechanisms. In: Neu J. *Gastroenterology and Nutrition, Neonatology Questions and Controversies*. Philadelphia, PA: Saunders Elsevier; 2008. pp. 3–27.

Montgomery RK, Mulberg AE, Grand RJ. Development of the human gastrointestinal tract: twenty years of progress. *Gastroenterology*. 1999; **116**(3): 702–31.

Moxey PC, Trier JS. Specialised cell types in the human fetal small intestine. *Anat Rec*. 1978; **191**(3): 269–85.

Neu J, Douglas-Escobar MD. Gastrointestinal development: implications for infant feeding. In: Dugan C, Watkins JB, Walker WA, editors. *Nutrition in Pediatrics: basic science, clinical applications*. Ontario: BC Decker; 2008. pp. 241–9.

Neu J, Douglas-Escobar M, Lopez M. Microbes and the developing gastrointestinal tract. *Nutr Clin Pract*. 2007; **22**(2): 174–82.

Parracho H, McCartney A, Gibson G. Probiotics and prebiotics in infant nutrition. *Proc Nutr Soc*. 2007; **66**(3): 405–11.

Pender J, Thijs C, Vink C, *et al*. Factors influencing the composition of the intestinal microbiota in early infancy. *Pediatrics*. 2006; **118**(2): 511–21.

Riordan SM, Williams MD. Gut flora and hepatic encephalopathy in patients with cirrhosis. *N Engl J Med*. 2010; **312**(12): 1140–2.

Sanderson IR. Dietary regulation of gene expresion. In: Neu J. *Gastroenterology and Nutrition, Neonatology Questions and Controversies*. Philadelphia, PA: Saunders Elsevier; 2008. pp. 28–41.

Seibert II, Byrne WI, Euler AR. Gastric emptying in children: unusual patterns detected by scintigraphy. *Am J Roentgenol*. 1983; **141**(1): 49–51.

Shiojiri N. Development and differentiation of bile ducts in the mammalian liver. *Microsc Res Tech*.1997; **39**(4): 328–35.

Siafakas CG, Anatolitou F, Fusunyan RD, *et al*. Vascular endothelial growth factor (VEGF) is present in human breast milk and its receptor is present on intestinal epithelial cells. *Pediatr Res.* 1999; **45**(5 Pt. 1): 652–7.

Taché Y, Wingate DL, Burks TF, *et al.* Functional and chemical anatomy of gastric vago-vagal reflex. In: Taché Y, Wingate DL, Burks TF, editors. *Innervation of the Gut: pathophysiological implications.* Boca Raton, FL: CRC; 1994. pp. 81–92.

Trier JS, Moxey PC. Morphogenesis of the small intestine during fetal development. *Ciba Found Symp.* 1979; (70): 3–29.

Whitehead WE, Holtkotter B, Enck P, *et al.* Tolerance for rectosigmoid distension in irritable bowel syndrome. *Gastroenterology.* 1990; **98**(5 Pt. 1): 1187–92.

Wood JD. Fundamentals of neurogastroenterology. *Gut.* 1999; **45**(2): 6–16.

Xu RJ. Development of the newborn GI tract and its relation to colostrum/milk intake: a review. *Reprod Fertil Dev.* 1996; **8**(1): 35–48.

3.1: Assessment resources

Michele H Maddux, Amanda D Deacy and Colleen Lukens

Developed by the Assessment Working Group of the Pediatric Gastroenterology Special Interest Group (American Psychological Association – Division 54, Society of Pediatric Psychology)

INTRODUCTION

The following is a comprehensive but not exhaustive list of assessment measures that are commonly used in clinical practice of youth with paediatric gastroenterological conditions. The list contains a summary of measures across the following paediatric gastroenterological conditions: inflammatory bowel disease (IBD), functional abdominal pain, encopresis and paediatric feeding disorders. These assessments of paediatric gastroenterological conditions can be conducted via self-report (child and/or parent), physical examination, questionnaires and behavioural observations. The most common assessments include those of disease severity/activity, diagnostic classification, quality of life and parental behaviours, most of which can be instrumental in guiding treatment planning and intervention. All measures are classified as (1) well-established assessment, (2) approaching well-established assessment or (3) promising assessment, according to the criteria detailed by Cohen *et al.* (2008).

INFLAMMATORY BOWEL DISEASE
Quality of life
- IMPACT-III (well established)
  - **Description**: the IMPACT-III is a 35-item self-report, IBD-specific measure of health-related quality of life. It assesses the extent to which an adolescent is affected by a particular issue (e.g. stomach pain, missing out on certain activities) using 5-point Likert scaling. Lower scores indicate poorer health-related quality of life.
  - **Psychometric properties**: the original IMPACT consisted of 33 items; Cronbach's alpha was 0.96 with test-retest reliability of 0.90 (Otley *et al.*, 2002). This also distinguished patients with quiescent versus active disease, with higher IMPACT scores among those with quiescent disease. The IMPACT-II and IMPACT-III (Loonen et al 2002; Otley *et al.*, 2002) reflect modifications of the original measure, with simplified wording, 35 items and a visual analogue scale. Originally, six domains – that is, (1) bowel symptoms, (2) systemic symptoms, (3) social and functional concerns, (4) body image, (5) test and treatment concerns and (6)

emotional concerns – were proposed. However, a recent examination of this measure's factor structure revealed four factors with good to excellent reliability: (1) general well-being, (2) emotional functioning, (3) social functioning and (4) body image.

▶ **Relevant references**: Otley *et al.* 2002; Hyams *et al.*, 2007.

Family responsibility

- **Inflammatory Bowel Disease Family Responsibility Questionnaire** (promising)
  ▶ **Description**: this is a new 23-item measure of family involvement in IBD management, with parallel youth, maternal and paternal report versions. Respondents rate family members' involvement in various tasks on a 4-point Likert scale, with higher scores indicating greater involvement of the family member.
  ▶ **Psychometric properties**: Preliminary psychometric properties demonstrate high internal consistency (αs > 0.80) and moderate to high intercorrelations among reporters (i.e. mothers, fathers, youth) (Greenley *et al.*, 2010). The Inflammatory Bowel Disease Family Responsibility Questionnaire also shows that youth involvement increases with youth age, while parental involvement of IBD-related tasks decreases with youth age.
  ▶ **Relevant reference**: Greenley *et al.*, 2010.

Disease activity: Crohn's disease

- **Partial Harvey-Bradshaw Index (PHBI)** (well established)
  ▶ **Description**: the PHBI is a three-item measure of disease severity for patients with Crohn's disease that allows patients to rate three categories of symptom severity over the last 7 days. Symptom categories include general well-being, abdominal pain and number of liquid stools. Scores range from 0 to 12, with a higher score indicating more active disease (i.e. 0 = inactive disease; 1–4 = mild disease; ≥5 = moderate to severe disease).
  ▶ **Psychometric properties**: the PHBI has demonstrated adequate reliability and validity in prior studies and is very feasible. Previous work also documents high correlations between this measure and physician global assessments of disease activity (Markowitz *et al.*, 2000). Internal consistency of the PHBI has ranged from 0.71 to 0.88 when used among adolescents with IBD (Hommel *et al.*, 2011a, 2011b).
  ▶ **Relevant references**: Greenley *et al.* 2010; Harvey and Bradshaw, 1980; Markowitz *et al.*, 2000; Hommel *et al.*, 2011a.
- **Pediatric Crohn's Disease Activity Index (PCDAI)** (well established)
  ▶ **Description**: the PCDAI assesses Crohn's disease activity using both subjective (e.g. pain) and objective criteria (e.g. physical exam), laboratory findings (e.g. haematocrit, erythrocyte sedimentation rate, albumin) and growth parameters. Scores range from 0 to 100 (≤10 = inactive disease; 11–30 = mild disease; >30 = moderate to severe disease activity).

▶ **Psychometric properties**: the PCDAI is well validated, has good reliability and demonstrates high correlations with physicians' global assessments ($r = 0.80$) (Hyams *et al.*, 1991). It has also been shown to be responsive to improvements in disease activity in Crohn's disease patients over a short interval (Kundhal *et al.*, 2003).

▶ **Relevant references**: Hommel *et al.*, 2011b; Hyams *et al.*, 1991, 2005; Shepanski *et al.*, 2004.

Disease activity: ulcerative colitis

● **Pediatric Ulcerative Colitis Activity Index (PUCAI)** (well established)

▶ **Description**: the PUCAI is a six-item measure of disease severity for patients with ulcerative colitis. An interview format allows patients to report on six typical symptoms of ulcerative colitis including abdominal pain, rectal bleeding, stool consistency of most stools, number of stools per 24 hours, nocturnal stools and activity level. A total score is obtained by summing the six items, resulting in a range of 0–85, with a higher score representing more severe disease (i.e. 0–9 = inactive; 10–34 = mild; 35–64 = moderate; ≥65 = severe disease).

▶ **Psychometric properties**: the PUCAI has demonstrated good reliability and validity in prior research, it is feasible and it can be used as a primary outcome measure of disease activity. In the original validation sample of 48 children with ulcerative colitis, the PUCAI demonstrated high correlations with physician global assessments ($r = 0.91$) and colonoscopic appearance ($r = 0.71$), and it significantly differentiated between disease severity (none, mild, moderate, severe) (Turner *et al.*, 2007). A re-evaluation of the PUCAI's psychometric properties on 215 young patients with ulcerative colitis demonstrated similar findings (Turner *et al.*, 2009).

▶ **Relevant references**: Kundhal *et al.*, 2003; Turner *et al.*, 2007.

● **Lichtinger Ulcerative Colitis Clinical Activity Index (LCAI)** (approaching well established)

▶ **Description**: the LCAI uses both subjective and objective criteria to assess eight ulcerative colitis symptoms (score 0–21): daily stool frequency, nocturnal diarrhoea, visible blood in stool, faecal incontinence, abdominal pain or cramping, general well-being, abdominal tenderness and need for anti-diarrhoeal medication, with higher scores representing more severe disease. LCAI scores range from 0 to 21. Scores ≤2 indicate quiescent disease; <10 indicate a response to therapy; ≥10 indicate active disease and no response to therapy.

▶ **Psychometric properties**: among the small number of published manuscripts that have used the LCAI, very few provide psychometric data; available data suggest good reliability (e.g. $\alpha = 0.85$). The LCAI is easy to administer and relies largely on subjective criteria of disease activity.

▶ **Relevant references**: Turner *et al.*, 2009; Lichtiger *et al.*, 1994.

FUNCTIONAL ABDOMINAL PAIN

Diagnosis and classification

- **The Questionnaire on Pediatric Gastrointestinal Symptoms – Rome III version (QPGS-RIII)** (approaching well established)
  - ▶ **Description**: the QPGS is an instrument used to diagnose functional gastrointestinal disorders (FGIDs) in children and adolescents, using the Rome III paediatric criteria originally put forth in 1999. Using parallel parent and child reports, the measure assesses the frequency (i.e. never to everyday) and duration (i.e. less than an hour to all day) of abdominal pain occurring in the past 2 weeks and produces a specific, descriptive FGID diagnosis (functional dyspepsia, irritable bowel syndrome, abdominal migraine and functional abdominal pain).
  - ▶ **Psychometric properties**: in general, content validity of the QPGS has been established. The parent form appears to be a reliable measure for parents of children 4–9 years of age; the companion child self-report appears to be more reliable for 10- to 18-year-olds. Fair to moderate agreement in Rome criteria diagnosis of FGIDs has been found between child and parent reports of symptoms.
  - ▶ **Relevant references**: Lichtiger *et al.*, 1994; Fanjiang *et al.*, 2007.

Symptom severity

- **Abdominal Pain Index (API)** (well established)
  - ▶ **Description**: the API is a five-item scale used to assess the frequency, duration and intensity of abdominal pain episodes occurring within the previous 2 weeks.
  - ▶ **Psychometric properties**: standardised scores have been used effectively to differentiate children with chronic abdominal and their pain-free peers (Walker *et al.*, 1997). The API, in general, has been found to have good concurrent and predictive validity as well as acceptable internal consistency (e.g. 0.93) (Greco *et al.*, 2007) and test–retest reliability.
  - ▶ **Relevant references**: Caplan *et al.*, 2005; Helgeland *et al.*, 2009; Walker *et al.*, 1997; Walker and Greene, 1989.

Coping

- **Pain Response Inventory (PRI)** (well established)
  - ▶ **Description**: the PRI is a child-report measure of pain-coping strategies comprising three subscales: passive coping (15 items), active coping (24 items) and accommodative coping (16 items). Passive items include self-isolation, activity restriction, and catastrophising. Active coping strategies include problem-solving, social support seeking and distraction. Accommodative coping strategies include acceptance and self-encouragement.
  - ▶ **Psychometric properties**: reliability and validity have been determined to be adequate (e.g. Walker *et al.*, 1997). Example alpha reliabilities for

the three subscales ranged from 0.87 to 0.89 (i.e. P = 0.88; Act = 0.87; Acc = 0.89) (Kaczynski *et al.*, 2009).
▸ **Relevant references**: Caplan *et al.*, 2005; Greco *et al.*, 2007; Walker and Greene, 1989.

Parental responses to child pain behaviour

● **Illness Behavior Encouragement Scale (IBES)** (well established)
  ▸ **Description**: assesses provision of parental attention and special privileges and relief from normal responsibility during abdominal pain episodes.
  ▸ **Psychometric properties**: preliminary validation of the measure was demonstrated through significant correlations with abdominal pain-related behaviours (Walker and Zeman, 1992).
  ▸ **Relevant references**: Walker *et al.*, 2005; Kaczynski *et al.*, 2009; Walker and Zeman, 1992.
● **Adult Responses to Children's Symptoms (ARCS)** (approaching well established)
  ▸ **Description**: the ARCS is a parent-report measure that includes three analytically derived subscales assessing parents' responses to their children's pain – (1) parent protectiveness, (2) minimisation of pain and (3) encouraging and monitoring responses.
  ▸ **Psychometric properties**: the measure was developed and initially validated in parents of children aged 8–18 years (Van Slyke and Walker, 2006).
  ▸ **Relevant references**: Bijttebier and Vertommen, 1999; Schurman *et al.*, 2013.

Functional disability and impairment

● **Functional Disability Inventory (FDI)** (well established)
  ▸ **Description**: the FDI is a child-report measure that assesses children's reported difficulty in physical and psychosocial functioning due to their physical health. The measure contains items concerning perceptions of activity limitations during the previous 2 weeks, which children rate from 'no trouble' to 'impossible'.
  ▸ **Psychometric properties**: the FDI has demonstrated reliability in children and adolescents (i.e. internal consistency of 0.85 to 0.92 and 2-week test–retest reliability of 0.74 for child-report and 0.64 for parent-report) (Claar and Walker, 2006). Evidence of validity was examined by correlations with school absence ($r = 0.44$; $p < 0.001$) and somatic symptoms ($r = 0.45$; $p < 0.001$) (Walker and Green, 1991). Alpha reliability has been adequate (e.g. 0.89 in Kaczynski *et al.*, 2009).
  ▸ **Relevant references**: Robins *et al.*, 2005; Van Slyke and Walker, 2006; Claar *et al.*, 2010.

ENCOPRESIS

Symptom assessment

- **Virginia Encopresis–Constipation Apperception Test** (promising)
  - ▸ **Description**: the Virginia Encopresis–Constipation Apperception Test is a picture-based test based on the biopsychobehavioural model and is utilised to evaluate theoretical and clinical parameters relevant to children with encopresis, including such constructs as pain; ignoring distension cues; toilet avoidance; resistance to parental instructions; parent–child conflict; and shame, deception and rejection. It is made up of nine pairs of bowel-specific and nine parallel generic drawings. Caregivers and children independently select the picture in each pair that best describes them or their child.
  - ▸ **Psychometric properties**: better internal consistency has been established for the bowel-specific items (0.68–0.70) than for the generic items (0.33–0.43). Test–retest reliability over 6 months has shown significant and positive correlations. Assessment of construct validity included pre- and post-treatment comparisons; encopretic children and their mothers reported more bowel-specific, but not more generic, problems at baseline. Bowel-specific scores improved significantly post-treatment only for those patients who demonstrated significant symptom improvement.
  - ▸ **Relevant references**: Walker and Greene, 1991; Claar and Walker, 2006.

Diagnosis and classification

- **Profile of Toileting Issues (POTI)** (approaching well established)
  - ▸ **Description**: the POTI is a 56-item caregiver checklist assessing diagnostic criteria for enuresis and encopresis, as well as potential functions of these disorders including pain, avoidance, internal cues, non-compliance, shame/deception, aversive parenting, peer rejection and medical problems. Caregivers indicate presence or absence of a problem, and a total score is derived by summing response, with a higher score being reflective of more significant toileting problems. It can be used with individuals between the age of 4 years and adulthood.
  - ▸ **Psychometric properties**: psychometric properties of the POTI were evaluated using a sample of patients between the ages of 16 and 89 years. Internal consistency as measured by Cronbach's alpha was 0.79 when the original 56 items were included. The authors then removed any item with a coefficient of 0.30, given an increase in Cronbach's alpha; 21 items were subsequently removed. Cronbach's alpha was 0.83 for the remaining 32 items. Evaluation of inter-rater reliability indicated a significant positive correlation between raters ($r = 0.44$; $p < 0.05$).
  - ▸ **Relevant references**: Cox et al., 2003; Ritterband et al., 2006; Matson et al., 2011a, 2011b.

PAEDIATRIC FEEDING DISORDERS

Observational coding systems

- **Mealtime Observation Schedule (MOS)** (approaching well established)
  - ▸ **Description**: the MOS is a direct observation measure of children's eating behaviour and parental management of mealtime behaviour. The MOS requires that users review videotaped meals and code the presence of parent and child behaviours during 10-second intervals over the course of a 20-minute meal.
  - ▸ **Psychometric properties**: inter-rater reliability has demonstrated kappa coefficients ranging from 0.71 to 0.99 for parent behaviours and from 0.50 to 0.99 for child behaviours. In the evaluation of the validity of the measure, the authors (Sanders *et al.*, 1993a) found significant and positive correlations between in-home parent-reported assessment of mealtime behaviour difficulties and observations of mealtime behaviour as assessed by the MOS.
  - ▸ **Relevant references**: Belva *et al.*, 2011;Berlin *et al.*, 2010; Matson *et al.*, 2010; Sanders *et al.*, 1993a,b.
- **Dyadic Interaction Nomenclature for Eating (DINE)** (well established)
  - ▸ **Description**: the DINE is a behavioural coding system used in the assessment of caregiver and child mealtime behaviours and interactions through direct observation. The DINE was created to examine the occurrence of mealtime behaviour problems in children with cystic fibrosis as compared with children without cystic fibrosis. The DINE requires the user to review mealtimes that are video-recorded. Most behaviours on the DINE are coded as to their occurrence or non-occurrence during 10-second intervals; however, the overall frequency of a few behaviours is recorded as well. The DINE comprises three categories: (1) parent behaviour, (2) child behaviour and (3) child eating behaviour.
  - ▸ **Psychometric properties**: reliability of coding was calculated using kappa coefficients (examining agreement of raters on the occurrence of each behaviour in a 10-second interval). The average kappa coefficient was 0.79 (0.72–0.86) for parent behaviours, 0.83 (0.79–0.92) for child behaviours and 0.97 (0.86–0.95) for child eating behaviours. In a study utilising the DINE for observation of mealtime behaviour in children with type 1 diabetes mellitus (Patton *et al.*, 2006), inter-rater reliability coefficients were 0.65 for parent behaviours, 0.76 for child behaviours and 0.90 for child eating behaviours.
  - ▸ **Relevant references**: Sanders *et al.*, 1993a; Sanders and Le Grice, 1989; Stark *et al.*, 1995, 1997; Piazza-Waggoner *et al.*, 2008; Patton *et al.*, 2006.

Standardised caregiver report inventories

- **Behavioral Pediatrics Feeding Assessment Scale (BPFAS)** (well established)
  - ▸ **Description**: the BPFAS is a caregiver-report instrument that examines patterns of parent and child behaviour around mealtimes. The authors

(Crist & Nappier-Philips, 2001) originally created the measure to evaluate mealtime behaviour problems commonly observed in young children with cystic fibrosis as compared with children with no health concerns. This 35-item standardised caregiver report inventory is designed to obtain information on the mealtime behaviour of children between the ages of 9 months and 8 years of age. Twenty-five items are descriptions of childhood mealtime behaviours, while the remaining 10 items describe caregiver strategies for managing mealtime behaviour problems. Caregivers indicate how often the child engages in a particular eating behaviour or how often the caregiver uses a particular management strategy, using a 5-point Likert scale ranging from 'Never' to 'Always'. Responses to the Likert scale items are summed to create a total frequency score. As well, a total problem score is obtained from caregiver responses regarding whether a particular child behaviour or parental strategy is a problem, indicating 'Yes' or 'No'.

▶ **Psychometric properties**: internal consistency using Cronbach's alpha indicates values between 0.76 and 0.88 for the full scale, 0.84 for the child section and 0.74 for the parent section. As well, test–retest reliability over a 2-year interval revealed significant correlations, ranging from 0.82 to 0.85 for each of the subscales and the total score. The BPFAS is shown to discriminate between children referred to clinics for feeding problems and a normative sample. A factor analysis of the 25 child-related items of the BPFAS identified a five-factor structure in each of three independent samples. The interpretable factors identified included picky eaters (items related to a child's willingness to try new foods), toddler refusal – general (items describing disruptive mealtime behaviour), toddler refusal – textured foods (refusal behaviour specific to chewable foods), older children refusal – general (items unique to older children) and stallers (items such as letting food sit in the mouth, preference for drinking over eating, and not coming readily to the table).

▶ **Relevant references**: Sanders and Le Grice, 1989; Patton *et al.*, 2006; Stark *et al.*, 2000.

● **Children's Eating Behavior Inventory (CEBI)** (promising)

▶ **Description**: the CEBI was designed to evaluate the presence of eating and mealtime behaviour problems in children with medical and developmental disorders as well as to evaluate the level of caregiver stress related to mealtime behaviour. It contains 40 items: 28 items are related to food preference, motor skills and mealtime behaviour in young children, while 12 items evaluate caregiver emotion and interactions related to mealtime behaviour. A caregiver indicates how often a child engages in a particular eating behaviour or how often the caregiver experiences a particular emotion at mealtimes using a 5-point Likert scale to create a total eating problem score. As well, a total problem score is obtained from caregiver responses regarding whether a particular child behaviour or parental strategy is a problem, indicating 'Yes' or 'No'.

▶ **Psychometric properties**: in the combined sample, internal consistency has been assessed for four subgroups: (1) two parents with two or more children, (2) two parents with one child, (3) one parent with two or more children and (4) one parent with one child. Alphas ranged from 0.71 to 0.76 (all groups) and 0.58 (one parent and two or more children). Test–retest reliability over a 4- to 6-week period revealed reliability coefficients of 0.87 for the total problem score and 0.84 for percentage of items perceived by caregivers as problematic. The total eating problem score of the CEBI and the proportion of items perceived as a problem are found to discriminate between children referred for treatment of feeding difficulties and children not referred.

▶ **Relevant references**: Crist *et al.*, 1994; Crist and Napier-Phillips, 2001.

● **Screening Tool of Feeding Problems (STEP)** (approaching well established)

▶ **Description**: the STEP was designed to assist in the early identification and subsequent treatment of feeding problems observed specifically in individuals with mental retardation. Twenty-three items assess mealtime behaviour problems related to aspiration risk, food selectivity, feeding skills, disruptive mealtime behaviour and nutrition-related feeding problems. Individuals rate the frequency and severity of a behaviour. The STEP utilises a 3-point Likert scale: 0 = behaviour never occurs; 1 = occurrence between 1 and 10 times over the past month; and 2 = occurrence more than 10 times over the past month. If the response is 1 or 2, a follow-up question requires the responder to rate the severity of the behaviour on a scale of 0–3.

▶ **Psychometric properties**: a factor analysis in the initial validation study revealed an eight-factor structure, with seven interpretable factors. Internal consistency for the full measure was 0.68. Alpha for the individual scales was variable, ranging from 0.19 to 0.70. Test–retest reliability over 3 weeks was 0.72 for the full scale and ranged from 0.26 to 0.79 for each of the subscales. Inter-rater reliability was 0.71 for the full scale and ranged from 0.55 to 0.81 for individual scales. A second validation study conducted in 2002 lent preliminary support for the validity of the STEP as a tool to facilitate diagnosis of two specific feeding disorders, rumination and pica.

▶ **Relevant references**: Archer and Streiner, 1994; Archer *et al.*, 1991; Crist and Napier-Phillips, 2001; Manson et al 2010a, b

● **Brief Autism Mealtime Behavior Inventory (BAMBI)** (well established)

▶ **Description**: the BAMBI was designed to evaluate the nature of mealtime behaviour problems in children with autism. The caregiver is asked to indicate how often his or her child engages in a particular eating behaviour, on a Likert scale ranging from 1 to 5. A total frequency score is derived from the sum of the items with higher scores representing more problematic mealtime behaviour.

▶ **Psychometric properties**: preliminary psychometric analyses have revealed a reliability coefficient of 0.61 for the full scale. A validation resulted in an 18-item measure with a three-factor model: eight items relate to eating a limited variety of foods, five items suggestive of food refusal and disruptive mealtime behaviour, and five items that are related to characteristics associated with autism. Internal consistency is 0.88 for the full scale, 0.87 for the Limited Variety factor, 0.76 for the Food Refusal factor, and 0.63 for the Features of Autism factor. Test–retest reliability coefficient over a 7-month period is 0.87. BAMBI has strong positive correlations with external criterion measures (e.g. dietary variety, caloric intake, subscales of the Gilliam Autism Rating Scale).

▶ **Relevant references**: Matson and Kuhn, 2001a; Kuhn and Matson, 2002; Gilliam,1995.

● **Feeding Strategies Questionnaire (FSQ)** (promising)

▶ **Description**: the FSQ is a 32-item parent-report measure that assesses strategies used to address or prevent feeding problems. Respondents indicate the extent to which they agree or disagree with each item using a Likert scale (1 = strongly disagree; 5 = strongly agree). The measure comprises six factors: (1) Mealtime Structure, (2) Consistent Mealtime Schedule, (3) Child Control of Intake, (4) Parent Control of Intake, (5) Between Meal Grazing and (6) Encourages Clean Plate. The measure is based on both feeding dynamics and biobehavioural approaches.

▶ **Psychometric properties**: alpha coefficients range from 0.70 to 0.89. Structural and content validity were supported by independent ratings by practitioners in the field as well as goodness of fit indices. Construct validity was assessed by examining the relationship among individual scales of the FSQ and between the scales of the FSQ and the About Your Child's Eating scale, an established measure that evaluates parent beliefs and concerns about children's eating behaviour. Correlations were all in the expected direction, with significant correlations observed among many of the scales.

▶ **Relevant reference**: Matson and Kuhn, 2001b.

● **About Your Child's Eating (AYCE)** (promising)

▶ **Description**: the AYCE is a 25-item parent report measure that assesses parent beliefs and concerns regarding their child's eating, specifically evaluating the frequency of child eating behaviours, parents' mealtime interactions with the child, and caregiver feelings about mealtimes using a Likert scale such that a rating of 1 indicates 'Never' and a rating of 5 indicates 'Nearly Every Time'. The AYCE is made up of three scales: (1) Child Resistance to Eating, (2) Positive Mealtime Environment and (3) Parent Aversion to Mealtime. A total score (Feeding Relationship Disturbance score) is calculated by averaging the sums for the three scales.

▶ **Psychometric properties**: internal consistency is as follows: 0.89 for the Child Resistance to Eating factor, 0.80 for the Positive Mealtime Environment subscale, and 0.72 for the Parent Aversion to Mealtime factor. Subsequently, a confirmatory factor analysis was run and reliability indices were as follows: 0.86 for Child Resistance to Eating,

0.80 for Positive Mealtime Environment, and 0.66 for Parent Aversion to Mealtime.

‣ **Relevant reference**: Lukens and Linscheid, 2008.
● **Parent Mealtime Action Scale (PMAS)** (approaching well established)
  ‣ **Description**: the PMAS was developed to identify child and parent mealtime behaviours. The PMAS is a 31-item scale with nine dimensions determined by factor analysis: snack limits (three items), positive persuasion (four items), daily fruits and vegetables availability (three items), use of rewards (four items), insistence on eating (three items), snack modelling (three items), special meals (four items), fat reduction (three items), many food choices (four items). Caregivers are asked to indicate how often they demonstrate each mealtime action in a typical week using a Likert scale such that 1 = never, 2 = sometimes and 3 = always. Norms were developed for children between the ages of 2 and 12 years.
  ‣ **Psychometric properties**: reliability indices for the 31-item scale suggested moderate to high internal consistencies (Cronbach alphas were 0.42 to 0.81) and moderate to high test–retest and inter-rater reliability (ranged from 0.51 to 0.78). Examination of the convergent validity for the nine PMAS subscales indicated a mean correlation of 0.69 (0.59–0.78). To assess construct validity, PMAS scores were examined in relation to dietary analysis (parent report of the frequency of their child's consumption of 20 fruits, 20 vegetables and 12 snack foods as compared with recommended daily servings). This assessment indicated that all subscales (with the exception of use of rewards) were correlated with healthier diets and weight.
  ‣ **Relevant references**: Hendy *et al.*, 2009;Hendy *et al.*, 2012; Berlin *et al.*, 2011; Davies *et al.*, 2007; Williams *et al.*, 2011.

REFERENCES

Archer LA, Rosenbaum PL, Streiner DL. The Children's Eating Behavior Inventory: reliability and validity results. *J Pediatr Psychol.* 1991; **16**(5): 629–42.

Archer LA, Streiner DL. The revised Children's Eating Behavior Inventory: further psychometric properties [unpublished manuscript]. 1994.

Belva B, Matson JL, Barker A, *et al.* The relationship between adaptive behavior and specific toileting problems according to the Profile on Toileting Issues (POTI). *J Dev Phys Disabil.* 2011; **23**(6): 535–42.

Berlin KS, Davies WH, Silverman AH, *et al.* Assessing children's mealtime problems with the Mealtime Behavior Questionnaire. *Child Health Care.* 2010; **39**(2): 142–56.

Berlin KS, Davies WH, Silverman AH, *et al.* Assessing family-based feeding strategies, strengths, and mealtime structure with the Feeding Strategies Questionnaire. *J Pediatr Psychol.* 2011; **36**(5): 586–95.

Bijttebier P, Vertommen H. Antecedents, concomitants, and consequences of pediatric headache: confirmatory construct validation of two parent-report scales. *J Behav Med.* 1999; **22**(5): 437–56.

Caplan A, Walker LS, Rasquin A. Development and preliminary validation of the Questionnaire on Pediatric Gastrointestinal Symptoms to assess functional gastrointestinal disorders in children and adolescents. *J Pediatr Gastroenterol Nutr.* 2005; **41**(3): 296–304.

Claar RL, Guite JW, Kaczynski KJ, *et al.* Factor structure of the Adult Responses to Children's Symptoms: validation in children and adolescents with diverse chronic pain conditions. *Clin J Pain.* 2010; **26**(5): 410–17.

Claar RL, Walker LS. Functional assessment of pediatric pain patients: psychometric properties of the Functional Disability Inventory. *Pain.* 2006; **121**(1–2): 77–84.

Cohen LL, La Greca AM, Blount RL, *et al.* Introduction to special issue: evidence based assessment in pediatric psychology. *J Pediatr Psychol.* 2008; **33**(9): 911–15.

Cox DJ, Ritterband LM, Quillian W, *et al.* Assessment of behavioral mechanisms maintaining encopresis: Virginia Encopresis-Constipation Apperception Test. *J Pediatr Psychol.* 2003; **28**(6): 375–82.

Crist W, McDonnell P, Beck M. Behavior at mealtimes and the young child with cystic fibrosis. *J Dev Behav Pediatr.* 1994; **15**(3): 157–61.

Crist W, Napier-Phillips A. Mealtime behaviors of young children: a comparison of normative and clinical data. *J Dev Behav Pediatr.* 2001; **22**(5): 279–86.

Davies WH, Ackerman LK, Davies CM, *et al.* About your child's eating: factor structure and psychometric properties of a feeding relationship measure. *Eat Behav.* 2007; **8**(4): 457–63.

Fanjiang G, Russell GH, Katz AJ. Short- and long-term response to and weaning from infliximab therapy in pediatric ulcerative colitis. *J Pediatr Gastroenterol Nutr.* 2007; **44**(3): 312–17.

Gilliam JE. *Gilliam Autism Rating scale.* Austin. TX: Pro-ED. 1995.

Greco LA, Freeman KE, Dufton L. Overt and relational victimization among children with frequent abdominal pain: links to social skills, academic functioning, and health service use. *J Pediatr Psychol.* 2007; **32**(3): 319–29.

Greenley RN, Doughty A, Stephens M, *et al.* Brief report: development of the inflammatory bowel disease family responsibility questionnaire. *J Pediatr Psychol.* 2010; **35**(2): 183–7.

Harvey RF, Bradshaw JM. A simple index of Crohn's disease activity. *Lancet.* 1980; **1**(8167): 514.

Helgeland H, Flagstad G, Grøtta J, *et al.* Diagnosing pediatric functional abdominal pain in children (4–15 years old) according to the Rome III criteria: Results from a Norwegian prospective study. *J Pediatr Gastroenterol Nutr.* 2009; **49**(3): 309–15.

Hendy HM, Williams KE, Camise TS, *et al.* The Parent Mealtime Action Scale (PMAS): development and association with children's diet and weight. *Appetite.* 2009; **52**(2): 328–39.

Hendy HM, Seiverling L, Lukens CT, *et al.* Brief Assessment of Mealtime Behavior in Children: psychometrics and association with child characteristics and parent responses. *Child Health Care.* 2012; **42**(1): 1–14.

Hommel K, Hente, EA, Odell S, *et al.* Evaluation of a group-based behavioral intervention to promote adherence in adolescents with inflammatory bowel disease. *Eur J Gastroenterol Hepatol.* 2011a; **24**(1): 64–9.

Hommel K, Herzer M, Ingerski L, *et al.* Individually-tailored treatment of medication non-adherence: a pilot study. *J Pediatr Gastroenterol Nutr.* 2011b; **53**(4): 435–9.

Hyams J, Crandall W, Kugathasan S, *et al.* Induction and maintenance infliximab therapy for the treatment of moderate-to-severe Crohn's disease in children. *Gastroenterology.* 2007; **132**(3): 863–73.

Hyams JS, Ferry GD, Mandel FS, *et al.* Development and validation of a pediatric Crohn's disease activity index. *J Pediatr Gastroenterol Nutr.* 1991; **12**(4): 439–47.

Hyams J, Markowitz J, Otley A, *et al.* Evaluation of the pediatric Crohn Disease Activity Index: a prospective multicenter experience. *J Pediatr Gastroenterol Nutr.* 2005; **41**(4): 416–21.

Kaczynski KJ, Claar RL, Logan DE. Testing gender as a moderator of associations between psychosocial variables and functional disability in children and adolescents with chronic pain. *J Pediatr Psychol.* 2009; **34**(7): 738–48.

Kuhn DE, Matson JL. A validity study of the Screening Tool of Feeding Problems (STEP). *J Intellect Dev Disabil.* 2002; **27**(3): 161–7.

Kundhal PS, Critch JN, Zachos M, *et al.* Pediatric Crohn Disease Activity Index: responsive to short-term change. *J Pediatr Gastroenterol Nutr.* 2003; **36**: 83–9.

Lichtiger S, Present DH, Kornbluth A, *et al.* Cyclosporine in severe ulcerative colitis refractory to steroid therapy. *N Engl J Med.* 1994; **330**(26): 1841–5.

Loonen HJ, Grootenhuis MA, Last BF, *et al.* Measuring quality of life in children with inflammatory bowel disease: the impact-II (NL). Quality of Life Research, 2002; **11**(1): 47–56.

Lukens CT, Linscheid TR. Development and validation of an inventory to assess mealtime behavior problems in children with autism. *J Autism Dev Disord.* 2008; **38**(2): 342–52.

Markowitz J, Grancher K, Kohn N, *et al.* A multicenter trial of 6-mercaptopurine and prednisone in children with newly diagnosed Crohn's disease. *Gastroenterology.* 2000; **119**(4): 895–902.

Matson JL, Dempsey T, Fodstad JC. *The Profile of Toileting Issues (POTI).* Baton Rouge, LA: Disability Consultants; 2010.

Matson JL, Kuhn DE. Identifying feeding problems in mentally retarded persons: Development and reliability of the screening tool of feeding problems (STEP). *Res Dev Disabil.* 2001a; **22**(2): 165–72.

Matson JL, Kuhn DE. *Screening Tool of Feeding Problems (STEP).* Baton Rouge, LA: Disability Consultants; 2001b.

Matson JL, Neal D, Hess JA, *et al.* Assessment of toileting difficulties in adults with intellectual disabilities: an examination using the Profile of Toileting Issues (POTI). *Res Dev Disabil.* 2011a; **31**(1): 176–9.

Matson JL, Horovitz M, Sipes M. Characteristics of individuals with toileting problems and intellectual disability using the Profile of Toileting Issues (POTI). *J Ment Health Res Intellect Disabil.* 2011b; **4**(1): 53–63.

Otley A, Smith C, Nicholas D, Munk M, Avoilo J, Sherman PM, Griffiths AM. The IMPACT questionnaire: a valid measure of health-related quality of life in pediatric inflammatory bowel disease. *J Pediatr Gastroenterol Nutr.* 2002; **35**(4): 557–63.

Patton SR, Dolan LM, Powers SW. Mealtime interactions relate to dietary adherence and glycemic control in young children with type 1 diabetes. *Diabetes Care.* 2006; **29**(5): 1002–5.

Piazza-Waggoner C, Driscoll KA, Gilman DK, *et al.* A comparison using parent report and direct observation of mealtime behaviors in young children with cystic fibrosis: implications for practical and empirically based behavioral assessment in routine clinical care. *Child Health Care.* 2008; **37**(1): 38–48.

Ritterband LM, Cox DJ, Gordon TL, *et al.* Examining the added value of audio, graphics, and interactivity in an Internet intervention for pediatric encopresis. *Childrens Health Care.* 2006; **35**(1): 47–59.

Robins PM, Smith SM, Glutting JJ, *et al.* A randomized controlled trial of cognitive-behavioral family intervention for pediatric recurrent abdominal pain. *J Pediatr Psychol.* 2005; **30**(5): 397–408.

Sanders MR, Le Grice B. Mealtime observation schedule: an observer's manual [unpublished technical manual]. Queensland: Herston; 1989.

Sanders MR, Le Grice B, Turner KMT. Mealtime observation schedule: an observer's manual. Rev ed [unpublished technical manual]. Queensland: Behaviour Research and Therapy Centre; 1993a.

Sanders MR, Patel RK, Le Grice B, *et al.* Children with persistent feeding difficulties: an observational analysis of the feeding interactions of problem and non-problem eaters. *Health Psychol.* 1993b; **12**(1): 64–73.

Sanders MR, Turner KMT, Wall CR, *et al.* Mealtime behavior and parent-child interaction: a comparison of children with cystic fibrosis, children with feeding problems, and nonclinic controls. *J Pediatr Pyschol.* 1997; **22**(6): 881–900.

Schurman JV, Hunter HL, Danda CE, *et al.* Parental illness encouragement behavior among children with functional gastrointestinal disorders: a factor analysis with implications for research and clinical practice. *J Clin Psychol Med Settings.* 2013; **20**(2): 255–61.

Shepanski MA, Markowitz JE, Mamula P, *et al.* Is an abbreviated Pediatric Crohn's Disease Activity Index better than the original? *J Pediatr Gastroenterol Nutr.* 2004; **39**(1): 68–72.

Stark LJ, Jelalian E, Mulvihill M, *et al.* Eating in preschool children with cystic fibrosis and healthy peers: behavioral analysis. *Pediatrics.* 1995; **95**(2): 210–15.

Stark LJ, Jelalian E, Powers SW, *et al.* Parent and child mealtime behavior in families of children with cystic fibrosis. *J Pediatr.* 2000; **136**(2): 1995–2000.

Stark LJ, Mulvihill M, Jelalian E, *et al.* Descriptive analysis of eating behavior in school-age children with cystic fibrosis and healthy control children. *Pediatrics.* 1997; **99**(5): 665–71.

Turner D, Hyams J, Markowitz J, *et al.* Appraisal of the pediatric ulcerative colitis activity index (PUCAI). *Inflamm Bowel Dis.* 2009; **15**(8): 1218–23.

Turner D, Otley AR, Mack D, *et al.* Development, validation, and evaluation of a pediatric ulcerative colitis activity index: a prospective multicenter study. *Gastroenterology.* 2007; **133**(2): 423–32.

Van Slyke DA, Walker LS. Mother's responses to children's pain. *Clin J Pain.* 2006; **22**: 387–91.

Walker LS, Greene JW. Children with recurrent abdominal pain and their parents: more somatic complaints, anxiety, and depression than other patient families? *J Pediatr Psychol.* 1989; **14**: 231–43.

Walker LS, Greene JW. The Functional Disability Inventory: measuring a neglected dimension of child health status. *J Pediatr Psychol.* 1991; **16**(1): 39–58.

Walker LS, Smith CA, Garber J, *et al.* Development and validation of the pain response inventory for children. *Psychol Assess.* 1997; **9**(4): 392–405.

Walker LS, Smith CA, Garber J, *et al.* Testing a model of pain appraisal and coping in children with abdominal pain. *Health Psychol.* 2005; **24**: 364–74.

Walker LS, Zeman JL. Parental response to child illness behavior. *J Pediatr Psychol.* 1992; **17**(1): 49–71.

Williams KE, Hendy HM, Seiverling LJ, *et al.* Validation of the Parent Mealtime Action Scale (PMAS) when applied to children referred to a hospital-based feeding clinic. *Appetite.* 2011; **56**(3): 553–7.

3.2: Children with toileting problems

3.2a: Constipation in children: flow chart example

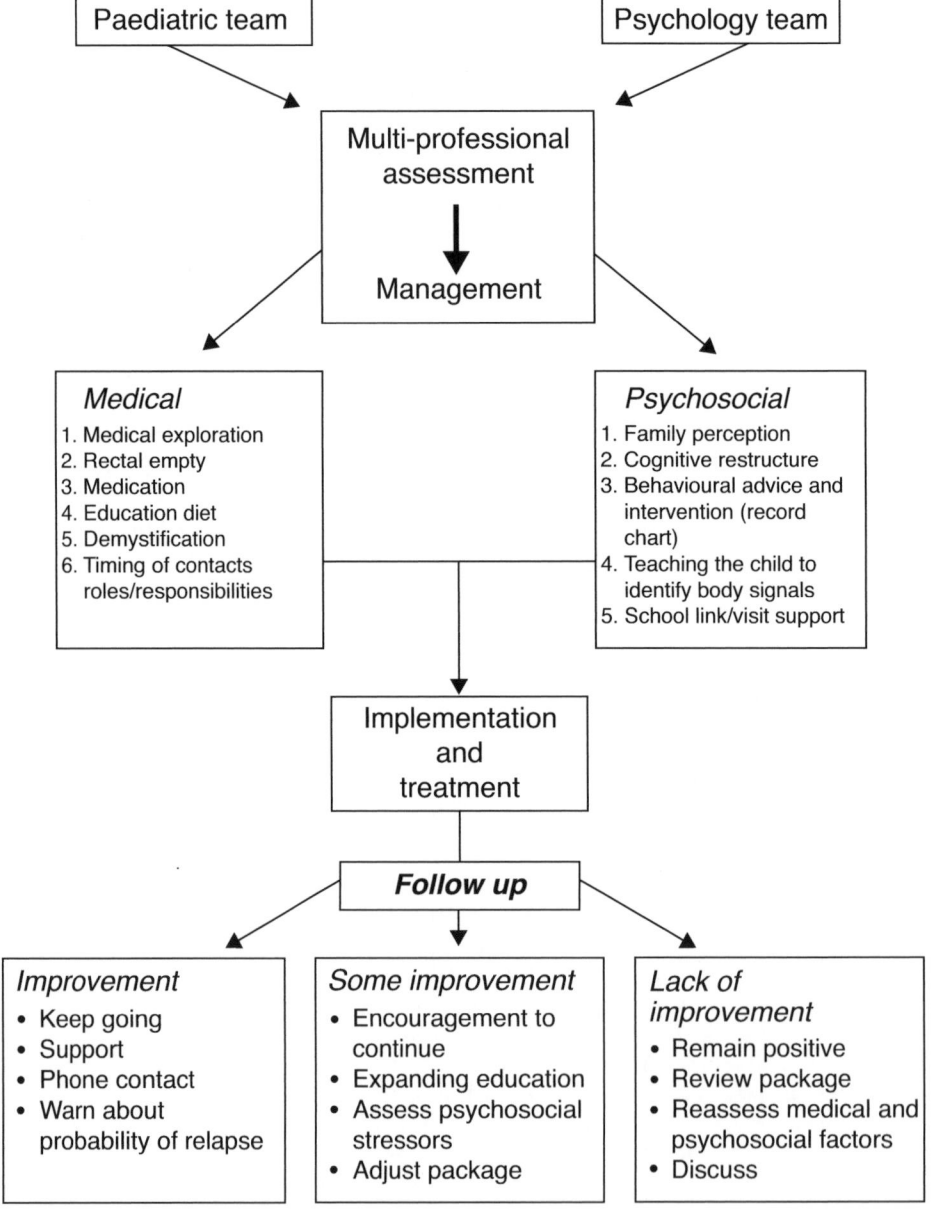

3.2b: Constipation in children: clinical interview

EXAMPLE OF CLINICAL INTERVIEW FOR CHILDREN WITH TOILETING PROBLEMS

NAME OF CHILD: _____ DoB:_____

Name of parent/guardian: _____

Address: _____

_____

_____

_____

Telephone No: _____

FIP/TCS No: _____

GP name: _____

Health Visitor/School Nurse: _____

DATE OF ASSESSMENT: _____

Name/profession of assessor: _____

General/medical

(NB If the child is under 1 year of age, see separate sheet)

1. **Do you have any concerns about the health of your child?**
    ❒ Yes   ❒ No
    If yes, obtain further details.

2. **Do you have any concerns about your child's growth or development?**
    ❒ Yes   ❒ No
    (NB check child's weight, height, growth chart)

3. **What is your child's toilet routine at present?**

4. **Does your child indicate his or her toilet needs?**   ❒ Yes   ❒ No

5. **Is your child's toilet routine the same in all environments?** (For example, school, home, friend's house)   ❒ Yes   ❒ No
    If no, obtain further details.

6. **Where does your child usually go to the toilet?**

7. **Describe your child's usual stool.**
    (NB use the Bristol Stool Scale)
    • **Consistency**
    • **Amount**
    • **Frequency**
    • **Any problems with flatulence or wind**

8. **Does your child ever soil?** ❑ Yes ❑ No
   If yes, obtain further detail (e.g. when, how often)

9. **Does your child have any accidents (e.g. soiling) at night?**
   ❑ Yes ❑ No
   If yes, obtain further details (e.g. frequency)

10. **Does your child have any other illness that might affect his or her toileting habits?** (For example, poor weight gain) ❑ Yes ❑ No
    If yes, obtain further details

11. **Does your child suffer with abdominal pain?** ❑ Yes ❑ No
    If yes, obtain further details (e.g. frequency, severity)

12. **Does your child ever bleed when passing a stool?** ❑ Yes ❑ No
    If yes, obtain further details (e.g. frequency, severity)

13. **Are you giving your child any medication to help him or her go to the toilet?** ❑ Yes ❑ No
    If yes, obtain further details (e.g. past and current medication)

14. **Is there any family history of toileting problems or constipation?**
    ❑ Yes ❑ No
    If yes, obtain further details

Fluid, diet, exercise

1. **How much fluid does your child drink in a day?**
   ❑ Less than 2½ to 3 pints a day ❑ More than 2½ to 3 pints a day

   Does your child have access to drinks at school?

   What types of drinks does your child usually have?

   ❑ Water   ❑ Fruit juice   ❑ Squash
   ❑ Fizzy drinks   ❑ Tea/coffee   ❑ Milk
   ❑ Other – obtain further details

2. **How much milk does your child usually drink in a day?**
   ❑ Less than 1 pint a day   ❑ 1 to 1½ pints a day
   ❑ More than 1½ pints a day

3. **Does your child eat fruit and vegetables?** ❑ Yes ❑ No
   If yes, how many portions a day?

4. **What type of bread does your child usually eat?**
   ❑ White   ❑ High-fibre white ❑ Granary
   ❑ Wholemeal   ❑ Mixture   ❑ Rarely eats bread

5. **What type of breakfast cereal does your child usually eat?**

6. **How much exercise does your child usually do in a week?**

7. **What type of exercise does your child usually do?**

Miscellaneous

1. **What type of toilet facilities do you have at home?**
   (For example, number of toilets, number in family using facilities)
   Can your child sit on the toilet him- or herself or does your child need
   help to get up?
   Can your child pull his or her pants or trousers down on his or her own?
   Can your child flush the toilet him- or herself?
   Can your child turn the light on in the toilet or does he or she need help?

2. **What type of washing facilities do you have at home?**
   (For example, washing machine or bathing facilities and number in family using facilities)

3. **Does your child have any attendance problems at school?**
   Is your child ever reluctant to go to school?

4. **Is your child's toileting resulting in any problems in the family?**
   (For example, teasing, sibling rivalry, tension or argument between family members)

5. **Who is the main person concerned about your child's toileting?**

6. **What other services are involved?**
   (For example, Social Services, Family Support Workers, psychologist, dietitian)

If other services are involved, obtain further details about why.

Summary of assessment
General/Medical
Fluid/Diet/Exercise
Miscellaneous

Action plan (agreed with parent/guardian and child)
Aim:
Specific goals:
Literature given:
Further review:

Other professionals involved:

Referral: Yes/No

If yes, further details

3.2c: Constipation in children: policy flow chart example

Tess Mobberley

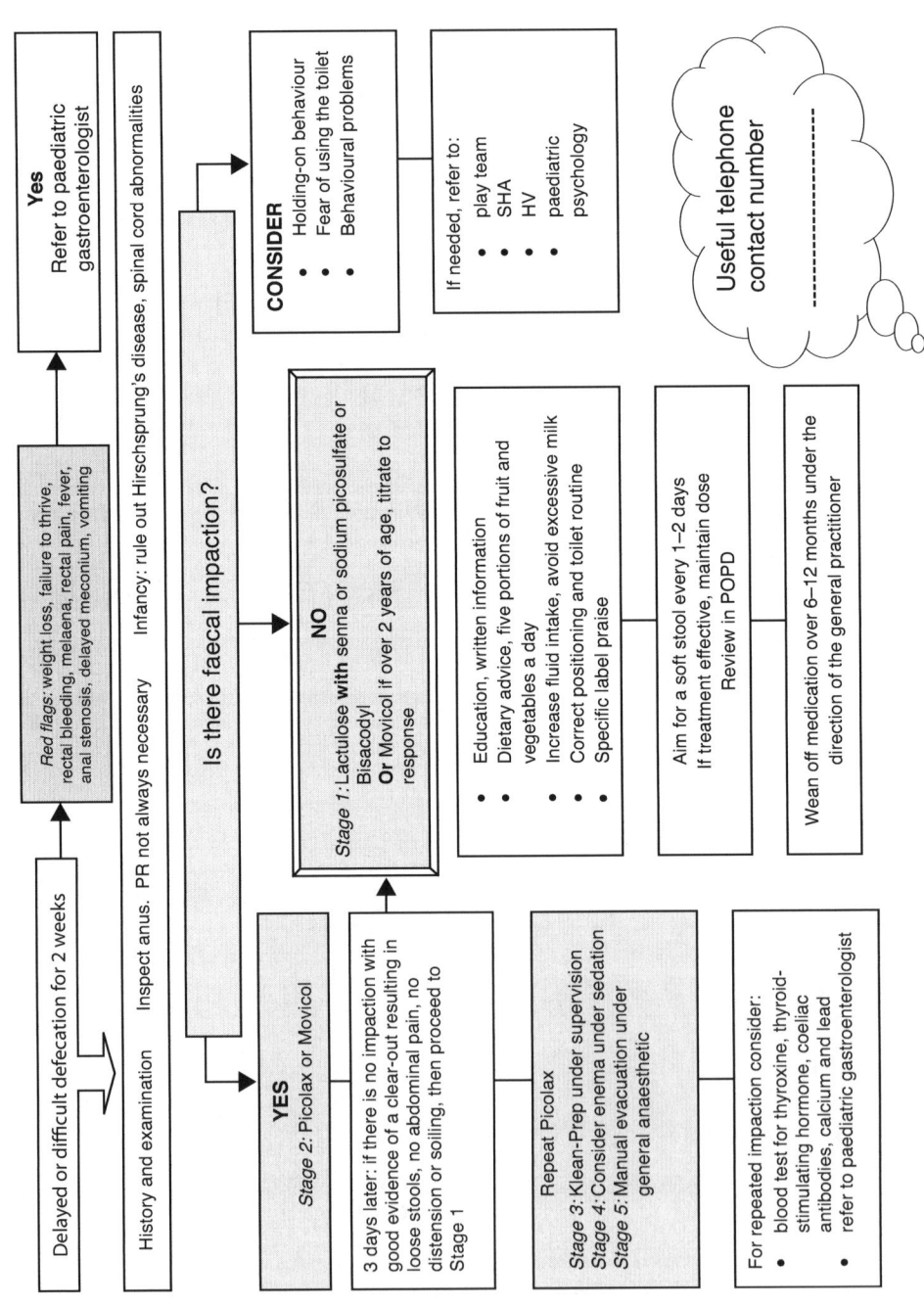

Delayed or difficult defecation for 2 weeks

History and examination   Inspect anus.   PR not always necessary   Infancy: rule out Hirschsprung's disease, spinal cord abnormalities

Red flags: weight loss, failure to thrive, rectal bleeding, melaena, rectal pain, fever, anal stenosis, delayed meconium, vomiting

Yes
Refer to paediatric gastroenterologist

Is there faecal impaction?

YES
Stage 2: Picolax or Movicol

3 days later: if there is no impaction with good evidence of a clear-out resulting in loose stools, no abdominal pain, no distension or soiling, then proceed to Stage 1

Repeat Picolax
Stage 3: Klean-Prep under supervision
Stage 4: Consider enema under sedation
Stage 5: Manual evacuation under general anaesthetic

For repeated impaction consider:
• blood test for thyroxine, thyroid-stimulating hormone, coeliac antibodies, calcium and lead
• refer to paediatric gastroenterologist

NO
Stage 1: Lactulose **with** senna or sodium picosulfate or Bisacodyl
Or Movicol if over 2 years of age, titrate to response

• Education, written information
• Dietary advice, five portions of fruit and vegetables a day
• Increase fluid intake, avoid excessive milk
• Correct positioning and toilet routine
• Specific label praise

Aim for a soft stool every 1–2 days
If treatment effective, maintain dose
Review in POPD

Wean off medication over 6–12 months under the direction of the general practitioner

CONSIDER
• Holding-on behaviour
• Fear of using the toilet
• Behavioural problems

If needed, refer to:
• play team
• SHA
• HV
• paediatric psychology

Useful telephone contact number
_____

3.2d: Medication management

Tess Mobberley

TABLE 3.2D.1 Medication for constipation

	Age of patient			
	Under 1 year	*1–5 years*	*5–10 years*	*12+ years*
Lactulose	2.5 mL BD	5 mL BD	10–15 mL BD	15–20 mL BD
Senna	0.5 mL/kg nocte	2.5–5 mL nocte	5–10 mL nocte	10–20 mL nocte
Sodium picosulfate	2.5 mL nocte	5 mL nocte	7.5 mL nocte	10–15 mL nocte
Bisacodyl (5 mg tablet)	....	1 tab nocte	1–2 tabs nocte	2–4 tabs nocte
Movicol Paediatric Plain sachet *(patient over 2 years old)*	....	1–4 sachets a day	2–4 sachets a day	....
Movicol sachet *(patient over 12 years old)*	....	....	....	1–3 sachets a day

TABLE 3.2D.2 Medication for disimpaction

	Age of patient			
	1–2 years	*2–5 years*	*5–9 years*	*9+ years*
Picolax sachet Give one dose and repeat after 6 hours	Quarter of sachet	Half of sachet	Three-quarters of sachet	Whole sachet
	Dissolve powder in 30 mL water Care should be taken to allow solution to cool, as it generates heat Can be mixed with juice Follow up with plenty of fluids			
Klean Prep sachet	....	....	500 mL	1 L
	Add one sachet to 1 L water Can be mixed with juice			
Movicol Paediatric Plain sachet *(patient over 5 years old)*	....	• Day 1 × four sachets • Day 2 × six sachets • Day 3 × eight sachets • Day 4 × ten sachets		....
Movicol sachet *(patient over 12 years old)*	....	....	....	Eight sachets in 1 L water over 6 hours for maximum of 3 days

3.2e: Talk about constipation

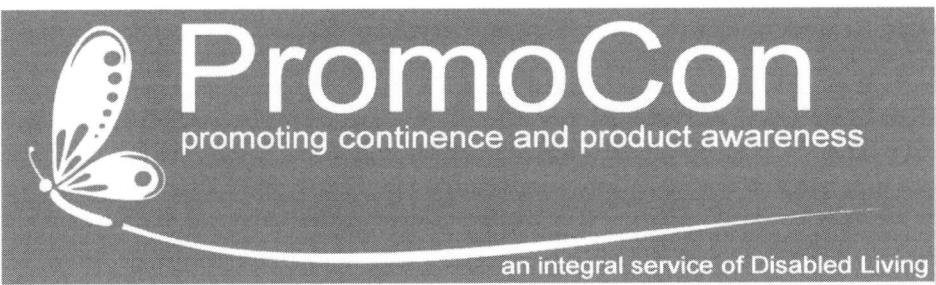

Talk about Constipation

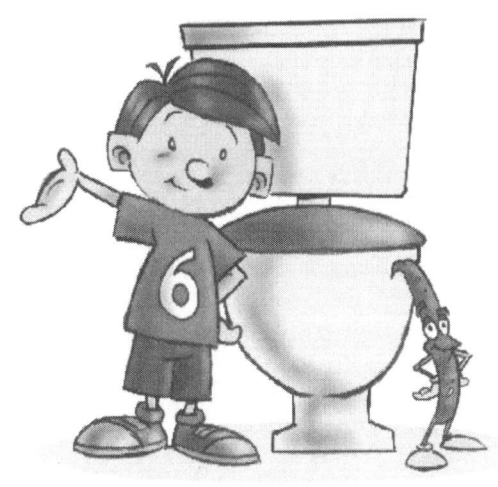

Reproduced with the kind permission of PromoCon/Disabled Living

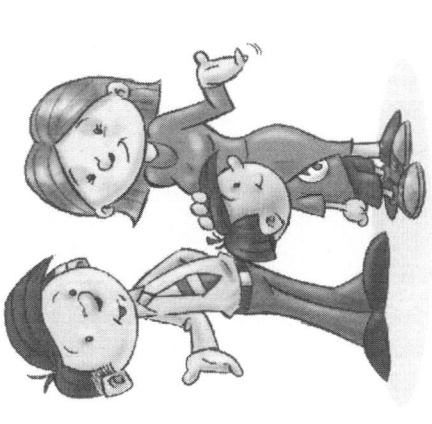

It is important to **talk** about the problem of **constipation** and **soiling**. Do **not** keep it a **secret**.

3

This book has been designed to help young children understand about constipation and soiling (having poo accidents in your pants).

It explains why it happens and what can help things get better.

It is important to remember that if a child is soiling they may have been constipated for many months without anyone knowing.

This problem can be helped. Treatment often takes a while to work. It should be continued for a long time (often more than 12 months) to stop it happening again.

2

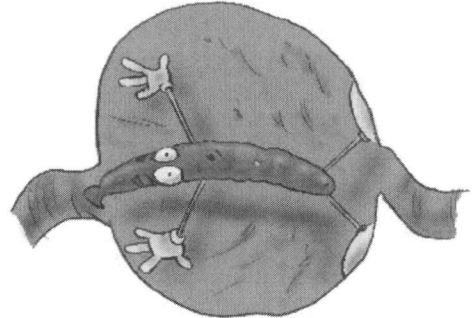

Poo sometimes gets 'stuck' in your bottom

5

Where does poo come from?

Everybody needs to poo and wee. All your friends, your mum and dad and even famous footballers, and pop stars.

When we eat there is always some part of the food that our body doesn't need. Our body gets rid of this part of the food. That is our poo!

4

What is 'constipation'?

Constipation means that you are not doing enough poos, we need to do at least 3 poos per week, or that your poo has become hard which can make it difficult to come out. It is often called 'Idiopathic Constipation' and that means the cause is unknown

How does constipation happen?

Although we don't always know why it happens, we know what things make poo hard:

- Not eating enough fruit and vegetables
- Not drinking enough
- Not sitting on the toilet for long enough
- Putting off going to the toilet when we need to poo

6

How can I stop the soiling?

We need to get rid of the poo that is sitting in your bottom as that is causing all the problems!

You can help this by:

- Taking medicine called 'laxatives'
- Make sure you sit on the toilet regularly, try to do a poo everyday
- Sit on the toilet for about 5-10 minutes and try and 'push' the poo out
- Don't hold on if you feel you need to poo!
- Have 6-8 water based drinks per day
- Eat more fruit and vegetables
- Have lots of exercise

7

Why does the poo come out by itself into my pants?

When you get constipated the poo sits in your bottom instead of coming out into the toilet. This poo gets bigger and harder and eventually 'wedges' open the top bit of your bottom. This normally acts as a 'special door' which keeps all your poo inside until you sit on the toilet!

Also there is a bendy bit at the end of your bowel which also helps to keep the poo inside. When you are constipated the poo sitting in your bottom keeps this bendy bit of your bowel straight so that the squidgy poo higher up can squeeze past into your pants ('sneaky poo!).

This happens without you doing anything - so it is not your fault!

9

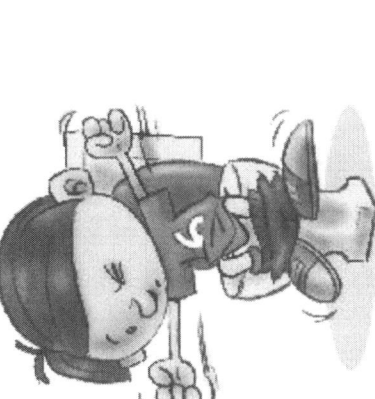

Constipation means that it is **difficult** for your **poo** to come **out!**

8

11

What else can I do to help?

- Decide which is the best time to sit on the toilet everyday to try and do a poo. After a main meal is best.
- Keep a note of when you do a poo on the toilet so you can tell the person helping you to get better
- Work out with your mum (or whoever is looking after you) what you need to do with any pants that have 'sneaky poo' in them

10

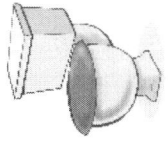
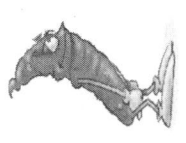
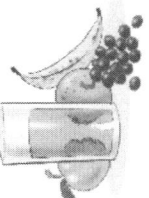
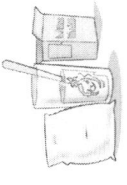

There are **lots of things** you can do to **help** things **get better**

Further information

PromoCon

Disabled Living

Tel: 0161 607 8219

Email: promocon@disabledliving.co.uk

Website: www.promocon.co.uk

PromoCon, working as part of Disabled Living Manchester, provides impartial advice and information regarding a whole range of products, such as musical potties and other toilet training equipment and swimwear and washable trainer pants for children who have delayed toilet training.

Information is also available regarding which services and resources are available for both children and adults with bowel and/or bladder problems

www.childhoodconstipation.com

Web site which is an information resource for parents, carers, health professionals and children.

13

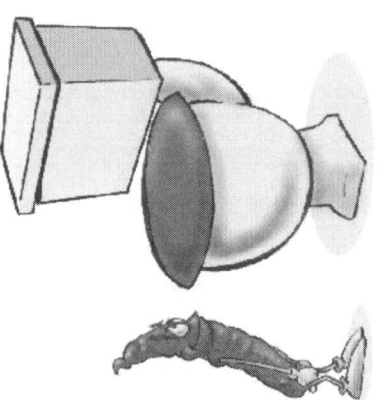

Poo wants to get to the **toilet!**

12

Further information

NICE has produced guidance regarding best practice in the assessment and treatment of idiopathic constipation in childhood. NICE made several recommendations including:

- Do not use dietary interventions alone as first-line treatment for idiopathic constipation
- Treat constipation with laxatives....
- Offer PEG 3350 + electrolytes (Movicol), as first line treatment

The following document has been produced specifically for families
CG99 Constipation in children and young people:
understanding NICE guidance. This can be downloaded from:
http://www.nice.org.uk/nicemedia/live/12993/48752/48752.pdf

14

Titles of other booklets currently available in this series:

Talk about going to the toilet

Talk about bedwetting

Talk about day time wetting

No part of this document may be photocopied or circulated without the authors permission

June Rogers MBE

Illustrations – Les Eaves

Copyright © PromoCon

Disabled Living. Registered Charity No: 224742

2004

Updated 2011

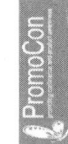

15

3.2f: Understanding Hirschsprung's disease: a guide for parents and carers

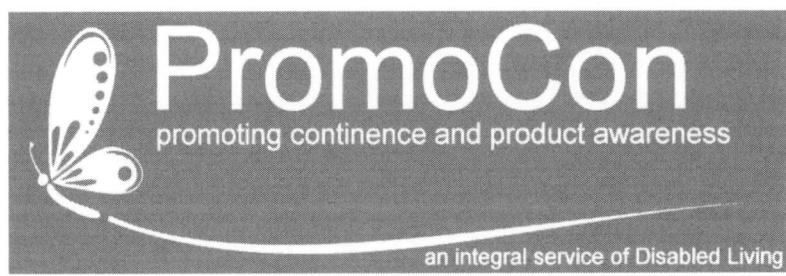

Understanding Hirschsprung's Disease

A guide for parents and carers

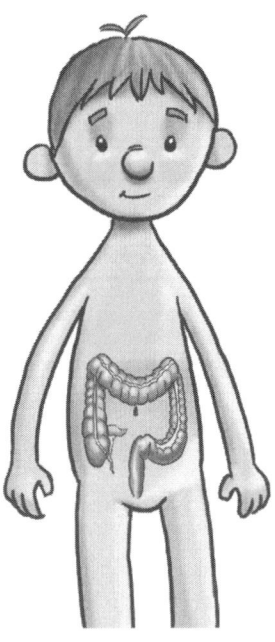

Reproduced with the kind permission of PromoCon/Disabled Living

What is Hirschsprung's disease ?

Hirschsprung's Disease is a rare congenital abnormality (from birth) which affects specific nerve cells, called parasympathetic ganglion cells, in the large bowel (colon).

Normally, as the baby is developing in the womb the nerve cells grow along the intestines towards the rectum. In children with Hirschsprung's Disease the nerve cells stop growing too soon. This happens before the 12th week of development and the reason for this is not yet known.

The result is the lack of these ganglion cells in the rectum and also in varying degrees along the length of the colon. Absence of the ganglion cells means that signals to the muscles are not sent and the colon is unable to relax - this prevents movement of stools (poo) along the colon resulting in constipation or in severe cases complete obstruction.

How severe the Hirschsprung's disease is depends on how much of the colon is affected. Short-segment Hirschsprung's Disease means only the last part of the colon is affected while long-segment Hirschsprung's means that most or all of the colon is affected

How common is it?

Hirschsprung's is a rare disease. The incidence is 1 in 5000 live births and it affects more boys than girls. However, for children with Down's Syndrome there is a 40% increased risk of Hirschsprung's Disease occurring

1

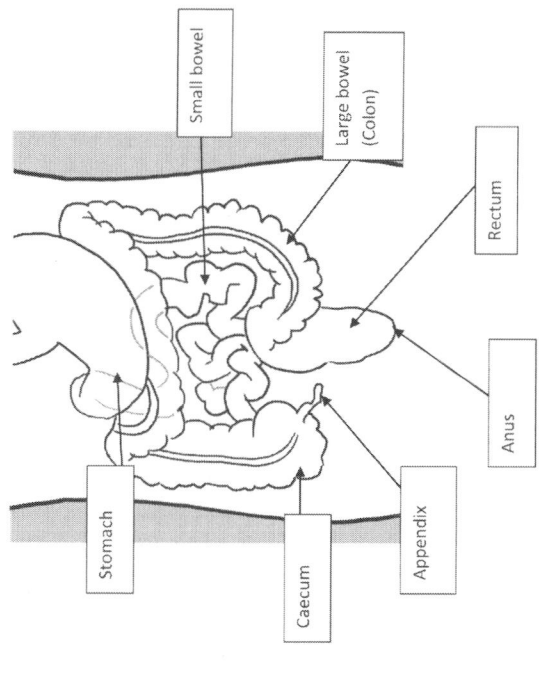

Stomach

Small bowel

Large bowel (Colon)

Caecum

Appendix

Rectum

Anus

Diagram of Digestive System

2

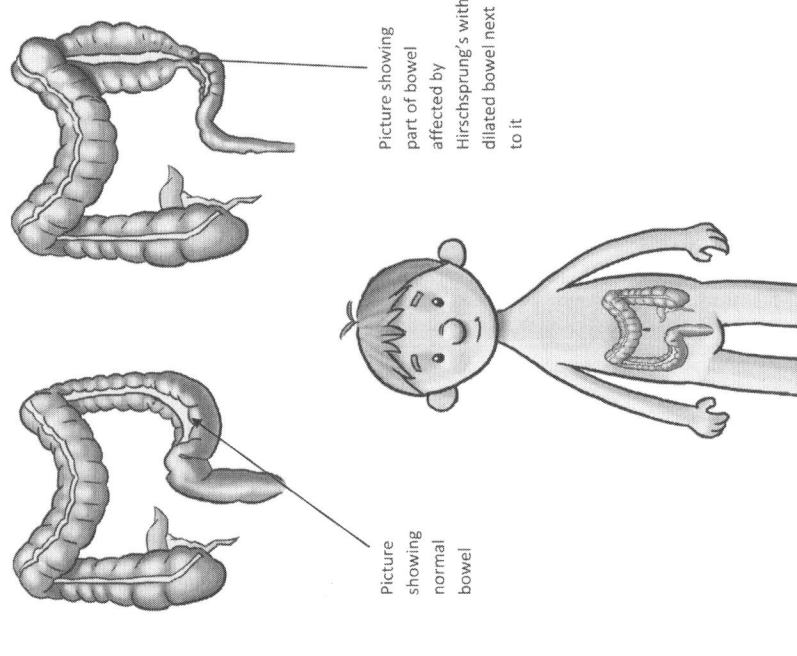

Picture showing part of bowel affected by Hirschsprung's with dilated bowel next to it

Picture showing normal bowel

Picture showing the position of the bowel in the body and how Hirschsprung's Disease affects it

4

What are the presenting symptoms?

Hirschsprung's disease is usually identified shortly after birth. Delay in the passage of meconium (the first sticky, black stool) which is usually passed in the first 48 hours following birth is a common symptom. A distended abdomen or vomiting may also occur.
Older infants and children with short-segment Hirschsprung's may present later with chronic constipation which is resistant to usual treatments, and is often accompanied by poor weight gain.

How is it diagnosed?

The doctor will usually carry out a physical examination, including feeling the babies' tummy and putting a finger in their bottom. However, the only definitive way to test for Hirschsprung's disease is a rectal biopsy – this involves taking a sample of cells from the rectum and looking at them under a microscope. If Hirschsprung's disease is present there will be an absence of ganglion cells in the sample biopsied. Other tests may include blood tests and X-rays. An abdominal x-ray will show a distended bowel above the affected section, but a barium enema may be used to determine the extent of the problem.

What is the long term outcome?

The majority of children who are born with Hirschsprung's disease do very well. However, a number of children may have ongoing problems with diarrhoea or constipation, soiling and abdominal pain. Some children may take longer to toilet train, because of the problems with bowel management. Sometimes long term medication and further interventions, including surgical, are needed to help with these problems.

3

How is it treated?

The immediate management of the baby will depend very much on the extent of the Hirschsprung's disease and the particular hospital unit the infant has been admitted to.

Some infants will be managed in the short term with rectal washouts before surgery is undertaken, to remove the affected bowel and attach the healthy bowel to the anus, called a 'pull through' operation . Sometimes the surgery needs to be done in 2 stages, with a colostomy or ileostomy being formed soon after birth, and the second stage of connecting the healthy bowel to the anus at a later stage.

A colostomy is where the large bowel is brought to the surface of the abdomen (tummy) and an opening is formed. An ileostomy is where the small bowel is brought to the tummy wall. In both cases the poo is collected in a special bag (stoma bag), stuck over the opening.

A stoma can be a scary thing to contemplate living with initially, but there is support available from stoma nurses or paediatric community nurses. They can show you how to look after a stoma and will also tell you how you can get the supplies, which you will need.

What happens when the stoma is reversed?

Following the reversal of a stoma, some children, especially those left with a short colon (because they have had a large part of their colon removed or it was absent), may initially have very loose, watery stool's. As stools are alkaline, if they come into prolonged contact with skin, they will 'burn' the skin and make it very sore. The use of specific barrier creams can help alleviate or prevent this from happening – your health care professional can advise you further

What is Enterocolitis?

The cause of enterocolitis is not fully understood but it is thought that poor movement of the intestinal contents and bacterial invasion are contributory factors. It presents as severe inflammation of the bowel and is often accompanied by explosive diarrhoea, foul smelling stool, vomiting, abdominal distension and fever. The risk for enterocolitis is higher in children with Down's Syndrome and any child suspected of being affected should be referred for urgent medical treatment.

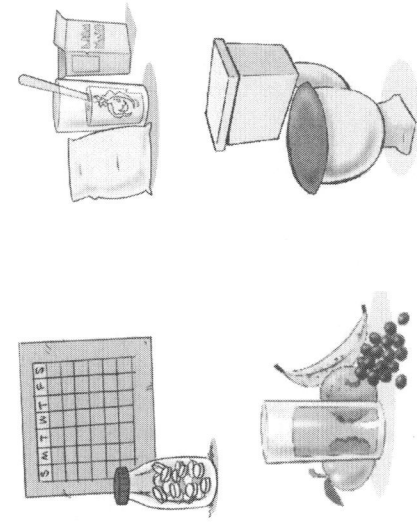

Laxatives, fluids, fibre intake and toileting programmes are all important in maintaining health bowels

Notes

Caring for children with Hirschsprung's disease.

It does depend on how much bowel has been affected, and the results of the surgery, as to what problems the child will have. Some children will be fully continent and toilet trained by the time they get to school age, but may still need laxatives and a structured bowel programme including easy access to the toilet, because their need to poo is so unpredictable.

Others may struggle with constipation and soiling until they are in their teens, and some may need further surgery to enable continence. Obviously there is a strong link between becoming continent of faeces and an improvement in quality of life. This makes it really important for these children to receive the practical support from schools, parents and carers, to stand the best chance in being successful at toilet training.

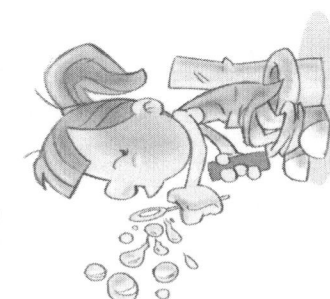

A structured bowel training programme should always be introduced

This booklet has been designed to help those involved with the care of children with Hirschsprung's disease to understand what it is, the treatment involved and why long term good bowel management is so important.

This booklet is part of a series for children with bowel problems.

Titles of other booklets currently available in this series:
'Talk about going to the toilet'
'Talk about constipation'
'Understanding constipation in infants and toddlers'
'Understanding toilet refusal – the child who will only poo in a nappy'
'Understanding Ano-Rectal Malformations '
'Understanding bowel management'
'Understanding Bowel problems in schools'

No part of this document may be photocopied or circulated without the authors permission.

June Rogers MBE, Team Director of PromoCon
Anna Turner, Paediatric Continence Advisor

Illustrations - Les Eaves

This booklet was developed with support from the Down's Syndrome Association and the Platinum Trust

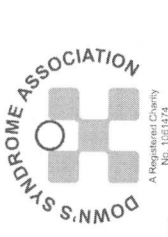

A Registered Charity No. 1061474

Diversions

Diversions is a support network, based in the North West of England, for families with a child or young person living with a bladder or bowel diversion/dysfunction

Contact:
Melissa – 07816513889
Rachael – 07814613669
Email: diversions@live.co.uk

Down's Syndrome Association

Provides information and support regarding all aspects of Down's Syndrome to all those who need it.

Langdon Down Centre
2a Langdon Park
Teddington
Middlesex
TW11 9PS
Tel: 0333 1212 300.
Email: info@downs-syndrome.org.uk

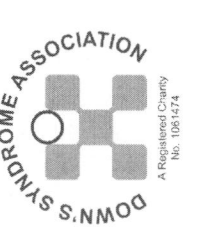

A Registered Charity No. 1061474

PromoCon

PromoCon, part of the charity Disabled Living, provides qualified impartial advice and information regarding products and services for children and adults with bowel and/or bladder problems

Disabled Living
Tel: 0161 607 8219
Email: promocon@disabledliving.co.uk
Website: www.promocon.co.uk

3.2g: Handouts from Chapter 8

Caroline E Danda and Paul E Hyman

HANDOUT 1: ENCOURAGING SUCCESSFUL TOILETING

We want to make it easier to help your child learn to use the bathroom appropriately. Following these tips will make it easier for your child to use the bathroom on his or her own.

- Make using the bathroom pleasant. Let your child to read books or listen to music while sitting on toilet.
- Do not let your child to sit on the toilet for longer than 5 minutes. Forcing your child to sit on the toilet any longer is like a punishment and is not necessary.
- Use a footstool or phone books on the floor so your child's feet are on a firm place while sitting on the toilet. Having a firm place for your child's feet makes it easier to push.
- Suggest trying to go to the bathroom after waking up in the morning or 30 minutes after meals. These are times that many people feel like they have to go. Make the suggestion brief and matter-of-fact (without any long explanations or urging). If your child does not want to go to the bathroom, *do not* force him or her and do not ask again. If your child agrees and sits on the toilet, praise your child, regardless of whether there is a bowel movement.

Dealing with soiling or accidents

- Deal with soiling using a matter-of-fact, non-angry tone of voice. For example, you might say, 'You've soiled your pants. You need to change your clothes now.'
- Do not force the child to admit soiling, and do not criticise. If you know your child has soiled, do not ask your child whether he or she has dirty pants. Rather, make a statement such as the one given here in the previous point.
- Have the child participate in cleaning up. For example, young kids can help put dirty clothes in the hamper and older children can help with the laundry. Participation in cleaning up should not be viewed as punishment. Cleaning up is a direct result (i.e. a logical consequence) of soiling, much like having to clean up after spilling a drink on the floor.
- Stop nagging, reminding, lecturing and punishing. These parenting behaviours give too much attention to the problems the child is having with toileting, which can make the problem worse and make the parents and the child feel bad (which is *not* necessary).

Use attention to encourage better behaviours

- Pay attention to your child's good behaviours. Catch your child being good. Ignore small problems and focus on what your child does right. Children naturally want to act in ways that get them noticed, whether it is 'good' attention, like praising, or 'bad' attention, like punishment and nagging. So pay less attention to problem toileting behaviour and deal with problem behaviours quickly and matter-of-factly (as already described). Pay more attention to your child's good behaviours – and not just those related to toileting. This helps your child feel better about him- or herself and takes the focus of attention away from toileting.
- Praise your child with words and touch. Describe and praise behaviours that you want your child to do more often. For example, if you want your child to follow directions better, then make a comment such as, 'Thanks for doing what I said right away' when you see your child do what you asked them to do. Other examples include 'I like the way you said please when you asked' and 'You're a great helper.'
- Use lots of pats and hugs, especially with younger children.

Look for and pay attention to small changes in your child's behaviour. Behaviour does not change overnight. Comment on small steps that your child makes towards going to the bathroom on his or her own. For example, your child telling you when he or she has an accident, changing clothes on his or her own, or sitting on the toilet are all steps to going to the bathroom on his or her own.

HANDOUT 2: EXAMPLE OF DAILY RECORDING

Monday	Tuesday	Wednesday	Thursday	Friday	Saturday	Sunday

Bowel movements or soiling

Time of day	Bowel movement	Consistency	Amount (approximate)	Where	Other notes
	Yes	Runny	¼ cup	On toilet	
	No	Soft	½ cup	In underwear	
	Soil only (not clean)	Semi-soft	¾ cup		
		Hard	1 cup		
			1¼ cup		
			1½ cup		

Time of day	Bowel movement	Consistency	Amount (approximate)	Where	Other notes
	Yes	Runny	¼ cup	On toilet	
	No	Soft	½ cup	In underwear	
	Soil only (not clean)	Semi-soft	¾ cup		
		Hard	1 cup		
			1¼ cup		
			1½ cup		

Time of day	Bowel movement	Consistency	Amount (approximate)	Where	Other notes
	Yes	Runny	¼ cup	On toilet	
	No	Soft	½ cup	In underwear	
	Soil only (not clean)	Semi-soft	¾ cup		
		Hard	1 cup		
			1¼ cup		
			1½ cup		

Time of day	Bowel movement	Consistency	Amount (approximate)	Where	Other notes
	Yes	Runny	¼ cup	On toilet	
	No	Soft	½ cup	In underwear	
	Soil only (not clean)	Semi-soft	¾ cup		
		Hard	1 cup		
			1¼ cup		
			1½ cup		

Miralax dose	Time of day

Exercise

Amount of time	Type of exercise	Activity level (low, medium, high)

Notes on food and liquid intake

Time of day	Food or liquid	Amount eaten or drunk

3.3: Notes on cyclical vomiting syndrome

Compiled by Clarissa Martin

BASIC CONCEPTS

- Cyclical vomiting syndrome (CVS) is a heterogeneous group of symptoms that constitute a rare disorder of unknown aetiology and pathogenesis (Sunku, 2009).
- CVS is characterised by recurrent episodes of vomiting followed by symptom-free intervals (Li *et al.*, 2008).
- CVS has an incidence in children of 3.15/100 000 children per year and affects 2% of the children. These children may require repeated hospitalisation and have their quality of life reduced (Drumm *et al.*, 2012; Forbes and Fairbrother, 2008; Lee *et al.*, 2012; Li *et al.*, 2008; Olson and Li, 2002).
- Delays on diagnosis have been found and have varied from 1.9 to 2.5 years (Abell *et al.*, 2008; Li, 2000a).
- CVS may increase the risk of dysphagic infant death (Talbert, 2009).
- Several working hypothesis:
  - CVS is associated with migraine headache (Li *et al.*, 1999)
  - CVS is a chronic idiopathic functional gastrointestinal disorder (Forbes and Fairbrother, 2008; Venkatesan *et al.*, 2010) with dysfunctional brain–gut interaction (Fleisher, 1997; Wood, 1999)
  - CVS is a mitochondrial dysfunction (Boles, 2011; Boles and Williams, 1999)
  - CVS is a rare abnormality of the endocrine system (Sato *et al.*, 1988).

CLINICAL DIAGNOSIS

Diagnosis for children must be based on special manifestations of CVS including symptom-free interval and excluding specific systemic diseases (Dong *et al.*, 2008).

NASPGHAN, the North American Society of Pediatric Gastroenterology, Hepatology, and Nutrition, has published a consensus statement detailing guidelines for the diagnosis and treatment of CVS in children (Li *et al.*, 2008), establishing criteria around:
- severe and constant nausea
- repeated and severe vomiting episodes
- violent retching.

Other associated symptoms are:
- pale skin
- photophobia and phonophobia
- motion sickness
- abdominal pain
- diarrhoea
- lethargy
- depression
- anxiety
- panic attacks.

CONTRIBUTING FACTORS

Gastrointestinal causes are:
- dysmotility / gastric dysrhythmia
- mucosal gastrointestinal injury
- anatomic gastrointestinal malformations
- gall bladder and pancreatic problems
- gastro-oesophageal reflux disease
- irritable bowel disease
- abdominal pain.

Other medical causes are:
- neurological
- metabolic
- endocrine
- renal
- allergies
- fasting
- ingestion of certain products (e.g. drugs).

Psychological factors are:
- stress
- anxiety
- environmental and family conflicts
- physical and emotional abuse
- internalising and somatisation patterns
- over-reactive and excited temperament.

MANAGEMENT AND TREATMENT

- There are empiric guidelines for the treatment of CVS (Fleisher, 2008) and the consensus statement from NASPGHAN (Li *et al.*, 2008)
- Currently, there is no treatment regimen for CVS with a strong evidence base (Lee *et al.*, 2012)

- Some research evidence has indicated that pharmacological therapies including anti-migraine, anti-emetic, prokinetic and anticonvulsant agents have been effective (Chow and Goldman, 2007; Fleisher, 1994; Fleisher and Matar, 1993)

Pharmacological therapy

Prophylactic inter-episodes:
- anti-migraine medication (Paul *et al.*, 2012; Hikita *et al.*, 2011)
- anticonvulsants (Olmez *et al.*, 2006)
- antidepressants (Kumar *et al.*, 2012; Ghosh *et al.*, 2009)
- supplements (Boles *et al.*, 2010; Boles, 2011).

Prodromal phase:
- abortive anti-emetics.

Acute phase:
- supportive admission for fluids provision, analgesia and sedation.

Psychological therapies

- Cognitive and behavioural therapy and biofeedback (Slutsker *et al.*, 2010)
- Relaxation training, guided imagery and hypnosis (Stein *et al.*, 1997; Fennig and Fennig, 1999)

REFERENCES

Abell TL, Adams KA, Boles RG, *et al.* Cyclic vomiting syndrome in adults. *Neurogastroenterol Motil.* 2008; **20**(4): 269–84.

Boles RG. High degree of efficacy in the treatment of cyclic vomiting syndrome with combined co-enzyme Q10, L-carnitine and amitriptyline, a case series. *BMC Neurol.* 2011; **11**: 102.

Boles R, Lovett-Barr MR, Preston A, *et al.* Treatment of cyclic vomiting syndrome with co-enzyme Q10 and amitriptyline, a retrospective study. *BMC Neurol.* 2010; **10**: 10.

Boles RG, Williams JC. Mitochondrial disease and cyclic vomiting syndrome. *Dig Dis Sci.* 1999; **44**(8 Suppl.): S103–7.

Chow S, Goldman RD. Treating children's cyclic vomiting. *Can Fam Physician.* 2007; **53**(3): 417–19.

Dong M, Li ZH, Li G. [Clinical characteristics of 41 children with cyclic vomiting syndrome] [Chinese]. *Zhonghua Er Ke Za Zhi.* 2008; **46**(6): 450–3.

Drumm BR, Bourke B, Drummond J, *et al.* CVS in children: a prospective study. *Neurogastroenterol Motil.* 2012; **24**(10): 922–7.

Fennig S, Fennig S. Diagnostic delays and dilemmas: management of affected patients in the psychiatric inpatient unit of a general children's hospital. *Gen Hosp Psychiatry.* 1999; **21**(2): 122–7.

Fleisher DR. Cyclic vomiting syndrome. In: Hyman P, DiLorenzo C, editors. *Pediatric GI Motility Disorders.* New York, NY: Academy Professional Information Services; 1994. pp. 89–104.

Fleisher DR. Cyclic vomiting syndrome: a paroxismal disorder of brain-gut interaction. *J Pediatr Gastroenterol Nutr.* 1997; **25**(Suppl. 1): S13–15.

Fleisher DR. *Empiric Guidelines for the Management of Cyclic Vomiting Syndrome*. Columbia, MO: author; 2008. Available at: www.cvsa.org.uk/downloads/Fleisherguidlines.pdf (accessed 14 January 2014).

Fleisher DR, Matar M. The cyclic vomiting syndrome: a report of 71 cases and literature review. *J Pediatr Gastroenterol Nutr*. 1993; **17**(4): 361–9.

Forbes D, Fairbrother S. Cyclic nausea and vomiting in childhood. *Aust Fam Physician*. 2008; **37**(1–2): 33–6.

Ghosh JB, Roy M, Peters T. Cyclic vomiting syndrome responding to amitryptiline. *Indian J Pediatr*. 2009; **76**(12): 1261–2.

Hikita T, Kodama H, Kaneko S, *et al*. Sumatriptan as a treatment for cyclic vomiting syndrome: a clinical trial. *Cephalalgia*. 2011; **31**(4): 504–7.

Kumar N, Bashar Q, Reddy N, *et al*. Cyclic vomiting syndrome (CVS): is there a difference based on onset of symptoms–pediatric versus adult? *BMC Gastroenterol*. 2012; **12**: 52.

Lee LY, Abbott L, Mahlangu B, *et al*. Management of CVS: a systematic review. *Eur J Gastroenterol Hepatol*. 2012; **24**(9): 1001–6.

Li BU. Cyclic vomiting syndrome. *Curr Treat Options Gastroenterol*. 2000a; **3**: 395–402.

Li BU, Lefevre F, Chelinsky GG, *et al*. North American Society for Pediatric Gastroenterology, Hepatology and Nutrition consensus statement on the diagnosis and management of cyclic vomiting syndrome. *J Pediatr Gastroenterol Nutr*. 2008; **47**(3): 379–93.

Li BU, Murray RD, Heitlinger LA, *et al*. Is cyclic vomiting syndrome related to migraine? *J Pediatr*. 1999; **134**: 567–72.

Olmez A, Köse G, Turanli G. Cyclic vomiting with generalized epileptiform discharges responsive to topiramate therapy. *Pediatr Neurol*. 2006; **35**(5): 348–51.

Olson A, Li BU. Diagnostic workup of children with cyclic vomiting: a cost-effectiveness analysis. *J Pediatr*. 2002; **141**(5): 724–8.

Paul SP, Barnard P, Soondrum K, *et al*. Antimigraine (low-amine) diet may be helpful in children with cyclic vomiting syndrome. *J Pediatr Gastroenterol Nutr*. 2012; **54**(5): 698–9.

Sato T, Igarashi M, Minami S, *et al*. Recurrent attacks of vomiting, hypertension, and psychotic depression: a syndrome of periodic catecholamine and prostaglandin discharge. *Acta Endocrinol (Copenh)*. 1988; **117**(2): 189–97.

Slutsker B, Konichezky A, Gothelf D. Breaking the cycle: cognitive behavioral therapy and biofeedback training in a case of cyclic vomiting syndrome. *Psychol Health Med*. 2010; **15**(6): 625–31.

Stein MT, Katz RM, Jellinek MS, *et al*. Cyclic vomiting. *J Dev Behav Pediatr*. 1997; **18**(4): 267–70.

Sunku B. Cyclic vomiting syndrome: a disorder of all ages. *Gastroenterol Hepatol*. 2009; **5**(7): 507–15.

Talbert DG. Cyclic vomiting syndrome: contribution to dysphagic infant death. *Med Hypotheses*. 2009; **73**(4): 473–8.

Venkatesan T, Tarbell S, Adams K, *et al*. A survey of emergency department use in patients with cyclic vomiting syndrome. *BMC Emerg Med*. 2010; **10**: 4.

Wood JD. Enteric nervous control of motility in the upper gastrointestinal tract in defensive states. *Dig Dis Sci*. 1999; **44**(8 Suppl.): S44–52.

3.4: Functional gastrointestinal disorders: a case example

Compiled by Clarissa Martin

Dear Mrs

Re: YP (a Young Person who is 14 years old)

Thank you for contacting us for advice regarding YP's longstanding abdominal pain.

You told us that YP had been seen by numerous doctors and specialists over a 2- to 3-year period. Medical tests conducted included MRI, scan, ultrasound scans and X-rays. However, all of them had returned clear, indicating that YP's pain was not a symptom of any identified medical illness. Your child was seen by a consultant paediatric gastroenterologist at the Hospital of North-East Area. During your conversation with this doctor our services were recommended mainly due to lack of paediatric psychology resources in your geographical area. We informed you that we only provide paediatric community support services for families living within the South-West area.

Understandably, you feel desperate, moving from one health professional to another while YP is in pain and YP's quality of life is deteriorating. YP has now been out of school since last Christmas and is no longer seeing friends. We then offered a complimentary and urgent appointment for you and your family. In our phone conversation I also stated that through listening to your narratives and in absence of underlined medical illness, my first thinking was that perhaps YP was suffering a functional gastrointestinal disorder (FGID). I sent you some web links for you to be familiar with this condition. I also stated that the pathophysiology of FGID was not well understood but research indicates that it may involve changes in the brain–gut axis, visceral hypersensitivity and abnormal gut motility, with stress being a contributory factor. You found this information helpful.

You attended the appointment with YP. We agreed that the aim for this appointment was for me to explore the background information of YP and discuss with you my first tentative formulation regarding YP's current difficulties, while also suggesting a potential initial management plan. You and YP agreed with this approach. No further appointments were booked and we agreed that all information gathered during this consultation was going to be sent to North-East health services.

Family background and early development
You family unit includes you, your husband and YP. Your pregnancy proceeded without complications. However, YP was born with the umbilical cord around

her neck. You also recall YP having had breathing difficulties. YP remained in the hospital neonatal unit for 1 week. YP was bottle-fed and struggled with feeding. YP presented problems during the weaning phase. You were concerned that YP emptied her bowels frequently as a baby and you sought medical advice for this. Later, when YP was a toddler she suffered from constipation, requiring hospital admission for a clearance of faecal impaction. I understand from you that YP also suffers some food allergies and intolerances.

YP found difficulties adapting to nursery and you stated that this seemed to be related to separation anxiety issues. This is a pattern that repeated when YP started school. However, YP was sociable and made friends. You describe YP as a child with good academic performance. You have always received very positive reports from YP's teachers. You feel YP has a tendency to be a perfectionist when completing homework. YP likes arts but owing to the abdominal pain YP has been absent from school for 6 months now.

Social relationships

You stated that social relationships were not a problem for YP in the past. However, YP is currently more focused on communicating only through social networks – mainly Twitter – rather than meeting friends face-to-face. You were concerned about YP's social isolation, which you felt is aggravated by YP's school absence. I was concerned about YP frequenting social networks beyond your control, as YP is a vulnerable minor (vulnerability that is exacerbated by her condition).

Observation

From the beginning and throughout all of our conversation YP remained listening and in silence. YP was seated with her back bent over forwards, forming a strong backbone curvature, and with the arms crossed over her belly. We agreed that this non-verbal language could be interpreted as saying, '*I am in pain*' and it was easy to feel sorry for YP. At some point and when I was questioning YP's access to Twitter YP turned her back towards us and we agreed that this attitude seemed an indication of feeling disappointed. We also agreed that if we ourselves maintained this physical position for a while we would inevitably feel pain.

Listening to your narratives, observing YP's behaviour during consultation and taking into account that no medical illness has been identified, I stated that my *tentative formulation* supported my initial hypothesis of YP potentially suffering a FGID.

Preliminary formulation

There were in YP's history predisposing biological factors that indicate the possibility of being at risk of suffering a FGID at later stages of development. YP found difficulties in feeding, passed liquid stools very frequently and suffered constipation. These could have been initial symptoms of gut motility dysfunction that may have impacted on the brain–gut axis. Visceral sensitivity could also have been present, as YP also suffers from food-related allergies. Obviously suffering physical discomfort from early stages of development makes children feel vulnerable to the environment and they learn to rely on parental presence to feel confident. These factors could explain YP's initial difficulties adapting to the nursery and school environment. It seems that these initial difficulties arose out of underlying emotional insecurity and attachment-related issues, as you have no doubt about YP's cognitive abilities and academic performance is of no concern. All of these things might have precipitated the emergence of personality traits aimed at enabling YP to take greater control of the environment – a response to feeling unsafe. Personality traits of perfectionism are also linked to low self-esteem and poor physical health.

Pain is a complex, multidimensional perception, which is mediated by psychological and situational factors. A critical contributory factor in the distress associated with it is what is known as *'emotional coping'*. It is not surprising therefore that an association between exposure to pain and depression has been reported in the research literature. YP seems to feel hopeless, with low energy and interest in activities and feeling pain. All these features may be symptoms of depression. Understandably, YP has developed an avoidance pattern of behaviour that could have provided YP with some so-called 'secondary gains', such as being at home and having lots of parental attention; secondary gains such as these often play a part in maintaining the behaviour. YP seems trapped in a vicious circle of this learnt avoidance pattern.

This vicious circle permeates the whole family system. You have described how you and your husband are afraid to wake YP up in the morning because she screams and cries; you therefore avoid a situation that is painful for you too. At the same time you also feel trapped, moving around among health professionals and feeling hopeless. However, you have managed to find a way for your family to move forwards and your support towards YP and your family's resilience serve as clear protective factors.

Recommendations
We discussed this tentative formulation and it seemed that it made sense for all of us. You also asked if it would be appropriate to ask the doctor to prescribe stronger pain medication, as YP had stopped taking the one initially prescribed on the grounds that it was not working. I stated that medication for pain and depression may help to alleviate symptoms but it does not change behaviour that contributes to the perception of pain. It is common in these cases to conclude that painkillers are not helping. They should be considered as a first step. This made sense for you, as this reflected your own experience.

Taking all of this into consideration my first recommendations were:
- for YP to have a full, in-depth assessment of all factors identified in the formulation to verify the initial hypothesis
- for YP's *depression symptoms to be evaluated* for mental health practitioners in your area as an *urgent matter*
- to complete a psychological assessment of YP to enable an appropriate

intervention and treatment programme to be designed tailored to YP's specific needs
- to set up a liaison and communication plan between health professionals and school staff in order to help YP to return to the school in a step-by-step format
- to deliver a Health Education intervention for YP and your family – this would help all of you to show consistency in supporting YP to move forwards
- to implement a psychological intervention for pain and depression symptoms
- this intervention in pain should follow current research findings and guidelines that recommend a combination of pain management strategies and cognitive behavioural therapy for the management of child and adolescent chronic pain.

We also agreed on the following *management strategies* recommended with the aim to stop the situation deteriorating. These strategies may be set in motion while waiting for arrangements for YP to have access to the psychological assessment and treatment.
- We agreed to write this letter for you with copies to be sent to health professionals in the North-East Area in order to facilitate discussion.
- You also are going to share this letter with YP's school head teacher to urgently apply for home tuition. This will help YP to maintain current academic level.
- You are also going to make arrangements with YP's school to facilitate YP's attendance at art classes, as YP enjoys this. In doing so we are maintaining a minimum baseline in order to help YP to return to full school attendance in the near future.
- You husband and you are going to discuss with YP a timetable according to what YP is able to do – for example. waking up in the morning, washing and self-grooming, coming downstairs instead of providing breakfast for YP in her bedroom, and so forth. This will provide YP with a minimum sense of purpose for every day.
- This timetable will include social activities – for example, inviting friends to spend Friday afternoons with YP and then they could enjoy social networks together, and so forth.
- Twitter would be allocated within family activities to allow parental control and mitigate social isolation.

At the end of our consultation you stated that it had been very useful for both of you and you felt helped. No further questions were raised at the time.
   I hope everything outlined here may be of help to you.

Yours sincerely,
Consultant Paediatric Clinical Psychologist

3.5: Example of tube-weaning feeding therapy at inpatient setting

3.5a: Inpatient behavioural protocol

Terence Dovey and Clarissa Martin

NOTES: FIRST OBSERVATION SESSION

C is a 5-year-old Caucasian child who loves socialising, attention from adults and craftwork. She also likes a lot of physical contact and 'roughhousing'.

C's natural behaviour profile throughout the day can be defined by periods of hyperactivity and calm engagement with activity. The mum reported that this behaviour was related to when she thought C was hungry. *It would appear that C has learnt that being hungry is related to hyperactivity.* This has become problem behaviour and is directly related to the 'slowness' of C drinking the PediaSure. The consumption of PediaSure takes anything between 10 and 90 minutes to drink a small bottle. While drinking, C has to be constantly reminded to take a sip. C appears to take in a normal amount of fluid and holds it in the mouth for a while before swallowing. Another behaviour noticed was that C also takes constant tiny sips of fluid. These all appear to be learnt behaviours. During this observation session, C's mum had to leave the room. C still had half a bottle left (around 60 minutes after our arrival). While the mother was out of the room, C wanted to hide from mum. The therapist stated that they could not play unless C had finished her drink. Although C failed to drink it all within the 3 minutes the mother was out of the room, C did finish it within a minute of her returning. Therefore, with motivation C could drink the PediaSure very quickly.

Consistent consumption of the PediaSure within 10 minutes seems a viable objective.

C has already developed *some preferences* towards tastes and foods and likes the taste of the following items:
- fish fingers (only the breadcrumbs around the outside – she will not eat the fish itself)
- toast (favourite item)
- wraps (anything can be put in a wrap and she will eat some of it.
- tomato soup
- bacon sandwiches
- BBQ sauce – only on Chinese ribs
- yogurt
- baked beans
- some vegetables

- crisps (Doritos, cheese and onion, flame grilled steak)
- apples
- sausages.

C does not like:
- ice cream
- carrots
- chocolate
- cheese.

The mum suggested that C's likes are defined by savoury tastes. Therefore, sweet foods may be avoided in the sessions.

C's daily cycle of activities is as follows: C is generally *tube-fed* three times a day: (1) at 7.30 a.m., (2) between 1.30 and 3 p.m. and (3) at 7 p.m. The daily hyperactive phase starts at 4.30 p.m. and ends at 6 p.m. This appears to coincide exactly with when C is given her PediaSure drink.

We would hypothesise at this point that after school C is hungry, as this is the longest duration that C goes while awake without calories. What we can learn here is that C is going to engage in hyperactivity when we start to lower her tube-feeds. This is going to be a problem in two ways: (1) she will be expending calories and (2) her hyperactivity will interfere with her eating behaviour.

We are unsure how C will respond to a 'no, no' command. According to the mother it is likely that C will not respond favourably. *Managing C's behaviour within the mealtime context is going to be through careful management of the contingencies.* The intervention is likely to work best if we allow C to win quickly at first and deliver the preferred activity very quickly. Craft activities or DVDs will provide sufficient motivation for the duration of the meal. It is important that C gets to choose the task. If C does not complete what is asked then the day should carry on without the preferred activity. C responds well to not achieving the tasks and the consequence of not getting what C wants. C also responds well to token reward systems. In C's school there is a gold star badge that is awarded each week to two students. Currently, C is the reigning gold badge owner and C likes that a lot.

There is a 'secret weapon' in terms of C's eating behaviour that we should also be aware of. C's food preference mirrors C's dad's. *It would appear that whatever the dad eats seems to be the foods that C will eat too.* C's preferences for food do appear to align with C's dad's favourite foods. C has learnt these preferences through imitation. C will readily take and ask for a selection of foods that C's dad eats. It may be beneficial to encourage C to eat the foods presented by telling her that these are now C's dad's favourite foods and to involve C's dad in choosing foods especially for her. If this is coupled with someone else to mimic then C could be likely to try the food. However, some foods are incongruent here, such as preference for savoury items and liking tomatoes, BBQ sauce and bacon. All of these foods are strong flavours and are hard to eat. Dad turned up right at the end of the session and we wonder if it might be worth taking his preferences and aim at these?

In terms of a functional diet then, we would like to run a programme of at least six opportunities per day. The choice at breakfast would be toast, cereal or bacon sandwiches. C can and has eaten toast in the past. Therefore, this should be the starting breakfast food. Mid-morning snack could be either yogurt or fruit. Lunch would be sandwiches or soup (tomato). We could start with tomato soup. We would like to add croutons or bread to this meal over the first few days as well as increase the quantity of the fluid. The mid-afternoon snack should be crisps (McCoy's or Doritos). The evening meal could be a variety of different foods including casseroles or lasagne. We like the idea of the casserole, as it is easy to consume, the food can be overcooked and therefore be soft for C to cope with. C's mum struggled to define what would be a good evening snack. We think that this could be adapted to perhaps a hot calorific milky drink such as hot Ovaltine with something on the side.

The PediaSure is currently given to C before the evening meal. C only has one per day. This we believe is interfering with eating at the meal by filling C up and denying C natural motivators. We would like to allocate these after each meal. They should come after the preferred activity and can be done in other classes. We should aim for a functional diet first and use the PediaSure as a back-up. If we go for the PediaSure first, then we will find it difficult to achieve oral eating, as she will be full of the sugary liquid.

Our initial thoughts would be a **changing criterion design**. With C having to eat progressively more food each session (by day) that coincides with the decrease in the tube-feeds. If C achieves the replacement of the calories through oral eating then C gets the reward activity. We would like to check her chewing ability though before we write more about this intervention.

Problem behaviours that have been observed in the past that might interfere with the intervention:
- oral sensitivity on the sides of her mouth and back teeth
- gagging and retching
- defiance.

We will need to come with a routine to stop each of these behaviours as they arise. Just in case we have these as escape-maintained behaviours.

NOTES: SECOND OBSERVATION SESSION

C's jaw strength and ability to chew was checked.

C can bite using either the sides (back teeth) or the front of the mouth (using front teeth). This was tested this with Haribo jelly sweets. Therefore, C has shown to have the strength to chew tough foods, but C has not shown having the stamina to eat for long periods of time. In terms of tongue control, we learnt two things in this session. First, C will now freely touch the sides of the mouth with the tongue and will get little bits of food out of the sides of the mouth (between teeth and cheek). C's mother has worked on this as asked and C shows large improvements. The second thing was that C will engage in behaviours that C has previously refused to exhibit, as long as you give C a little time to think about it. On the first try of asking C to use the tongue to touch the sides of the mouth C refused. After a couple of minutes playing, C was asked in a tone of 'about to ask a question' and C automatically did it. This suggests that to request a behaviour from C will require patience and soft tone to get positive outcomes without having to reprimand. C is very willing to please and, therefore, giving her a little time to think about things that C does not necessarily want to do can prove dividends for control of C's behaviour.

Additional problem behaviours observed during the second assessment session was that C will 'secret away' foods that C is asked to eat. C will spit them into the hand and will hold them until C can put them somewhere when C thinks you are not looking. This can be readily countered and is frequently observed in all clinically relevant eating problems from anorexia nervosa to feeding disorders. Careful observation and subtle checking around where C is eating will eliminate this behaviour, as long as the right contingencies are in play.

QUANTITIES OF FOODS TO EAT BASED ON THE SPEED OF THE WEANING
Based on the information provided by C's mother, C will start the tube-weaning process in an energy deficit of 250 cals. *C's usual feeding regimen* is:
- through the tube: two 260 mL bolus (260 cals each) daily and 150 cals at night
- PediaSure: one 200 mL bottle (300 cals)
- Total Habitual Calorie Intake = 970 cals.

Upon presentation she will have had her feeds decreased to:
- 160 cals twice daily and 100 cals at night
- PediaSure: one 200 mL bottle (300 cals)
- Total Presentation Calorie Intake = 920 cals.

That would be an initial deficit of **250 cals** against habitual intake.
    The energy density of the initial target foods is as follows:
- white bread (toasted), 267 cals per 100 g
- tomato soup, 52 cals per 100 g
- mashed potato (5 g butter, 7 g milk), 104 kcals per 100 g.

That would leave a target for Day 1 as:
- 25 g of bread (half a slice of thick-cut bread)
- 100 g of tomato soup (quarter of a can)
- 150 g of mashed potato (total intake of 269 cals).

Of course, this is based solely on the target foods. C will be given the opportunity to eat other food items, however, these will be deemed as extra calories outside of the target. The energy values are based on the average branded food items available in the United Kingdom. It is expected there might be some minor variation in the energy content of the foods. For every 250 cals of food removed from C's diet, the target that day will increase to accommodate. This will be worked out at the end of each day to ensure that C has a balanced energy equation for the day (balanced is defined as compared to habitual calories rather than against activity).

INTERVENTION FOR PROBLEM BEHAVIOUR WHEN OBSERVED
Oral sensitivity on the sides of her mouth and back teeth
The behaviours observed in oral sensory sensitivity are expressed in the following sequence:

> C becomes distressed; C tries to get your attention; C puts her hand in her mouth; C sticks her tongue out and starts scraping it with her finger (even if the food is stuck in the teeth); C gags and retches; C vomits.

To counter this problem behaviour
A behavioural protocol to get C using her tongue more is already set in place. This was to place small items of food in the sides of C's mouth between the back teeth and the cheek. C was then asked to use the tongue to 'get them out' from there. C is getting better at this. As C gets better, C should have the skill to effectively (1) desensitise and (2) get the food out from wherever it is 'stuck'.

This problem has also manifest in C's teeth cleaning regimen. I have asked C's mum to increase the duration of teeth cleaning and to use the brush (and get C to use the brush) on C's back teeth more. This will also be worked on in the hospital by the play specialists focusing specifically on the very back of C's teeth. As C engages in this behaviour more, C should readily accept foods on her back teeth, which will help to chew it thoroughly.

If this appears during a meal
Interruption routine: C will become distressed and so a calm approach will be necessary. In a calm tone simply state '*show me where it is stuck*' and inform her that she should use her tongue first to get it out. If that does not work then tell C to use the fingers to pick it out. If that also fails then it may be worth showing C how to use a toothpick. By teaching this alternative and functionally appropriate behaviour, it should stop all future episodes of the behavioural escalation. I would like the hospital play specialists to have a session in addition to the tooth brushing on how to use a toothpick. If they are unable then prior to starting on any foods that have the possibility to get stuck in C's teeth, then it would be appropriate to task analyse this and have a session teaching C the behaviour.

An example task analysis for this intervention can be found in Table 3.5A.1. The psychologist can do this.

Summary

- Play therapist to teach tooth brushing
- Play therapist or psychologist to teach how to use a toothpick
- Psychologist to interrupt behavioural escalation by stating, 'it's OK, use your tongue, then use your finger, then use a toothpick'.

TABLE 3.5A.1 Task analysis for using a toothpick with C

Task analysis for using a toothpick

Step	Command	Topography to achieve
1	Open container	Open container (use finger to push the middle of the box on one side to reveal contents)
2	Select	Select toothpick (remove one toothpick from the container)
3	Check it	If any damage/faults can be seen with the selected toothpick then discard (throw toothpick in bin)
		If completely straight without any faults then continue
4	Hold it correctly	Hold toothpick at one end using thumb and forefinger
5	Put in mouth	Place toothpick on the front tooth of the offending jaw
6	Find the food	Lightly move toothpick along the teeth until it rests on the tooth closest to the trapped food
7	Put the toothpick next to your gum	Lightly move the toothpick to the top of the gum line where gum and tooth meet
8	Put the toothpick on the trapped food	Lightly slide the toothpick until it rests in the gap between the teeth and rests on the gum line
9	Scrape the food out	Using the end of the toothpick, try to dislodge the food item by scraping the gap between the teeth in a downward motion
10	Repeat	Repeat the last step five times
11	Push the food through to the other side	If this fails to remove the offending item then gently insert toothpick between the gap of the teeth to try to push the trapped item through to the other side
12	Spit it out or swallow it	Spit out or swallow the freed food item
13	Ok let's go brush your teeth	If this fails go brush teeth.

Gagging and retching

C's gagging and retching behaviours are functional in nature and are probably related to escape. It is important that we view this as a multifaceted behaviour and not confuse it between one of three different situations. These are (1) as part of the previous behavioural escalation, (2) as escape from mealtime and (3) as a functional behaviour for when food is stuck in the throat. It is important to spot which behaviour it is. In all situations, do not allow C to escape from the mealtime.

The first function should not occur as long as the interruption routine is in place and C has not got food stuck in the mouth. The second should be stopped through escape extinction – C is not allowed to leave the table or the mealtime if gagging or retching. If C gags to escape the mealtime, then the therapist will interrupt the behaviour through a 'no, no' routine. The third potential explanation of the behaviour is that food gets stuck in her throat. This is a functional outcome and should not be responded to at all. C has got scarring in her oesophagus that has caused some narrowing. We are not sure at this time how it will affect C's ability to swallow. This will be considered later in more detail; however, at this point, it is important that every time C has a solid piece of food to also encourage C to drink a sip of cola in order to aid in pushing the food down.

Summary
- To be aware that this behaviour is multifunctional.
- To respond with either a 'no, no' routine or the instruction to 'drink a sip of cola'.

Defiance
This is a rare behaviour for C, but it is likely to surface at some point in the protocol. C engages in this behaviour generally when scared or wants to do something else. It is important that C understands that oral eating comes before all activities. This will take some time to instil and will also require a generalisation routine beyond the hospital stay. During the hospital stay this can be dealt with through an escalation routine of our own. This would be:
- redirection back to task with the contingency that we will do what she wants after the meal
- 'no, no' routine with the statement that C is being naughty
- remove all social attention until C sits back down and starts eating again. Upon which time C immediately gets lots of attention again.

Summary
- To redirect, 'no, no' then ignore and turn away from C if defiant.

TABLE 3.5A.2 Schedule of daily activities with indicative time

Time of day	Activity
8–9 a.m.	Cystic fibrosis treatment
9–9.10 a.m.	Breakfast
9.10–9.25 a.m.	Reward time
9.25–9.30 a.m.	Brushing teeth
9.30–10.30 a.m.	Tube-feed and play therapist time
10.30–11.30 a.m.	School

(continued)

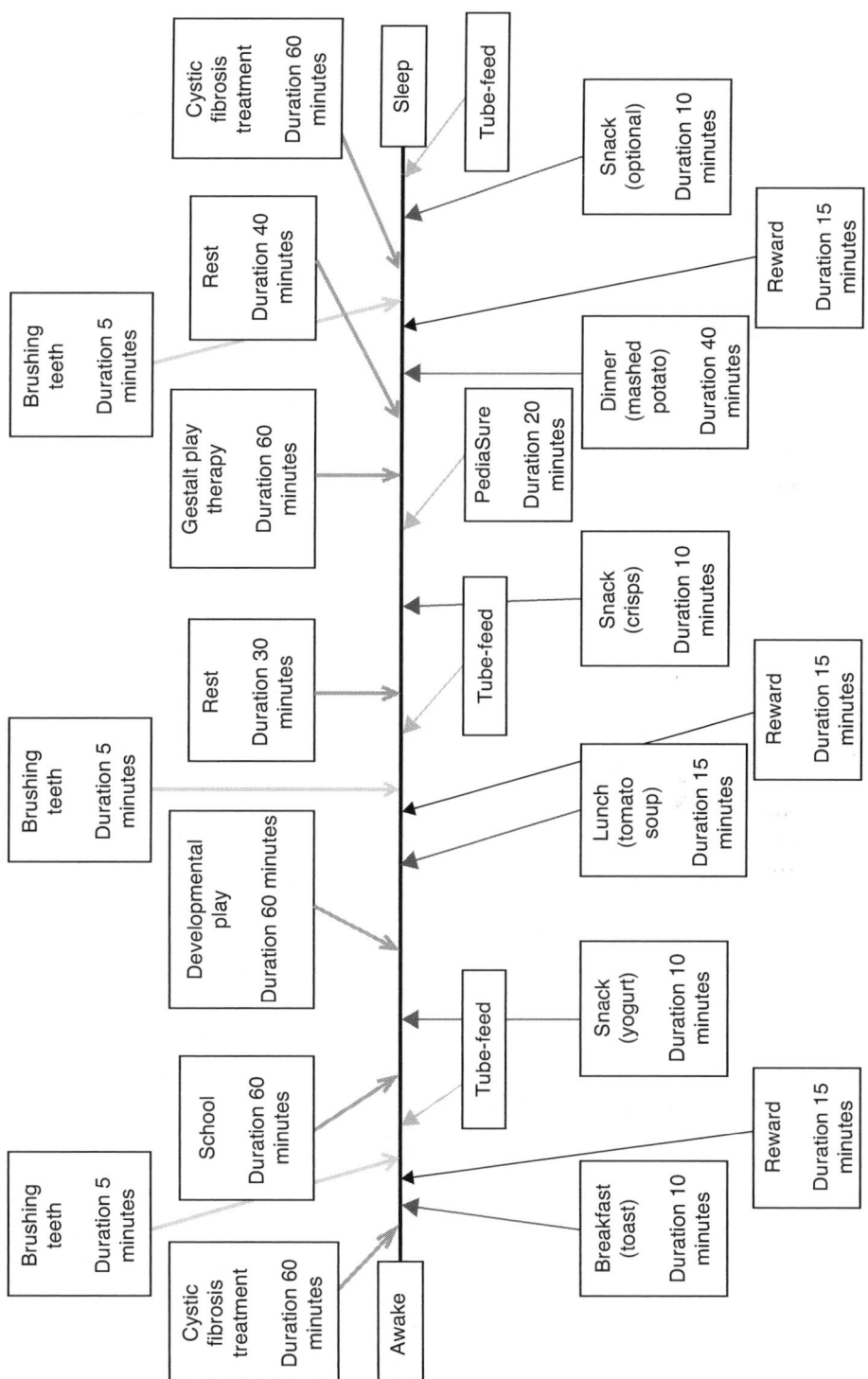

FIGURE 3.5A.1 The daily schedule for C

Time of day	Activity
11.30–11.40 a.m.	Snack
11.45 a.m.–12.45 p.m.	Developmental play
1–1.15 p.m.	Lunch
1.15–1.30 p.m.	Reward time
1.30–1.35 p.m.	Brushing teeth
1.35–2.35 p.m.	Tube-feed and play therapist time
2.35–3 p.m.	Rest
3–3.10 p.m.	Snack
3.10–3.30 p.m.	PediaSure
3.30–4.30 p.m.	Gestalt play therapy
4.20–5 p.m.	Rest
5–5.40 p.m.	Dinner
5.40–5.55 p.m.	Reward time
5.55–6 p.m.	Brushing teeth
6–7 p.m.	Cystic fibrosis treatment
7–7.30 p.m.	Optional snack with mum
7.30–8.30 p.m.	Tube-feed

THE INTERVENTION

Based on all of the information gathered about C and relating this to a 'real world' set of contingencies then we would like to use a Kinder Surprise-style intervention for C. What I mean by Kinder Surprise-style intervention is that C will get a tangible reward related to 'making' something using 'arts and crafts' if C achieves a preset amount of food designated at the beginning of the meal. The reference to the Kinder Surprise egg is that the child has to eat the chocolate first before receiving a toy that more often than not they have to build. This should play into activities that C finds naturally rewarding and by making these contingent on eating behaviour should increase the likelihood that C will eat larger quantities of food. The amount required to eat during the first meal will be offset by the amount C is receiving through her tube – this is important, as C will struggle to eat if she is already receiving calories through the tube. A discussion with hospital dietitian is necessary to set the exact amount required while feeds are being delivered. Until then, the amounts offered are only indicative. For this intervention to work effectively, it is important that all other arts and craft activities are limited during C's stay in the hospital. We need to make sure that C understands that activities that C likes happen after eating. C must understand the contingency of the arrangement. If C is given an art and craft activity at other time points then the reward routine may not work. The art and craft will be limited to the main meal of the day. C's strongest desires will need to link to the situation when the most calories are available.

Breakfast

Day 1: 7 a.m. (or 30 minutes before first tube-feeding)

C is asked to complete a preference test before the meal. Provide C with a list of three activities and place them on the table. The list of activities that C can draw upon for breakfast is a 15-minute DVD or one episode (Peppa Pig, Scooby-Doo, Thomas the Tank Engine), 15 minutes of playing whatever game C would like to or drawing/colouring.

The target food for breakfast in the first week is toast.

The rules for breakfast on Day 1 are as follows.

- C must eat half a slice of toast in 10 minutes
- After every bite C must take a sip of drink (cola or juice – C gets to choose)
- If C does this then C gets the chosen reward
- If C does not achieve the target then C does not get the reward and the day continues on from that point (i.e. going for tube-feeding and then to hospital school).

ADDITIONAL NOTE

I would also like C to wear a badge depending on how well she did on the last meal. The badges are based on what C likes at school. C loves getting gold stars. So this is what we will do too. There will be three levels of stars: Bronze, Silver and Gold. Gold is for C to wear if meets the objective. Silver is if C manages to meet the target amount of food outside of the time limit (so if the time runs out we can tell C that we are still playing for a silver star). Bronze is for if C manages to eat some of the food but not enough quantity. At the beginning of each meal/snack, C will be asked to give back the star and C has to 'win' it back. These 'stars' are very important, because I would like everyone who meets C to make a really big fuss if they see the gold star, a little fuss if they see the silver and no-fuss if they see the bronze. So how this will look is that staff members who meet C will greet C first before anyone else if they see a gold star. They will tell C, *'wow, gold star, you must have eaten all of your food and in time. You are a really good.'* If the silver then staff will greet C second after the therapist or whoever is with C and say, *'silver, you must have eaten all your food – that's good. Next time you just have to eat a little faster for the gold.'* And when bronze, then staff will acknowledge S but will not give C any praise. If C tries to interact with you, say, *'ah well, bronze star, I guess you ate some. I hope you can try harder next time, you'll do that for me won't you, C?'* If there are no stars at all then everyone must ignore C completely. If C persists then say, *'we only talk to children with stars'.*

It is important that everyone involved in this intervention is aware of these requirements, as we need to explain this protocol to C. We need to be able to control the quality of the interaction between C and hospital staff. This plays on C's preference for attention from adults.

Day 2: 7 a.m.

- *C must eat half a slice of toast in 10 minutes*
- After every bite C must take a sip of drink (cola or juice – C gets to choose)
- If C does this then C gets the chosen reward
- If C does not achieve the target then C does not get the reward
- Star awarded depending on outcome

Day 3: 7 a.m.

- *C must eat three-quarters of a slice of toast in 10 minutes*
- After every bite C must take a sip of drink (cola or juice – C gets to choose)
- If C does this then C gets the chosen reward
- If C does not achieve the target then C does not get the reward
- Star awarded depending on outcome

Day 4: 7 a.m.

- *C must eat a slice of toast in 10 minutes*
- After every bite C must take a sip of drink (cola or juice – C gets to choose)
- If C does this then C gets the chosen reward
- If C does not achieve the target then C does not get the reward
- Star awarded depending on outcome

ADDITIONAL NOTE

The amount that C is required to eat within the breakfast environment will be adapted based on performance. C can only move on to the next target when completing the last. So C can only move on to half a slice if C has a gold star from the previous day's breakfast where C ate a quarter of a slice.

One slice of toast for breakfast is a functional and socially acceptable breakfast. C should easily be able to accomplish this target. After the second day of achieving a whole slice of toast the reward choice at the beginning of the meal will be thinned to a FR3 scale (fixed ratio 3: to provide reinforcement for every three times she eats the whole slice) and just the stars will remain on a FR1. C will also now be offered a choice of which food she would like for breakfast from a choice of three (toast, cereal, bacon sandwich). When a new food is offered then a reward schedule comes back for a large target quantity. There is no need to increase the amount C is required to eat. This is because C is not being tube-fed at this time and has chosen the target food.

If we get an 'amazing' day then we must not go off this reward routine. C will always be rewarded for achieving the increments laid out here and not based on the previous behaviour. For example, if on Day 1 C eats all of the toast in 10 minutes, then this does not mean the next day that C has to replicate it. If C eats the preset amount then C is rewarded with the star at that point. Feel free to encourage C to continue to eat until 10 minutes are up and after that point give C the reward task.

PediaSure

The PediaSure is only to be introduced following the meal and only when the tube-feeds are at zero. C will take one PediaSure a day in the first instance at 4.30 p.m. When the tube-feeds stops altogether then this will increase to three times a day to be given at the same time instead of the tubes. We could 'replace' the tube routine with a PediaSure routine. A child dependent on PediaSure is not the preferred outcome from a behaviourist perspective; therefore, PediaSure should be treated as a supplement to the diet rather than a replacement for it. C already has a routine of tube-feeding. Once the tube-feeds have stopped then we will put in place an intervention to speed up C's drinking behaviour. Currently it is very slow. I would like C to drink the PediaSure within a 20-minute time limit, while engaged in other tasks – this could be school ones or any activity. C must learn to multitask with the drinking behaviour, as currently the tube-feeding routine means C is removed from the social environment. I do not want C to be removed to drink the PediaSure. I think this is because C drinks small quantities of liquid and does not connect the suck, hold in the mouth, and swallow very well. C will suck a little bit, hold it in the mouth for a few seconds and then eventually swallow. C then does other things until prompted to take a drink again. C needs to be encouraged to engage in these three behaviours in a cycle rather than just once through.

Routine to increase speed of drinking behaviour

The routine for speeding up C's drinking behaviour is relatively simple.

C can and has drunk fluids in the past. The only observable difficulty C has is that C has not managed to link the behaviour together very well and appears to get distracted from it. To engage C in the task, I would like to set this up as a race. The task is to last for a maximum of twenty minutes. The race is to finish the bottle. However, within the context of the race, there is an opportunity to show C how to drink faster. C does not develop a rhythm when drinking and this is the target to achieve. By using a metronome, get C to be drinking to a half second rhythm. The half seconds are defined by three sips (total 1.5 seconds) through the straw, then swallow (0.5 seconds), then breath (0.5 seconds) and then repeat. I believe this may be too quick for C, so we will start off slow with 1.5-second intervals and speed this up across three sessions. Feel free to push C to speed up if doing well. However, within the 'context' of the race, C should naturally do this, as C is about to chain together the individual behaviours. Of course if C wins then 'C is the best!' After three sessions with the therapist we will change the rules so C is racing against a previous time.

SUMMARY
- Sip, sip, sip, swallow, [breath] Sip, sip, sip, swallow [breath], Repeat until finished
- First session (afternoon, Day 1) on a 1.5-second interval
- Second session (afternoon, Day 2) on a 1-second interval
- Third session (afternoon, Day 3) on a 0.5-second interval

Lunch

Day 1: 12 p.m.

The target food for lunch in the first week will be tomato soup (with added ProCal if in calorie deficit from breakfast).

- C must eat quarter of a can of soup within 15 minutes
- If C does this then C gets the chosen reward
- If C does not achieve the target then C does not get the reward
- Star awarded depending on outcome

Day 2: 12 p.m.

- C must eat quarter of a can of soup and quarter of a slice of bread with butter within 15 minutes
- If C does this then C gets the chosen reward
- If C does not achieve the target then C does not get the reward
- Star awarded depending on outcome

Day 3: 12 p.m.

- C must eat quarter of a can of soup and half a slice of bread with butter within 15 minutes
- If C does this then C gets the chosen reward
- If C does not achieve the target then C does not get the reward
- Star awarded depending on outcome

Day 4: 12 p.m.

- C must eat half a can of soup and half a slice of bread with butter within 15 minutes
- If C does this then C gets the chosen reward
- If C does not achieve the target then C does not get the reward
- Star awarded depending on outcome

Day 5: 12 p.m.

- C must eat half a can of soup and three-quarters of a slice of bread with butter within 15 minutes
- If C does this then C gets the chosen reward
- If C does not achieve the target then C does not get the reward
- Star awarded depending on outcome

Day 6: 12 p.m.

- C must eat half a can of soup and three-quarters of a slice of bread with butter within 15 minutes
- If C does this then C gets the chosen reward
- If C does not achieve the target then C does not get the reward
- Star awarded depending on outcome

Day 7: 12 p.m.

- C must eat half a can of soup and one slice of bread with butter within 15 minutes
- If C does this then C gets the chosen reward
- If C does not achieve the target then C does not get the reward
- Star awarded depending on outcome

Dinner

This is the meal when people in the United Kingdom consume the most calories and as such this is the target meal where all of our best reward activities will be placed. All rewards that result in the largest quantity of food eaten in a given meal will be found as the rewards in the evening meal at a higher rate of consistency as the intervention progresses.

The target food for C in the main meal will be mashed potato in the first instance. This is for us to *texture fade* the foods that are 'harder' to eat. Mashed potato provides us with two major advantages: (1) it does not require chewing and (2) we are able to manipulate the calorie content of this food item very easily. Additional foods that C chooses each day should be added to this meal. C has some strong food preferences and this should be encouraged. However, the reward will be dependent on the eating of the mashed potato only for the first 3 days. This is to ensure that we are getting as much calories as possible within the smallest volume.

- C must eat all of the potato presented within 40 minutes
- If C does this then she gets her chosen reward
- If C does not achieve the target then C does not get the reward
- Star awarded depending on outcome; star taken home at the end of the day

After Day 3 and if C has got three gold stars for this meal, then we would move on to other carbohydrate-dense foods. The family eat pasta and this should become a target at some point in the intervention. Employing this as a later target allows us to help C to work on chewing. The target in the meal or snack time is to provide C with someone to imitate chewing the foods presented. C struggles with this and will watch mum chew. C has yet to master this and so it is clear that C is not manipulating food in the mouth very well. It may be necessary to do some 'open-mouth chewing' with C to observe the chewing and let C observe the therapist chewing too. Every time that C chews with the back teeth, therapist will praise C on an FR1 (Fixed ratio 1: continuous reinforcement) schedule. Once C is doing this consistently then we need to move this to an FR3 then FR7 (fixed ratio 3/7: every three/seven times that behaviour is presented)and finally remove it altogether. C must be encouraged to chew using back teeth as much as possible. Success at chewing toast and mashed potato will help for the more complex textures that we can potentially introduce within the intervention. Usually, people chew between 10 and 30 times per mouthful. This number can be used as a guide.

Snacks

Snacks will be one of three items delivered three times a day. The items will be yogurt, an item of fruit or a packet of crisps. C will hand back the star and will be asked to eat the entire amount of food presented in the snack time. No rewards other than the star will be delivered with the snack time. This is for two reasons: (1) snacks are for extra calories and are not the same as a meal. I would like C to learn this and (2) to observe the value C places on the star as currency/control of the behaviour. The reward routine surrounding the snack time may change depending on the value C places on the star. The quantity of the snack time will be increased concomitant with the decrease in the tube-feeds given. Exact quantities will be discussed with the dietitian.

In the first three afternoon snack sessions C will have crisps. This is where we will teach her to chew. Chewing is not an easy process and difficulties are common even in otherwise typically developing children with feeding problems. The chewing routine will be set out through a series of commands and a task analysis (*see* Table 3.5A.3). C will be praised only in this session. There is evidence that praise works in this protocol and I do not want C's behaviour to be overly rewarded in the hospital. The target is eating calories and these will receive the tangible rewards. The task analysis that is offered in Table 3.5A.3 is not entirely complete. It may be required to shape this behaviour through gradually increasing the complexity of this routine.

TABLE 3.5A.3 Task analysis for chewing

Step	Command	Topography to achieve
1	Take a crisp	Select a crisp
2	Put it in the side of your mouth	Place a Dorito crisp on the back molar teeth of the dominant side
3	Bite	Using the back teeth, break a portion of the crisp between the upper and lower jaws
4	Chew	Move jaw up and down in a chewing motion such that the upper and lower teeth make contact once every 1.5 seconds
5	Show me	Open the mouth to inspect the end result and whether it is suitable to swallow
6	Keep chewing or swallow	Depending on the outcome of step 5
7	Repeat steps 1–6 for non-dominant side	Alternate dominant and non-dominant sides
8	Swap it over	Once mastered on both sides add in this command and get C to use her tongue to swap the crisp to the other side of the mouth.

The first step would be to get C to simply crush the food with the back teeth while the feeding therapist holds the food in place. C would be praised every time an audible sound is made as the food is crushed. The second step would be to follow the routine in Table 3.5A.3. Finally, in order to create a functional chewing behaviour, C would have to bite the food off with the front teeth, move the food with the tongue to the back teeth, chew it and then swallow it. This chewing protocol has evidence base behind it and works with children with congenital delay. I expect C to master this very quickly.

TEXTURE FADING WITHIN THE PROTOCOL

Concomitant with the increase in chewing behaviour and endurance, C will be asked to tackle increasingly more difficult textures of the same food item. These will be delivered alongside the previous texture in the first instance. Using potatoes as an example for how this will work in the intervention would be as follows:
- first – mashed potato
- second – baked potato (no skin)
- third – chips
- fourth – roasted.

Therefore, on Days 1–3 C will be asked to consume ever-increasing amounts of mashed potato. Once C is able to successfully chew through a packet of crisps, the potatoes will be phased through the levels offered here. It is important that the food is offered in a scenario of 'as well as' rather than 'as instead of'. We want C to make the link between the products to understand that the word 'potato' comes in different forms and can taste slightly different. This will aid in the script-based categorisation of foods.

In relation to the intervention, C will be given mashed potato until C chews adequately, and then offered baked potato together with the mashed potato. Once C is readily consuming the baked potato the mashed potato will be faded out and replaced with chips alongside the baked potato. The end goal will be to offer C roasted potatoes, although it is not expected that this will be achieved in the inpatient setting. It is likely to require an extended intervention in order to achieve this variety.

A secondary texture fading protocol within the intervention is to transition from soup to sandwiches in the following order:
- first – soup
- second – soup with bread
- third – soup with bread and ham
- fourth – ham sandwiches.

If successful, then C can be readily exposed to other sandwich fillings in order to add variety into the diet. Furthermore, the sandwich will serve as a medium to deliver exposure routines to salad-type food items to eventually work on micronutrient intake.

MEASURABLE DEFINITION OF SUCCESS

Measureable targets to assess within this intervention to 'prove' successful tube-weaning are:

- amount of food consumed (grams)
- amount of liquid consumed (millilitres)
- amount of bites taken and swallowed (count)
- amount of chews per bite of food (average per meal).

This data will be taken for every single item of food that she is presented with. All food must be weighed before it is presented to C and weighed before it is thrown out. A recording sheet will be provided and the feeding therapist in the room will be expected to do this. A measuring cylinder will be available for the fluids too. The bites and chewing behaviour will be recorded from observing the video recording.

Criteria for discharge

The intervention appeared to be successful during the intensive phase. Some minor transitional difficulties were observed and rectified.

Criteria in place for discharge:

- the continuation of the oral eating to meet calorie needs
- the continued spontaneous acceptance of need foods into the diet
- to continue to eat through at least one major insult (acute respiratory infection).

Advice for the tube:

- to leave in place until the criteria for discharge have been met
- six months' duration of oral eating or to continue to eat through two major insults.

TABLE 3.5A.4 Materials: example of record sheet for food intake

Day	Target food	Meal	Fat	Carbohydrate	Protein	Energy	Amount served (g)	Amount left over (g)	Amount ingested (g)	Ingested (kcal)	Bites
1	Toast	Breakfast	8.77	15.2	2.65	146					
	Yogurt	Snack									
	Soup	Lunch	3	5.9	0.8	52					
	Crisps	Snack									
	Mashed potato	Dinner	4.3	15.5	1.8	104					
		Optional									

TABLE 3.5A.5 Example task analysis record sheet for chewing (first two sessions completed at assessment)

Step	Command	Achieved							
		Session 1	Session 2	Session 3	Session 4	Session 5	Session 6	Session 7	Session 8
1	Take a crisp	+	+	+	+	+	+		
2	Put it in the side of your mouth	-	+	+	+	+	+		
3	Bite	-	+	+	+	+	+		
4	Chew	-	-	+	+	+	+		
5	Show me	-	-	+	+	+	+		
6	Keep chewing or swallow	-	-	+	+	+	+		
7	Repeat steps 1–6 for non-dominant side	-	-	+	+	+	+		
8	Swap it over	-	-	+	+	+	+		
				R12	R32	R40	Completed		

3.5b: Tube-weaning feeding therapy

EXAMPLE OF TUBE-FEED REDUCTION, CALORIC RECOUNT AND FOOD SELECTION

Enteral tube-feed nutrition reduction management

Discussion among parents, dietitian and psychologists/feeding therapists allowed to establish a schedule for reduction of feeds, to identify the child's food preferences and to create menus following the child's preferences and a careful counting of calories. A record chart that included 'food offered and consumed' allowed caloric count every day and established the need for introduction of caloric supplements at the end of the day. Target foods and menus were established for every day and behavioural protocol for its consumption was implemented.

TABLE 3.5B.1 Reduction scheduled by dietitian

Days	Reduction of enteral tube-feeds	Notes
Sunday	From ×2 260 mL to 160 mL and ×1 150 mL to 100 mL	
Monday	From ×2 160 mL to 60 mL and ×1 100 mL to 0 mL	First day of admission
Tuesday	Will be 0 mL tube-feeds	To continue with one 200 mL PediaSure a day orally (>300 calories)

TABLE 3.5B.2 List of child's food preferences

Likes	Dislikes
Fish fingers (only the breadcrumbs around the outside)	Ice cream
Tomato soup	Carrots
Toast and **butter**	Chocolate
Yogurt	Cheese
Mashed potato	
Baked beans	
Sausages	

Note: bold indicates selection

Caloric recount

Current feeding regimen

Enteral tube nutrition or tube-feeds:
- two 260 mL bolus (260 cals each) daily and 150 cals at night
- Oral: one 200 mL PediaSure bottle (600 cals)

- Total habitual calorie intake = 1270 cals.

Upon admission

Upon presentation she will have had her feeds decreased to:
- 160 cals twice daily and 100 cals at night
- Oral: one 200 mL PediaSure bottle (600 cals)
- Total presentation calorie intake = 1020 cals.

Summary

That would be an initial deficit of 250 cals against habitual intake.

The initial target foods' energy density for eating orally would be as shown in the table here.

TABLE 3.5B.3 Admission: Day 1

Food	Amount	Kilocalories
White bread (toasted)	25 g (half a slice of thick-cut bread)	267 kcals per 100 g
Tomato soup	100 g (quarter of a can)	52 kcals per 100 g
Mashed potato	150 g (+5 g butter, +7 g milk)	104 kcals per 100 g
		Total: 423 kcals

Menu:
- breakfast – toast and butter
- lunch – tomato soup
- dinner – mashed potato.

3.5c: Results of the inpatient intervention and treatment outcomes

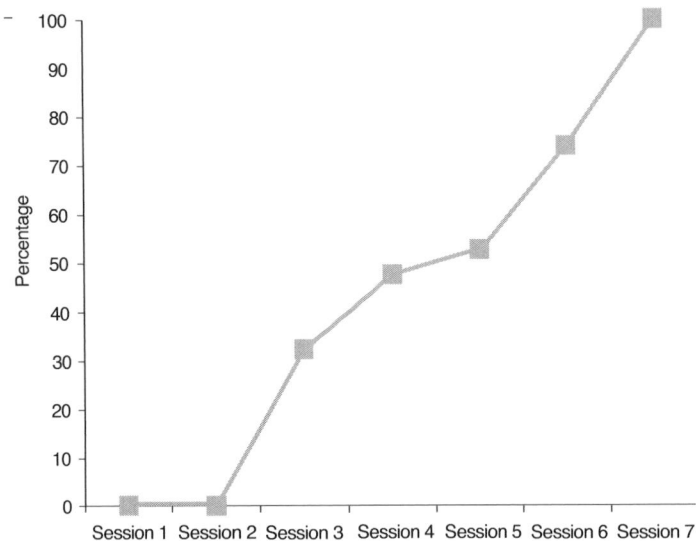

FIGURE 3.5C.1 Results of the chewing task through the percentage consumed of a packet of crisps

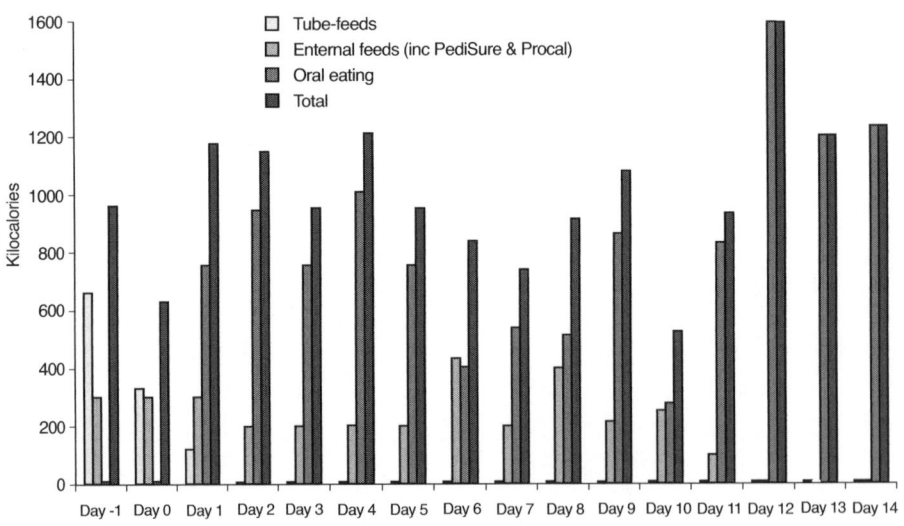

FIGURE 3.5C.2 Total food consumed in kilocalories by the method in which the food was consumed

TABLE 3.5C.1 Novel acceptance of foods after 1 month following intervention

Licked before intensive phase and consumed in sufficient quantity after intervention to sustain growth trajectory	*Novel acceptance 1 month after intensive intervention*
Yogurt	Toast
Sausage	Fish fingers
Mashed potato	Ice cream
Tomato soup	Melon
Bread	Sausage rolls
Doritos	Pasty
McCoy's (steak flavour)	Dairylea Dunkers
Pom Bears (cheese and onion flavour)	Garlic
Bread crumbs	Mini-malted milk biscuits
Wrap	Chocolate
Chicken	Cheese
BBQ sauce	Chicken casserole
Pork ribs	Heinz spaghetti
Spaghetti bolognaise	Pancake
Haribo jelly sweets	Frubes yogurt tube
Bacon	Fish cake
Apples	Carrot stick
Baked beans	Chicken nuggets with BBQ sauce
	Cheese and chive crisps
	Chicken pasties

3.5d: Follow-up: school report

Tania Emiliou

WEANING FROM TUBE-FEEDS: INTEGRATED INTENSIVE INTERVENTION – FOLLOW-UP REPORT

Introduction

Child is a 5-year-old Caucasian child diagnosed with cystic fibrosis who has received nutritional support from birth through artificial feeds (nasogastric and percutaneous endoscopic gastrostomy tubes). *Child* was referred to our Feeding Centre, which offers specialist services to children with complex feeding disorders.

At the Feeding Centre, health professionals assessed her for readiness for tube weaning. This was carried out in the following ways: making a summary of psychological intervention from the outpatient setting, carrying out a parental clinical interview, having discussions with the multidisciplinary team at the cystic fibrosis clinic, doing an updated direct assessment of *Child's* feeding behaviour and by undergoing pre-admission preparations in the form of child psychotherapeutic sessions to support her paediatric traumatic stress residual symptoms.

The results from the assessment indicated that inpatient intensive intervention for tube weaning was appropriate at the current stage. This was judged based on *Child's* ability to eat and drink at the minimum baseline for the intervention; *Child's* family being willing to participate with intensive treatment; having the medical condition stable; feeding behaviour being observable at baseline level; and consensus achieved to aim for oral caloric intake prioritising high-caloric foods. Following admission, *Child's* medical, nutritional, educational, developmental, social-emotional and family needs were all taken into account and cared for.

The intervention carried out involved different psychological techniques used to encourage *Child's* behaviour change. In summary, these were:
- *behaviour intervention* – these were applied at mealtimes to increase independence and age-appropriate self-feeding behaviour using positive reinforcement
- *psychoeducation* – cognitive behavioural techniques such as problem-solving or role play allowed to learn about human body functioning and needs
- *emotional support* – anxieties and fears were able to be expressed in a safe therapeutic context using Gestalt play therapy.

Within these techniques, specific intervention methods were applied in order to suit *Child's* current lifestyle and behaviour. Targets and goals were set for how much *Child* should eat daily. These challenges were reinforced using a reward system involving gold stars. Methods used for this intervention were described as a Kinder Surprise-style intervention, in that she will need to eat the food in order to receive the reward. *Child* was also encouraged to drink more and to increase the speed of drinking behaviour by learning to drink in a rhythm and by taking part in her own drinking race. These types of methods encouraged *Child* to gain confidence and change behaviours around feeding.

Child was discharged from the ward with '*normalised*' eating behaviour and results of intervention were presented to the cystic fibrosis team.

Follow-up sessions took place at *Child's* home and school to monitor generalisation of eating behaviour learnt. At the school, staff were extremely supportive in collecting observable measures of her progress.

Results of follow-up in school setting

At school daily records in the form of a worksheet were completed. The worksheet involved recording meals consumed at school and included information on:

- mealtime (e.g. break or lunch)
- type of food (e.g. crisps)
- food offered (measured in grams)
- food left (measured in grams)
- staff comments on *Child's* behaviour and mood (e.g. happy mood).

The school documented this during a 15-day period. Information was included for break (11.15–11.30 a.m.) and lunchtime (12.30–1.30 p.m.). Data from the 15 days were collected and gathered to create charts displaying *Child's* eating behaviour.

The amount of food that *Child* had been offered and then left was recorded in grams for both break and lunch (e.g. a sausage roll is 160 g). This was then calculated to show how much she had consumed during that time (e.g. she was offered 160 g but she left 20 g, therefore overall she ate 140 g).

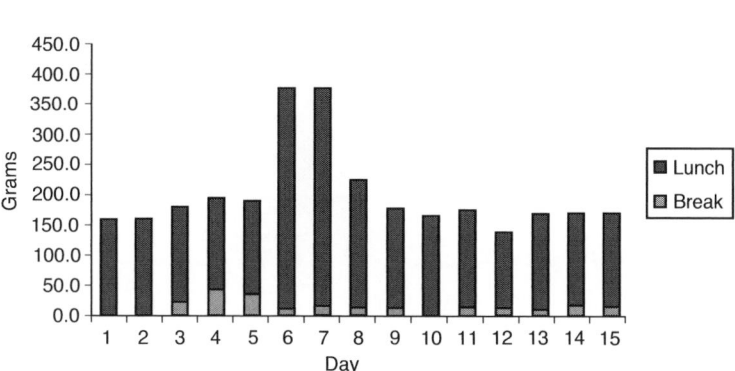

FIGURE 3.5D.1 Amount eaten break and lunch

As shown in the graph, *Child* **managed to eat every day at lunchtime in school** and almost every day at break time. The amount in grams of food consumed overall during both break and lunch varied between 140 and 382 g.

The types of food eaten were also recorded. This was collected and included in the data as the number of different items eaten. This displays the variety of food in *Child's* diet during the period of time the data were collected.

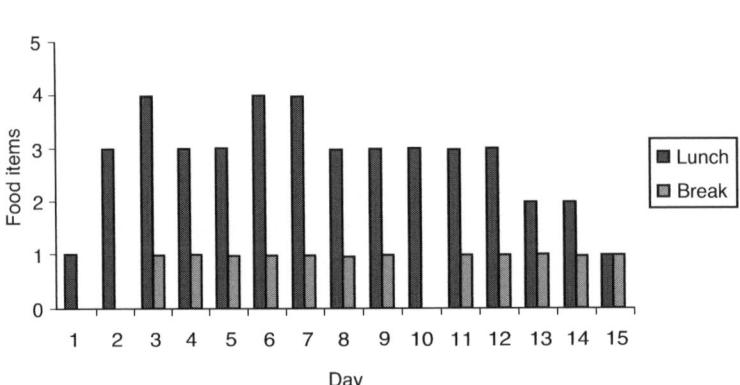

FIGURE 3.5D.2 Number of different types of food eaten

This graph shows that throughout the days *Child* was willing to eat numerous different foods. Break time usually complied with the recommended suggestion of toast. Lunch varied from on certain days having one food type and other days having up to four different types of food. This included a range of different foods such as sausage rolls, yogurt and crisps.

Food offered, eaten and left was recorded and she allowed observation to be made on how much food has been refused or left at the end of the mealtime.

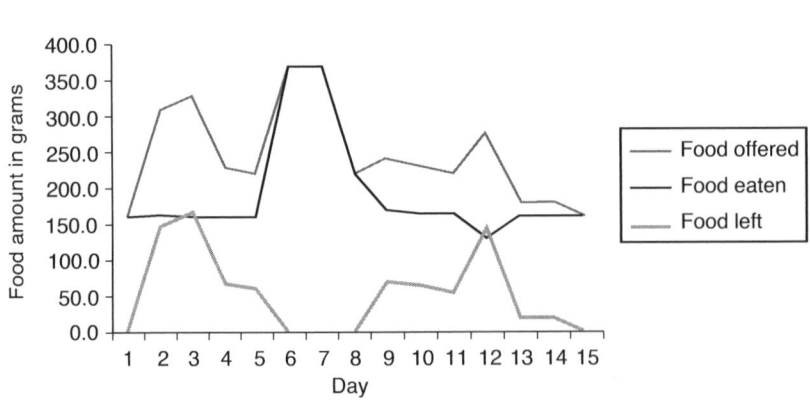

FIGURE 3.5D.3 Food offered, eaten and left at lunch

The line graph for lunch shows that in the majority of mealtimes *Child* was able to eat more food than she left. It also shows that on Days 1, 7, 8 and 9, *Child* finished eating all the food she was offered. The improvement and change in feeding behaviour is clear from the lowest line in the chart indicating food left.

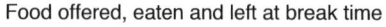

Food offered, eaten and left at break time

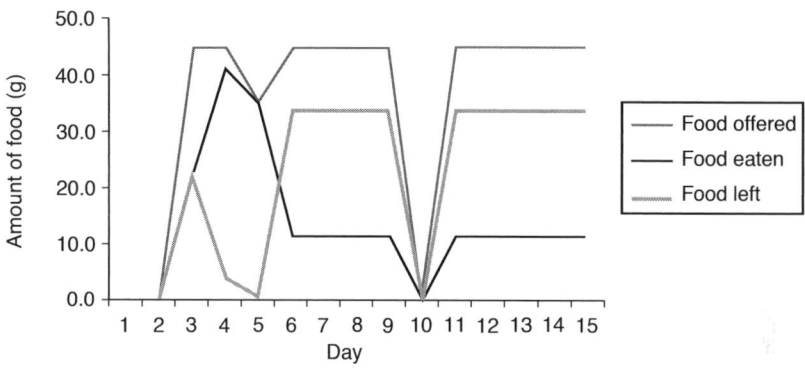

FIGURE 3.5D.4 Food offered, eaten and left at break time

As shown in this graph, eating the amount offered during break time appeared to be more difficult. On most days *Child* left more food than eaten; however, *Child* was still able to eat one-third of the offered toast. On Days 1, 2 and 10 no food was offered or eaten, sometimes because of absence. On some occasions *Child* ate the majority of the food offered. In one case *Child* requested to have a particular type of food (pancake) and ate the entire offered amount.

Total amount eaten recorded per day

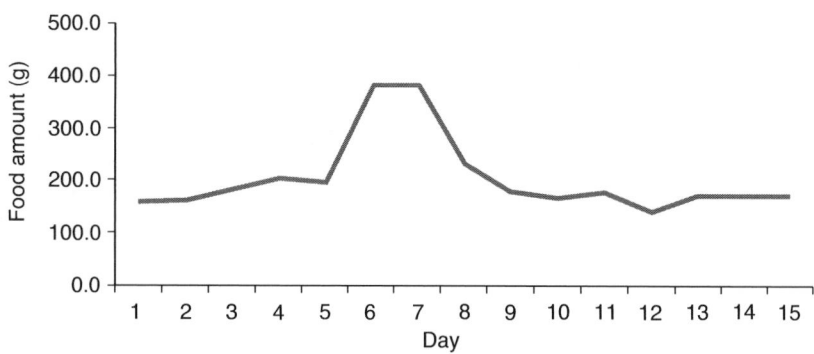

FIGURE 3.5D.5 Total amount eaten recorded per day

The final line graph shows the total amount that was recorded in school as eaten per day. Eating behaviour seems fairly consistent with an increase during Days 6, 7 and 8. Overall, over 100 g was consumed each day during school mealtimes, and in some cases she exceeded this by eating over 300 g of food, displaying a great improvement in feeding behaviour and an ability to eat independently during school time.

Summary

The follow-up showed that the intensive inpatient intervention was successful in teaching *Child* developmental age-appropriate eating behaviour. Furthermore, the behaviours learnt with the implementation of the inpatient feeding programme were generalised outside the hospital environment. *Child* displayed an ability to eat at home and in a school environment, demonstrating feeding behaviour that reflects behaviour considered close to the 'norm' for eating within her age group of reference.

The school *Child* attends was excellent in assisting and reporting mealtime behaviours, making it possible to report the outcome of the intervention and get a good perspective of how *Child's* behaviour has changed. The follow-up report allows furthering appreciation of differences in *Child's* eating behaviour before and after psychological intervention to be clearly defined. Prior to the intervention, *Child* had never eaten at her school premises, as *Child* was being tube-fed. Being unable to eat at school with other children was indeed affecting *Child's* quality of life and relationships with peers. Consistently eating every day at school alongside the other children has increased *Child's* quality of life.

Child has achieved the aims set out for the intervention and this is demonstrated in the follow-up period. The intervention has assisted *Child* in overcoming dependence on bolus feeding, as *Child* is now able to eat normally without the use of artificial feeds or added nutritional supplements. It has also helped to increase confidence in developing age-appropriate feeding behaviour to an extent where *Child* is able to eat normally in different environments such as school and home.

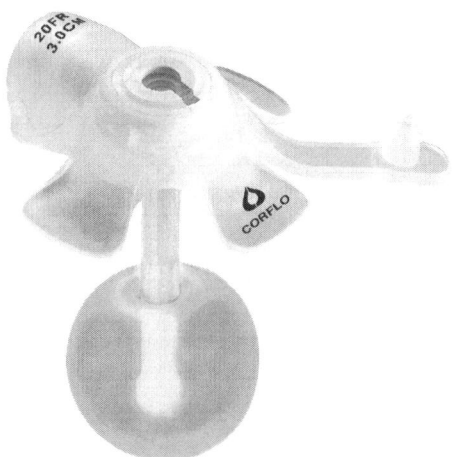

FIGURE 3.5D.6 CORFLO cuBBy Low-Profile Gastrostomy Device (LPGD) (reproduced with the kind permission of CORPAK MedSystems, Buffalo Grove, IL)

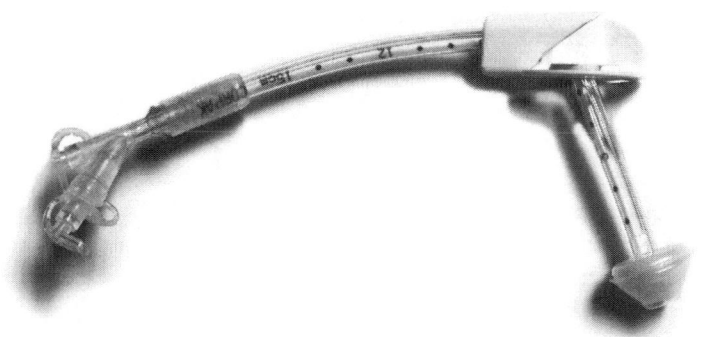

FIGURE 3.5D.7 CORFLO Max Percutaneous Endoscopy Gastrostomy System (PEG) (reproduced with the kind permission of CORPAK MedSystems, Buffalo Grove, IL)

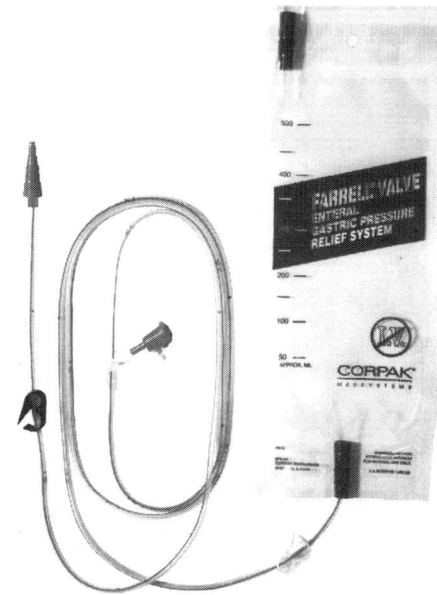

FIGURE 3.5D.8 CORFLO Farrell Valve Equipment (reproduced with the kind permission of CORPAK MedSystems, Buffalo Grove, IL)

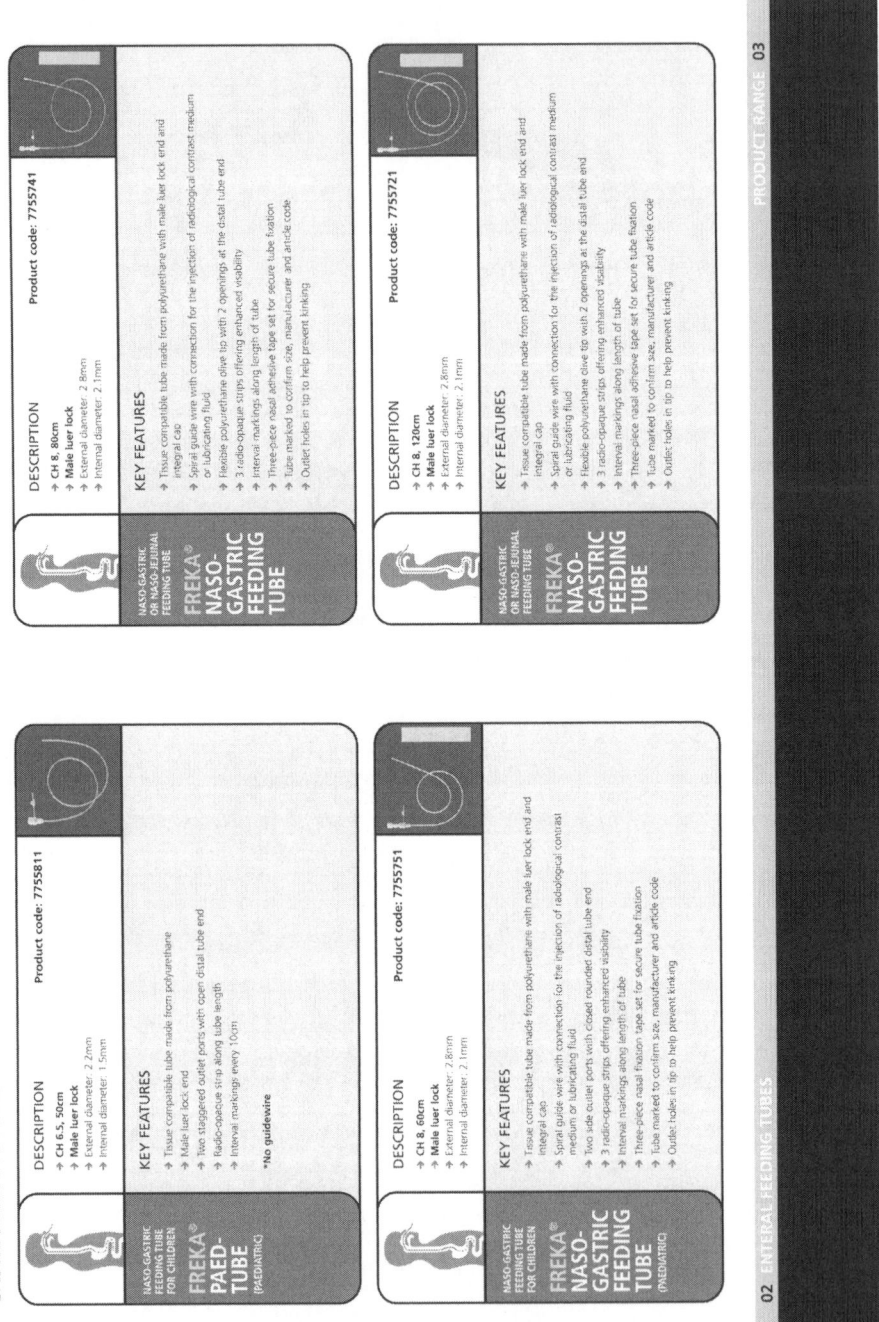

FIGURE 3.5D.9 Freka Enteral Feeding Tube (reproduced by kind permission of Fresenius Kabi. Whilst the information was correct at the time of publication clinicians should refer to the Fresenius Kabi website, www.fresenius-kabi.co.uk, for the most up-to-date information as this may change over time).

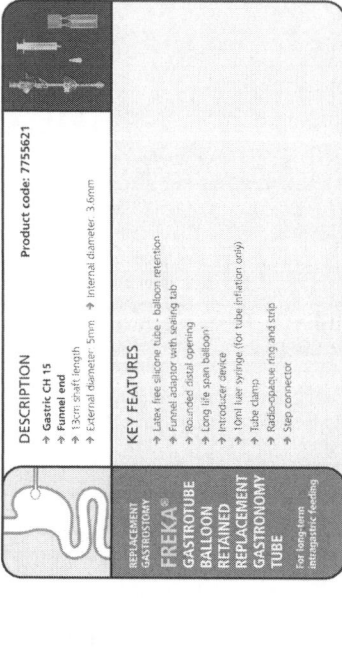

NASO-GASTRIC OR NASO-JEJUNAL FEEDING TUBE
FREKA® NASO-GASTRIC FEEDING TUBE

DESCRIPTION   Product code: 7755731
→ CH 10, 120cm
→ **Male luer lock**
→ External diameter: 3.4mm → Internal diameter: 2.2mm

KEY FEATURES
→ Tissue compatible tube made from polyurethane with funnel end
→ Spiral guide wire with connection for the injection of radiological contrast medium or lubricating fluid
→ Flexible polyurethane olive tip with 2 openings at the distal tube end
→ 3 radio-opaque strips offering enhanced visibility
→ Interval markings along tube length
→ Three-piece nasal fixation tape set for secure tube fixation
→ Tube marked to confirm size, manufacturer and article code
→ Outlet holes in tip to help prevent kinking

NASO-GASTRIC OR NASO-JEJUNAL FEEDING TUBE
FREKA® NASO-GASTRIC FEEDING TUBE (FUNNEL END)

DESCRIPTION   Product code: 7755731
→ CH 12, 120cm
→ **Funnel end**
→ External diameter: 3.9mm → Internal diameter: 2.9mm

KEY FEATURES
→ Tissue compatible tube made from polyurethane with funnel end
→ Spiral guide wire with connection for the injection of radiological contrast medium or lubricating fluid
→ Flexible polyurethane olive tip with 2 openings at the distal tube end
→ 3 radio-opaque strips offering enhanced visibility
→ Interval markings along tube length
→ Three-piece nasal fixation tape set for secure tube fixation
→ Tube marked to confirm size, manufacturer and article code
→ Outlet holes in tip to help prevent kinking

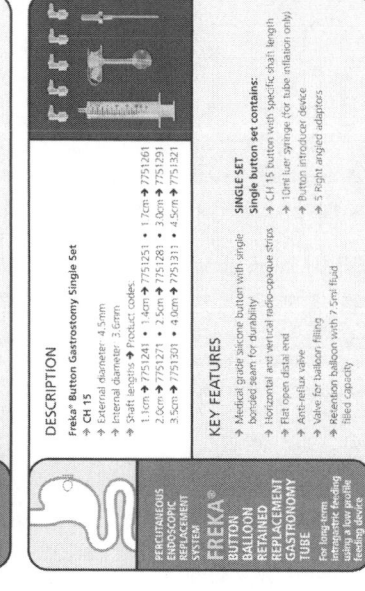

REPLACEMENT GASTROSTOMY
FREKA® GASTROTUBE BALLOON RETAINED REPLACEMENT GASTRONOMY TUBE
For long-term antragastric feeding

DESCRIPTION   Product code: 7755621
→ Gastric CH 15
→ **Funnel end**
→ 13cm shaft length
→ External diameter: 5mm → Internal diameter: 3.6mm

KEY FEATURES
→ Latex free silicone tube - balloon retention
→ Funnel adaptor with sealing tab
→ Rounded distal opening
→ Long life span balloon'
→ Introducer device
→ 10ml luer syringe (for tube inflation only)
→ Tube clamp
→ Radio-opaque ring and strip
→ Step connector

PERCUTANEOUS ENDOSCOPIC REPLACEMENT SYSTEM
FREKA® BUTTON BALLOON RETAINED REPLACEMENT GASTRONOMY TUBE
For long-term intragastric feeding using a low profile feeding device

DESCRIPTION
Freka® Button Gastrostomy Single Set
→ CH 15
→ External diameter: 4.5mm
→ Internal diameter: 3.6mm
→ Shaft lengths → Product codes:
1.1cm → 7751241 • 1.4cm → 7751251 • 1.7cm → 7751261
2.0cm → 7751271 • 2.5cm → 7751281 • 3.0cm → 7751291
3.5cm → 7751301 • 4.0cm → 7751311 • 4.5cm → 7751321

KEY FEATURES
→ Medical grade silicone button with single bonded seam for durability
→ Horizontal and vertical radio-opaque strips
→ Flat open distal end
→ Anti-reflux valve
→ Valve for balloon filling
→ Retention balloon with 7.5ml fluid filled capacity

SINGLE SET
Single button set contains:
→ CH 15 button with specific shaft length
→ 10ml luer syringe (for tube inflation only)
→ Button introducer device
→ 5 Right angled adaptors

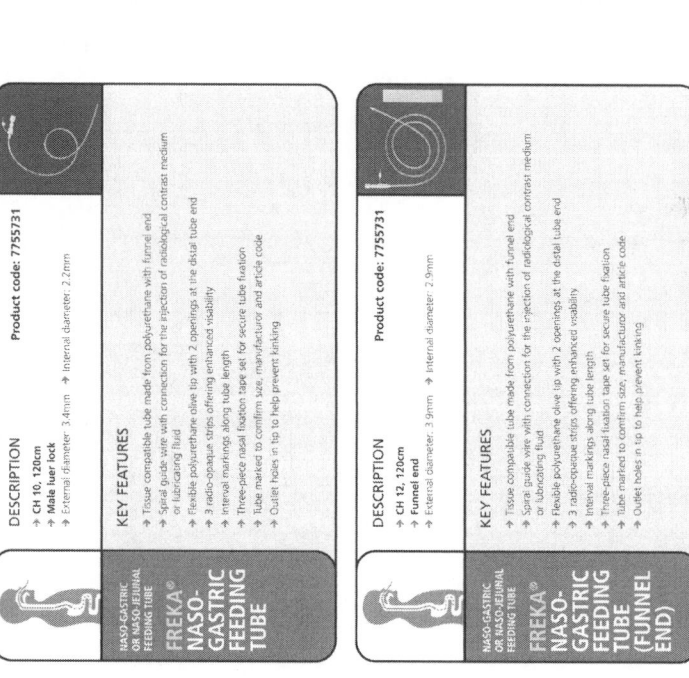

Index

Entries in **bold** refer to figures, tables and boxes.

CPD with Radcliffe

You can now use a selection of our books to achieve CPD (Continuing Professional Development) points through directed reading.

We provide a free online form and downloadable certificate for your appraisal portfolio. Look for the CPD logo and register with us at: www.radcliffehealth.com/cpd

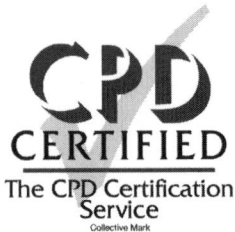

CPD
CERTIFIED
The CPD Certification
Service
Collective Mark

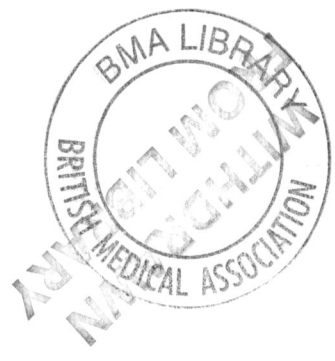